Pediatric Gastroenterology

A Color Handbook

John F. Pohl, MD
Professor of Pediatrics
Department of Pediatric Gastroenterology
Primary Children's Hospital
University of Utah, Salt Lake City, UT, USA

Christopher Jolley, MD
Professor and Chief
Division of Pediatric Gastroenterology,
Hepatology and Nutrition
Shands Children's Hospital
University of Florida, Gainesville, FL, USA

Daniel Gelfond, MD
Assistant Professor of Pediatrics and Pediatric Gastroenterology
Digestive Diseases and Nutrition Center
Women and Children's Hospital of Buffalo
Buffalo, NY, USA

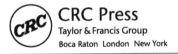

CRC Press
Taylor & Francis Group
Boca Raton London New York

CRC Press is an imprint of the
Taylor & Francis Group, an **informa** business

CRC Press
Taylor & Francis Group
6000 Broken Sound Parkway NW, Suite 300
Boca Raton, FL 33487-2742

© 2014 by Taylor & Francis Group, LLC
CRC Press is an imprint of Taylor & Francis Group, an Informa business

No claim to original U.S. Government works

Printed on acid-free paper
Version Date: 20140115

International Standard Book Number-13: 978-1-84076-202-0 (Paperback)

Visit the Taylor & Francis Web site at
http://www.taylorandfrancis.com

and the CRC Press Web site at
http://www.crcpress.com

Contents

Preface

Pediatric gastroenterology is a relatively young field in the overarching discipline of pediatrics. Over the past 20 years, there has been an explosion of clinical, basic science, and translational research leading to a better understanding of the physiology and disease processes in the gastrointestinal system of children. Endoscopic techniques have improved, correlation of radiographic and biopsy findings with disease have become better defined, and advances in transplant care have led to markedly improved survival, even in the smallest of infants.

Pediatric Gastroenterology: A Color Handbook was compiled with the intent to explore the entirety of pediatric gastro-enterology, including the gastrointestinal tract, liver, pancreas, and associated nutrition, radiographic, and endoscopic considerations. A large number of diverse topics are covered in this book in order to provide a basic overview of pediatric gastrointestinal disease. We have included a multitude of endoscopic, histologic, and radiographic images as well as illustrations and metabolic pathways to convey a better understanding of disease processes. The book ends with a list of recommended readings provided by the chapter authors. We hope that this book provides a solid introduction to pediatric gastroenterology for the reader, whether one is a gastroenterologist, general pediatrician, house staff, or medical student.

We would like to thank the Publisher, in particular Jill Northcott, Clair Chaventre, Paul Bennett, and Ruth Maxwell, for their helpful insight while we compiled our chapters. They were instrumental in making sure we had a firm understanding as to how the book would be put together as well as providing advice about image quality. We also want to thank our authors who worked so very hard in making sure that chapters were clear and concise while containing appropriate information. Finally, we wish to thank our spouses and children who were patient with us while we put this book together.

John Pohl
Christopher Jolley
Daniel Gelfond

Contributors

Razan Alkhouri, MD
Assistant Professor of
Pediatrics and Pediatric
Gastroenterology
Digestive Diseases and
Nutrition Center
Children's Hospital of Buffalo
Buffalo, NY, USA

Achiya Amir, MD
Division of Pediatric
Gastroenterology,
Hepatology, and Nutrition
The Hospital for Sick
Children
Toronto, ON, Canada

Robert Baker, MD, PhD
Professor of Pediatrics
Digestive Diseases and
Nutrition Center
Women and Children's
Hospital of Buffalo
Buffalo, NY, USA

Susan S. Baker, MD, PhD
Professor of Pediatrics
Digestive Diseases and
Nutrition Center
Women and Children's
Hospital of Buffalo
Buffalo, NY, USA

Douglas C. Barnhart, MD
MSPH
Primary Children's Hospital
University of Utah
Salt Lake City, UT, USA

Bradley A. Barth, MD,
MPH
Center for Pediatric
Gastroenterology
Children's Med Center of
Dallas
UT Southwestern
Dallas, TX, USA

Mark Bartlett, MD
Department of Pediatrics
Mayo Clinic
Rochester, MN, USA

Mirza B. Beg, MD, FAAP
Assistant Professor of Pediatrics
SUNY Upstate Medical
University
Pediatric Gastroenterology,
Hepatology, and Nutrition
Golisano Children's Hospital
Syracuse, NY, USA

Samra S. Blanchard, MD
Division Head, Pediatric
Gastroenterology and
Nutrition
University Maryland Medical
Center
Associate Professor of
Pediatrics
University of Maryland,
School of Medicine
Baltimore, MD, USA

Samuel Bitton, MD
Cohen Children's Medical
Center
North Shore-Long Island
Jewish Medical Center
New Hyde Park
New York, NY, USA

Rajasekhar Bodicharla, MD
Pediatric Gastroenterology
Marshfield Clinic System
Marshfield, WI, USA

David Brumbaugh, MD,
MSCS
Digestive Health Institute
Children's Hospital Colorado
University of Colorado
Aurora, CO, USA

Karolina Maria Burghardt,
MD, PhD
Division of Gastroenterology,
Hepatology, and Nutrition
The Hospital for Sick Children
Toronto, ON, Canada

Ricardo Caicedo, MD
Associate Professor of Pediatrics
Division of Pediatric
Gastroenterology,
Hepatology, and Nutrition
Levine Children's Hospital,
Carolinas HealthCare
System
Charlotte NC, USA

Kathy D. Chen, MD
St Christopher's Hospital for
Children
Drexel University College of
Medicine
Philadelphia, PA, USA

Amber Daigre, MD
Assistant Professor of Clinical
Pediatric Gastroenterology
University of Miami, Leonard
Miller School of Medicine
Miami, FL, USA

Anil Darbari, MD
Associate Professor of
  Pediatrics
George Washington School of
  Medical Health Sciences
Director, Comprehensive
  GI Motility Center
Pediatric Gastroenterology,
  Hepatology, and Nutrition
Children's National Medical
  Center
Washington DC, USA

Mark Davenport, ChM
FRCS (Paeds)
Professor of Paediatric Surgery
King's College Hospital
London, UK

Alan Delamatar, PhD
Director of Clinical Psychology
Professor of Pediatrics and
  Psychology
University of Miami Health
  System
Miami, FL, USA

Mark Deneau, MD, MPH
Assistant Professor
Department of Pediatrics and
  Child Health
Section of Pediatric
  Gastroenterology
University of Manitoba
Winnipeg, MB, Canada

Sonal Desai, MD
Assistant Professor of
  Pediatrics
Division of Pediatric
  Gastroenterology
Children's Hospital of San
  Antonio
San Antonio, TX, USA

Michael Docktor, MD
Instructor in Pediatrics
Division of Gastroenterology,
  Hepatology, and Nutrition
Boston Children's Hospital
Boston MA, USA

Debora Duro, MD, MS
Medical Director, Institute
  for Children's Advanced
  Nutrition (iCan) and
  Gastroenterology
Miami, FL
Associate Professor in
  Pediatrics at University of
  North Carolina
Chapel Hill, NC
Associate Professor in
  Pediatrics at Florida
  International University
Miami, FL
Instructor in Pediatrics at
  Harvard Medical School
Boston, MA, USA

David Easley, MD
Specially for Children
1301 Barbara Jordan Blvd
Suite 200
Austin, TX, USA

Katharine Eng, MD
Department of Pediatric
  Gastroenterology
Cleveland Clinic Foundation,
  Children's Hospital
Cleveland, OH, USA

Alessio Fasano, MD
Chief of Pediatric
  Gastroenterology and
  Nutrition
Massachusetts General
  Hospital for Children
Director of the Center for
  Celiac Research and
Director of the Mucosal
  Immunology and Biology
  Research Center
Massachusetts General
  Hospital East
Charlestown, MA, USA

Elizabeth A. Fialkowski,
  MD
Department of Surgery
Washington University School
  of Medicine
Division of Pediatric Surgery
St. Louis Children's Hospital
St Louis, MO, USA

Laura S. Finn, MD
Associate Professor of
  Pathology
Seattle Children's and
University of Washington
  School of Medicine
Seattle, WA, USA

James Franciosi, MD
Associate Chief, Division
  of Gastroenterology,
  Hepatology, and Nutrition
Nemours Children's Hospital
Associate Professor of
  Pediatrics
University of Central Florida
  College of Medicine
Orlando, FL, USA

Karen Francolla, MD
Office of Pediatric
  Gastroenterology and
  Nutrition
Hackensack University
  Medical Center
Hackensack, NJ, USA

Jose M. Garza, MD, MS
Children's Center for
  Digestive Healthcare, LLC
Atlanta, GA, USA

Louis Ghanem, MD, PhD
Division of Gastroenterology,
  Hepatology, and Nutrition
The Children's Hospital of
  Philadelphia
Philadelphia, PA, USA

Tanja Gonska, MD
Division of Gastroenterology,
  Hepatology, and Nutrition
The Hospital of Sick Children
Toronto, ON, Canada

Jose Greenspon, MD
Department of Surgery
Washington University School
  of Medicine
Division of Pediatric Surgery
St. Louis Children's Hospital
St Louis, MO, USA

Melanie Greifer, MD
Assistant Professor of
  Pediatrics
Cohen Children's Medical
  Center
North Shore-Long Island
  Jewish Medical Center
New Hyde Park
New York, NY, USA

Rohit Gupta, MD
Fellow, Gastroenterology and
  Hepatology
Seattle Children's and
University of Washington
  School of Medicine
Seattle, WA, USA

Sanjiv Harpavat, MD, PhD
Assistant Professor of
  Pediatrics
Gastroenterology,
  Hepatology, and Nutrition
Baylor College of Medicine
Texas Children's Hospital
Houston, TX, USA

Humaira Hashmi, MD
Digestive Diseases and
  Nutrition Center
Women and Children's
  Hospital of Buffalo
Buffalo, NY, USA

Justin Hollon, MD
Division of Pediatric
  Gastroenterology and
  Nutrition
John Hopkins University
  School of Medicine
Baltimore, MD, USA

Tara Holm, MD
Divison of Radiology
Amplatz Children's Hospital
University of Minnesota
Minneapolis, MN, USA

Sohail Z. Husain, MD
Children's Hospital of
  Pittsburgh of UPMC
Division of Pediatric
  Gastroenterology
Pittsburgh, PA, USA

Saleem Islam, MD, MPH
Department of Pediatric
  Surgery
University of Florida
Gainesville FL, USA

Kyle Jensen, MD, MPH
University of Utah
Primary Children's Hospital
Salt Lake City, UT, USA

Candi Jump, DO
Fellow, Department of
  Pediatric Gastroenterology,
  Hepatology, and Nutrition
The Children's Hospital of
  Philadelphia
Philadelphia, PA, USA

Ian Kang, MD
Assistant Professor of Clinical
  Pediatrics
University of Illinois College
  of Medicine-Peoria
Children's Hospital of Illinois
Peoria, IL, USA

Ajay Kaul, MD
Professor of Clinical Pediatrics
Director,
  Neurogastroenterology
  and Motility Disorders
  Program
Cincinnati Children's Hospital
  Medical Center
Cincinnati, OH, USA

Marsha Kay, MD
Chair, Department of
  Pediatric Gastroenterology
Director Pediatric Endoscopy
Pediatric Institute
Cleveland Clinic
Cleveland, OH, USA

Khalid Khan, MD
Associate Professor
Transplant Institute and
  Department of Pediatrics
MedStar Georgetown
  University Hospital
Washington, DC, USA

Anne C. Kim, MD, MPH
Clinical Assistant Professor of
  Surgery
University Hospitals
Cleveland, OH, USA

Katja Kovacic, MD
Division of Pediatric
  Gastroenterology,
  Hepatology, and Nutrition
Department of Pediatrics
Medical College of Wisconsin
Milwaukee, WI, USA

Rafal Kozielski, MD
Department of Pathology
Women & Children's
  Hospital of Buffalo
Buffalo, NY, USA

Daniel Leung, MD
Assistant Professor of
  Pediatrics
Baylor College of Medicine
Gastroenterology,
  Hepatology, and Nutrition
Texas Children's Hospital
Medical Director, Viral
  Hepatitis Clinic
Houston, TX, USA

B U.K. Li, MD
Program Director, Cyclic
  Vomiting Program
  and Pediatric Fellow's
  Education, Children's
  Hospital of Wisconsin
Professor of Pediatrics,
  Division of Pediatric
  Gastroenterology,
  Hepatology, and Nutrition
Medical College of
  Wisconsin
Milwaukee, WI, USA

Petar Mamula, MD
Director of Endoscopy
Division of Gastroenterology,
  Hepatology, and Nutrition
The Children's Hospital of
  Philadelphia
Philadelphia, PA, USA

Katie McDonald, PhD, RD,
  CSP
Clinical Dietitian
Primary Children's Hospital
Salt Lake City, UT, USA

Douglas Moote, MD
Digestive Diseases,
  Hepatology, and Nutrition
Connecticut Children's
  Medical Center
Hartford, CT, USA

Zohreh Movahedi, MD
University of Arizona
Tucson, AZ, USA

Karen F. Murray, MD
Professor of Pediatrics
Chief, Division of
  Gastroenterology and
  Hepatology
Seattle Children's and
University of Washington
  School of Medicine
Seattle, WA, USA

Vicky Ng, MD
Division of Pediatric
  Gastroenterology,
  Hepatology, and Nutrition
The Hospital for Sick
  Children
Toronto, ON, Canada

Molly O'Gorman, MD
University of Utah
Primary Children's Hospital
Salt Lake City, UT, USA

Niraj Patel, MD, MS
Assistant Professor of
  Pediatrics
Division of Infectious Disease
  and Immunology
Levine Children's Hospital
Carolinas Medical Center
Charlotte, NC, USA

Raza A. Patel, MD, MPH
University of Utah
Primary Children's Hospital
Salt Lake City, UT, USA

Adam Paul, MD
Pediatric Gastroenterology
Children's Hospital at Lehigh
  Valley Health Network
Allentown, PA, USA

Simon S. Rabinowitz, PhD,
  MD, FAAP
Professor of Clinical Pediatrics
Vice Chairman, Clinical
  Practice Development,
Pediatric Gastroenterology,
  Hepatology, and Nutrition
SUNY Downstate College of
  Medicine
The Children's Hospital at
  Downstate
Brooklyn, NY, USA

Archana Ramaswami, MD
Pediatrics
SUNY Upstate Medical
  University
Syracuse, NY, USA

Yuliya Rekhtman, MD
Associate Professor
Georgetown University
  Hospital
Children's Hospital
Washington DC, USA

Benjamin A. Sahn, MD
Division of Gastroenterology,
  Hepatology, and Nutrition
The Children's Hospital of
  Philadelphia
Philadelphia, PA, USA

Cathy Sampert
Division of Pediatric
  Gastroenterology,
  Hepatology, and Nutrition
Department of Pediatrics
Tripler Army Medical Center
Honolulu, HI, USA

Wael N. Sayej, MD
Digestive Diseases,
  Hepatology, and Nutrition
Connecticut Children's
  Medical Center
Hartford, CT, USA

Sarah Jane Schwarzenberg,
MD
Division of Pediatric
   Gastroenterology
Amplatz Children's Hospital
University of Minnesota
Minneapolis, MN, USA

Ami N. Shah, MD
Instructor of Surgery
Rush University Medical
   Center
Chicago, IL, USA

Slava Shapiro, DDS, MD,
PC
Woodbury Oral Surgery
167 Froehlich Farm Blvd
Woodbury, NY, USA

Mitchell Shub, MD
Division of Gastroenterology
Phoenix Children's Hospital
Professor and Vice-Chair,
   Department of Child
   Health
University of Arizona College
   of Medicine-Phoenix
Phoenix, AZ, USA

Thomas L. Sutton, MD
Rock Canyon Pediatric
   Specialists
University of Utah
Provo, UT, USA

David M. Troendle, MD
Pediatric GI Fellow
Children's Medical Center of
   Dallas
UT Southwestern
Dallas, TX, USA

Laurie A. Tsilianidis, MD
Division of Pediatric
   Endocrinology
Cleveland Clinic
Cleveland, OH, USA

William Twaddell, MD
Assistant Professor of
   Pathology
University of Maryland
   Medical School
Baltimore, MD, USA

Aliye Uc, MD
Professor of Pediatric
   Gastroenterology
University of Iowa Children's
   Hospital
Iowa City, IA, USA

Raghu U. Varier, DO
Pediatric GI Fellow
University of Utah
Primary Children's Hospital
Salt Lake City, UT, USA

Ghassan Wahbeh, MD
Associate Professor, Pediatric
   Gastroenterology
Director, Inflammatory Bowel
   Disease Program
Seattle Children's Hospital,
   University of Washington
Seattle, WA, USA

Brad W. Warner, MD
Jessie L. Ternberg MD, PhD
   Distinguished Professor of
   Pediatric Surgery
Washington University School
   of Medicine
Surgeon-in-Chief
St. Louis Children's Hospital
St. Louis, MO, USA

David A. Weinstein, MD,
MMSc
Professor of Pediatrics
Director, Glycogen Storage
   Disease Program
Associate Program Director
   for Research
University of Florida
Gainesville FL, USA

Robert Wyllie, MD
Associate Chief of Staff
Systemwide Medical
   Operations
Professor, Lerner College of
   Medicine
Department of Pediatric
   Gastroenterology
Cleveland Clinic
Cleveland, OH, USA

Shamila Zawahir, MD
Assistant Professor
Pediatric Gastroenterology
   and Nutrition
University of Maryland
   Children's Hospital
Baltimore, MD, USA

Roberto Zori, MD
Professor, Department of
   Pediatrics and of Pathology
Chief, Division of Clinical
   Genetics and Metabolism
Department of Pediatrics
University of Florida
Gainesville, FL, USA

Abbreviations

6-MMP 6-methylmercaptopurine
6-MP 6-mercaptopurine
6-TG 6-thioguanine
A1AT alpha-1 antitrypsin
ACA adenocarcinoma
AFP alpha-fetoprotein
AGA antigliadin antibody
AIDS acquired immunodeficiency syndrome
AIH autoimmune hepatitis
ALT alanine aminotransferase
ANA antinuclear antibody
ANCA antineutrophil cytoplasmic antibody
APBU anomalous pancreatobiliary union
APC argon plasma coagulation
ARM anorectal malformation/anorectal
   manometry
ASA aminosalicylic acid
ASC autoimmune sclerosing cholangitis
ASCA anti-*Saccharomyces cerevisiae* antibody
ASM acid sphingomyelinase
AST aspartate aminotransferase
ATP adenosine triphosphate
AVM arteriovenous malformation
AXR abdominal X-ray

BA biliary atresia
BRBNS blue rubber bleb nevus syndrome
BRRS Bannayan–Riley–Ruvalcaba
   syndrome

CBC complete blood count
CCK cholecystokinin
CD Crohn disease
CE capsule endoscopy
CF cystic fibrosis
CFA coefficient of fat absorption
CFTR cystic fibrosis transmembrane
   conductance regulator
CGD chronic granulomatous disease
CHF congestive heart failure
CM choledochal malformation
CMPE cow's milk protein enteropathy

CMV cytomegalovirus
CNI calcineurin inhibitor
CNS central nervous system
CRS congenital rubella syndrome
CS Cowden syndrome
CT computed tomography

DCI distal contractile integral
δ-ALA delta-aminolevulinic acid
DHE dihydroergotamine
DILI drug-induced liver injury
DNA deoxyribonucleic acid
DPPHR duodenum-preserving pancreatic
   head resection

EA esophageal atresia
EBNA Epstein–Barr nuclear antigen
EBV Epstein–Barr virus
EEC ectrodactyly-ectodermal clefting
EGD esophagogastroduodenoscopy
EGE eosinophilic gastroenteritis
EGG electrogastrography
EGJ esophagogastric junction
EHE epithelioid hemangioendothelioma
EHEC enterohemorrhagic *Escherichia coli*
ELISA enzyme-linked immunosorbent assay
EN enteral nutrition
EMA endomysial antibody
EMLA eutectic mixture of local anesthetics
EN enteral nutrition
ENS enteric nervous system
EPI exocrine pancreatic insufficiency
EPT esophageal pressure topography
EoE eosinophilic esophagitis
EPEC enteropathogenic *Escherichia coli*
ERCP endoscopic retrograde
   cholangiopancreatography
ESL embryonic (undifferentiated) sarcoma of
   the liver
ETEC enterotoxigenic *Escherichia coli*
EUS endoscopic ultrasound
EVL endoscopic variceal ligation

FAA fumarylacetoacetate
FAH fumarylacetoacetate hydrolase
FAP functional abdominal pain/familial
  adenomatous polyposis
FDA Food and Drug Administration
FE-1 fecal elastase-1
FGF fibroblast growth factor
FGID functional gastrointestinal disorder
FLC fibrolamellar carcinoma
FIP focal intestinal perforation
FNH focal nodular hyperplasia

gal-1-P galactose-1-phosphate
GALK galactokinase
GALT galactose-1-phosphate-uridyltransferase
GAVE gastric antral vascular ectasia
GE gastroesophageal
GERD gastroesophageal reflux disease
GES gastric emptying scintigraphy
GG granulomatous gastritis
GGT gamma-glutamyl transferase
GI gastrointestinal
GIST gastrointestinal stromal tumors
GLP glucagon-like peptide
GLUT-1 glucose transporter-1
GM-CSF granulocyte macrophage-colony
  stimulating factor
GMS Gomori methenamine silver nitrate stain
GSD glycogen storage disease
GvHD graft versus host disease

H&E hematoxylin and eosin
H2RA histamine-2-receptor antagonist
HA hepatocellular adenoma
HAT hepatic artery thrombosis
HB hepatoblastoma
HCC hepatocellular carcinoma
HD Hirschprung disease
HFI hereditary fructose intolerance
HHT hereditary hemorrhagic telangiectasia
HIV human immunodeficiency virus
HPD hydroxyphenylpyruvate dioxygenase
HPRT hypoxanthine phosphoribosyl
  transferase
HRM high-resolution manometry
HRS hepatorenal syndrome
HSP Henoch–Schönlein purpura
HSV herpes simplex virus
HT1 hereditary tyrosinemia type 1
HTLV human T-lymphotropic virus
HUS hemolytic uremic syndrome

IAS internal anal sphincter
IBD inflammatory bowel disease
IBS irritable bowel syndrome
ICC interstitial cells of Cajal
IFALD intestinal failure-associated liver
  disease
Ig immunoglobulin
IHH infantile hepatic hemangioma
IL interkeukin
INH isoniazid
INR international normalized ratio
IRT immunoreactive trypsinogen
IVIG intravenous immunoglobulin

JPS juvenile polyposis syndrome

KF Kayser–Fleischer
KIT tyrosine kinase receptor
KPE Kasai portoenterostomy
KTS Klippel–Trenaunay syndrome
KUB kidneys, ureters, bladder (X-ray)

LAD leukocyte adhesion deficiency
LCH Langerhans cell histiocytosis
LES lower esophageal sphincter
LGG *Lactobacillus rhamnosus* GG
LHM laparascopic Heller myotomy
LPJ lateral pancreaticojejunostomy
LTE laryngo–tracheo–esophageal
LTEC laryngo–tracheo–esophageal cleft

MALT mucosa-associated lymphoid tissue
MBS modified barium swallow
MCT medium-chain triglyceride
MDT multidisciplinary team
MELD Model for End-Stage Liver disease
MEN multiple endocrine neoplasia
MH mesenchymal hamartoma
MMF mycophenolate mofetil
MRCP magnetic resonance
  cholangiopancreatography
MRI magnetic resonance imaging

NAPQI N-acetyl-p-benzoquinoneimine
NBS newborn screening
NEC necrotizing enterocolitis
NG nasogastric
NLH nodular lymphoid hyperplasia
NO nitric oxide
NPC Niemann–Pick type C disease
NPO *nil per os*

NRH nodular regenerative hyperplasia (NRH)
NSAID nonsteroidal anti-inflammatory drug
NTBC 2-[2-nitro-4-fluoromethylbenzoyl]-1,
3-cyclohexanedione

OCP oral contraceptive pill
OG orogastric
OR odds ratio
ORT oral rehydration therapy

PAS periodic acid Schiff
PD pneumatic dilatation/pancreas divisum
PDGFR platelet-derived growth factor
receptor
PEG polyethylene glycol
PELD Pediatric End-Stage Liver Disease
(Score)
PERT pancreatic enzyme replacement therapy
PFT pancreatic function test
PHG portal hypertensive gastropathy
PJS Peutz–Jeghers syndrome
PLE protein-losing enteropathy
PMN polymorphonuclear
PN parenteral nutrition
POEM per oral endoscopic myotomy
PPI proton pump inhibitor
PSARP posterior sagittal anorectoplasty
PSC primary sclerosing cholangitis
PT prothrombin time
PTC percutaneous transhepatic
cholangiography
PTLD post-transplant lymphoproliferative
disorder
PUFA polyunsaturated fatty acid

RAA renin–angiotensin–aldosterone
RAIR rectoanal inhibitory reflex
RBC red blood cell
RICH rapidly involuting congenital
hemangioma
RMS rhabdomyosarcoma

SAAG serum-ascites albumin gradient
SBDS Shwachman–Bodian–Diamond
syndrome
SBS short bowel syndrome
SBP spontaneous bacterial peritonitis
SCC squamous cell carcinoma

SDS Shwachman–Diamond syndrome
SIADH syndrome of inappropriate
antidiuretic hormone
SIBO small intestine bacterial overgrowth
SLE systemic lupus erythematosus
SMA smooth muscle antibody
SNS specialized nutrition support
SSRI selective serotonin reuptake inhibitor
STEP serial transverse enteroplasty
SVR sustained viral response

TAT tyrosine aminotransferase
TBR tracheobronchial remnant
TCA tricyclic antidepressant
TEF tracheoesophageal fistula
TGF-β transforming growth factor-beta
TIPS transjugular intrahepatic portosystemic
shunt
TLESR transient lower esophageal sphincter
relaxation
TNF tumor necrosis factor
TPIAT auto-transplantation of islet cells
TPMT thiopurine methyltransferase
TPN total parenteral nutrition
tTG tissue transglutaminase

UC ulcerative colitis
UES upper esophageal sphincter
UGI upper gastrointestinal bleeding
US ultrasonography

VACTERL vertebrae, anal, cardiac,
tracheoesophageal, radial, renal, and limb
anomalies
VATER vertebrae, anal, tracheoesophageal,
and renal
VCA viral capsid antigen
VEGF vascular endothelial growth factor
VIP vasoactive intestinal polypeptide
VPA valproic acid
VZV varicella-zoster virus

WD Wilson disease

XO xanthine oxidase

ZES Zollinger–Ellison syndrome

CHAPTER 1

The Pediatric Gastrointestinal Physical Examination

David Easley

- **Introduction**
- **History**
- **Physical examination**
- **Examination of the pediatric patient with gastrointestinal disease**
- **Use of technology as adjunct to the history and physical examination**

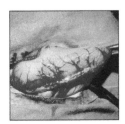 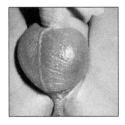 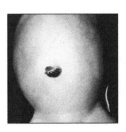 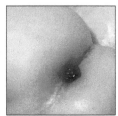

Introduction

As clinicians we have a vast array of tools at our disposal to evaluate for presence or absence of pathology in patients with potential gastrointestinal (GI) disease. It can be postulated that amongst the most important tools in the armamentarium available to us as clinicians, the patient's history and physical examination are among the most critical. Everything else typically flows from the historical and examination data obtained about the patient. This information provides direction and hones the areas that must be explored or may be ignored.

Pediatric providers should tailor history and physical examination details based upon the age and developmental status of the patient. Older adolescents may provide much or all of the history; this is certainly not the case in preverbal toddlers and infants.

Establishing a rapport in a safe, non-threatening environment whenever possible provides the best possible chance of obtaining

Table 1.1 Important findings on physical examination for gastrointestinal disease

1. Character/onset/location/changes of symptoms:
   - Sharp/dull/colicky
   - Any radiation
   - Acute versus chronic
   - Well localized/peritoneal signs
   - Significant change
2. Associated symptoms:
   - Change or loss of appetite
   - Weight loss or weight gain
   - Persistent or high fever
   - Bilious or persistent emesis
   - Presence of blood
   - Headaches, gait changes, seizures
   - Change in bowel or urinary habits
3. Significant medical history:
   - Prior hospitalizations or emergency visits
   - Predisposing factors (e.g. sickle cell disease)
   - Immunologic disease (HIV, immune deficiency)
   - Medications (e.g. corticosteroids, immunosuppressant agents)
   - Prior abdominal surgery
   - Congenital anomalies
   - Prior history of prematurity or extended NICU stay
4. Recent travel or exposures/ill contacts

HIV: human immunodeficiency virus; NICU: neonatal intensive care unit.

as much pertinent and relevant detail necessary to make an adequate assessment. Circumstances may dictate a more hurried approach in an emergent situation, for example, but should always be expanded to allow for more in depth questioning. There are a number of tools available that allow for prescreening such as history intake questionnaires.

Key elements that may be elucidated beyond the basic questions of a patient history intake will often be generated during questioning the patient and family. The timing around critical events in the family or chronicity of symptoms will often alter to a significant degree the potential etiologies of GI disease. It bears mentioning that the mere presence of symptoms for an extended period of time does not preclude the acute onset of new pathology.

Examples of historical details that may be of help are listed in *Table 1.1*. Pertinent physical examination findings in a patient with GI disease are listed in *Table 1.2*.

Table 1.2 Pertinent positive physical examination findings suggestive of gastrointestinal disease

Vital signs: Fever, tachycardia, hypotension

HEENT: Scleral icterus, oral/pharyngeal ulcerations, papilledema suggesting increased intracranial pressure

Cardiovascular: Tachycardia suggesting anemia

Lungs: Crackles/decreased airway sounds suggesting referred pain from pneumonia

Abdomen: Absent or increased bowel sounds, masses or umbilical hernias, tenderness (diffuse or localized), palpable organs (liver or spleen), ascites, rebound, guarding

Extremities: Clubbing to suggest anemia

Dermatologic: Rashes such as dermatitis herpetiformis

Anal/rectal examination: Presence of tags, tears, fissures, fistulas, or bleeding; presence of a transition zone to suggest Hirschsprung disease or capacious rectum as seen in chronic constipation

HEENT: head, ears, eyes, nose, and throat.

History

An example of historical data that would prompt specific evaluation on an abdominal physical examination would be the presence of vomiting (*Table 1.3*); for example, bilious emesis is indicative of obstruction distal to the ampulla of Vater.

A 1-month-old infant would more likely have a congenital abnormality such as malrotation such as that seen on an upper GI barium radiographic series (**1.1, 1.2**). The same age infant with persistent profuse nonbilious emesis would indicate an obstruction proximal to the ampulla of

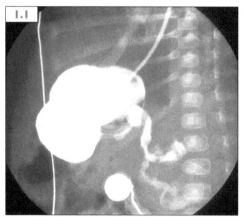

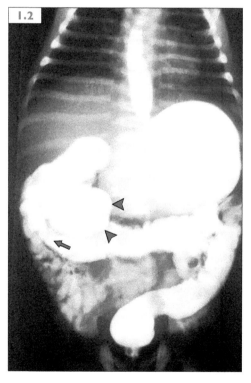

1.1 Upper gastrointestinal series demonstrating the 'corkscrew' pattern consistent with a midgut volvulus associated with intestinal malrotation.

1.2 Midgut volvulus with obstruction at the level of the duodenum. Note the position of the cecum in the right upper quadrant (arrow) and the termination of the duodenum, with the presence of 'beaking' (arrowheads) at the level of the obstruction.

Table 1.3 Causes of vomiting

Gastrointestinal
Esophagus (GERD, stricture, foreign body)
Stomach (gastric outlet obstruction, ulcer, foreign body, gastroparesis)
Intestine (atresia, malrotation, foreign body, inflammatory bowel disease, appendicitis)
Colon (imperforate anus, Hirschsprung disease, inflammatory bowel disease)

Infection
Helicobacter pylori
Infectious enteritis (viral, bacterial)

Renal
Urinary tract infection
Ureteropelvic junction obstruction

Neurologic
Brain tumor
Migraine variant (abdominal migraines, cyclic vomiting)
Chiari malformation
Seizure

Endocrine
Adrenal insufficiency
Diabetic ketoacidosis

Metabolic
Galactosemia
Hereditary fructosemia
Urea cycle defect
Lysosomal storage disorder
Peroxisomal disorder

Other
Bulimia
Psychogenic
Rumination
Drug toxicity
Superior mesenteric artery syndrome

GERD: gastroesophageal reflux disease.

Vater and could be pyloric stenosis at this age (**1.3–1.5**). Alternatively less common etiologies such as an antral or duodenal web would also present in similar fashion. The age of the patient will change the potential etiologies of GI disease dramatically. For example, a 2-year-old child with the same concerns of persistent emesis, especially if linked with colicky, episodic pain, could have an intussusception (**1.6**).

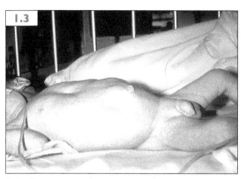

1.3 Giant peristaltic waves in the epigastrium associated with untreated pyloric stenosis.

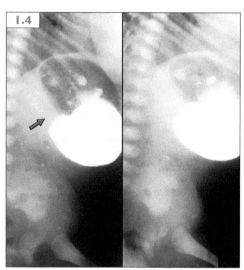

1.4 Upper gastrointestinal series demonstrating the 'string sign' (arrow), with pyloric stenosis visible at the level of the pylorus.

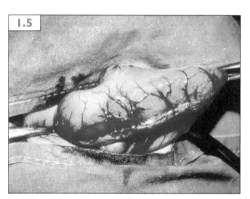

1.5 Pylorus immediately after pyloromyotomy for pyloric stenosis.

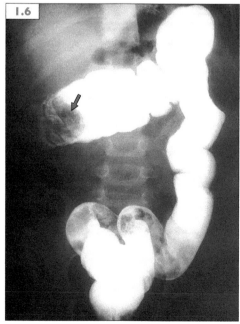

1.6 Intussusception to the level of the transverse colon. Note the filling defect at the level of the transverse colon (arrow).

Physical examination

It should be stated that a pediatric physical examination performed by a practitioner will differ from patient to patient; flexibility is often the key to obtaining subtle or otherwise hidden clues as to underlying pathology. Determining the presence of bowel sounds, palpating for organomegaly or the presence of ascites, and determining the location of abdominal pain are essential aspects of the pediatric GI examination.

Age plays a significant factor in what pathology may be present on physical examination. The younger the patient, the more likely congenital anomalies are a part of the differential diagnosis. Different ages will present with unique pathology. For example, a 1-week-old with severe constipation may have congenital hypothyroidism, imperforate anus, or Hirschsprung disease, all of which may be considered as part of the potential diagnoses. The same symptoms in a 16-year-old would yield vastly different potential etiologies and would more likely represent an acquired problem.

Of note, an interesting phenomenon has occurred in medicine in the last few decades. In the medical community's quest to diagnose and evaluate pathology as well as possible, there has been an effort to expand the diagnostic arsenal available to the clinician. The advent of increasingly complex laboratory evaluations and imaging, such as computed tomography, magnetic resonance imaging, and the advances in endoscopy, have irrevocably altered the landscape of medicine in many ways to the betterment of patient care. In this headlong rush to develop and embrace technology, however, it may be postulated that as clinicians there is a decreasing reliance on the physical examination.

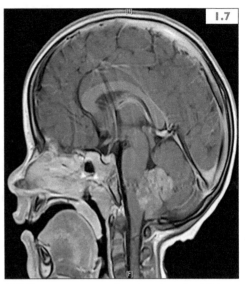

1.7 Brain tumor noted on imaging of a child who presented with occipital headaches and vomiting. She had significant vertigo noted during the physical examination.

Frequently, a test or image is used to replace clinical acumen. However, it should not be underestimated that a careful physical examination of the patient remains an invaluable tool. It is exceedingly rare for any portion of a careful physical examination, such as a rectal examination, to cause complications or harm. Also, it should be remembered that extraintestinal disease can cause GI symptoms, and such possibilities should be considered and evaluated for during physical examination (**1.7**).

Examination of the pediatric patient with gastrointestinal disease

The pediatric physical examination varies from that of the adult patient in significant ways. Due to the developmental needs of the pediatric patient, especially in the first few years of life, a careful approach is warranted. Distraction of the patient will allow for a better examination and closer evaluation of the patient's baseline clinical status.

A brusque, hurried approach typically will yield a less efficient examination in the long run as opposed to a slow, careful, measured examination, especially with younger children. The typical approach to examine an adult patient is to start at the head and proceed downward. Younger children may find this approach, especially with movement towards the face, intimidating or frightening. Adjusting the examination to what the child is comfortable with and proceeding as tolerated is a reasonable approach. Leaving the most uncomfortable parts towards the end, such as a rectal or genital examination, typically yields better results.

An old adage in pediatrics is that children are not 'little adults'. There is some definite wisdom to this statement, especially pertaining to the array of pathology that presents in children that may be rare or completely absent in the adult population. For example, the younger the patient, the more congenital anomalies may play a part. Certain physical findings that a complete examination may reveal can explain specific symptomatology. One example would be the young infant presenting with emesis in the immediate newborn period. A simple examination may reveal findings such as anal abnormalities or abdominal distention, that would point toward structural etiologies, such as an imperforate anus or Hirschsprung disease (**1.8–1.11**). A proximal bowel obstruction may present with distention of the epigastrium and a scaphoid appearance in the lower abdomen.

Alternatively, a more distal obstruction tends to present with delay in stooling or lack of stooling with more diffuse abdominal distention. Tympanic findings with percussion and hyperactive bowel sounds also may be part of the presenting features of a bowel obstruction. Hypoactive bowel sounds will be present if there is delay in diagnosis and obstruction has been present for some time.

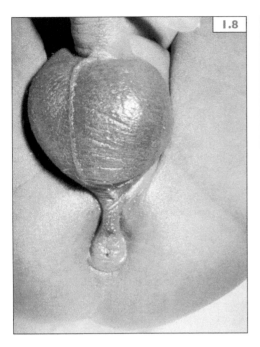

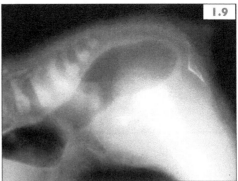

1.9 Plain film demonstrating absence of gas in the rectum consistent with a low-lying imperforate anus.

1.8 Imperforate anus visible with a dimple present at the site.

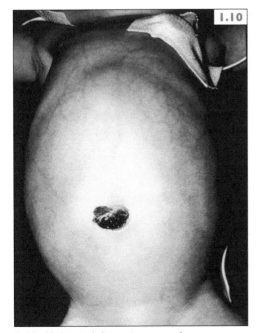

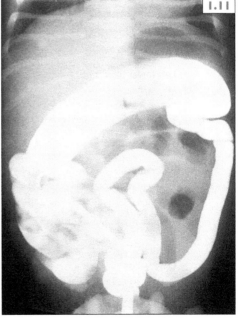

1.10 Abdominal distention secondary to Hirschsprung disease with significant distal bowel obstruction.

1.11 Narrowed segment in the distal colon and transition zone at the splenic flexure found in Hirschsprung disease. Distal narrowed bowel is consistent with the involved segment affected by Hirschsprung disease.

Table 1.4 Causes of abdominal pain based on location

Epigastric
GERD
Gastritis
Ulcer (gastric/duodenal)
Pancreatitis
Anatomic (volvulus, gastric outlet obstruction)

Right upper quadrant
Hepatitis
Gallbladder disease/dysfunction
Kidney disease
Pneumonia

Left upper quadrant
Splenic disease
Kidney disease
Pneumonia

Right lower quadrant
Appendicitis
Constipation
Crohn disease
Intussusception or other obstruction
Ovarian/testicular disease
Hernia
Infectious enteritis/mesenteric enteritis

Left lower quadrant
Constipation
Ovarian/testicular disease
Sigmoid volvulus
Colitis
Hernia

Perumbilical
Recurrent abdominal pain of childhood/functional gastrointestinal disorders
Constipation
Pancreatitis
Gastroenteritis

Diffuse
Constipation
Functional gastrointestinal disorder (irritable bowel syndrome)
Abdominal migraine
Sickle cell crisis
Acute porphyria

GERD: gastroesophageal reflux disease.

Abdominal examination of older children may yield findings such as abdominal tenderness that may be localized to the specific site of the pathology if there is peritoneal involvement (*Table 1.4*). Presence or absence of specific findings, such as rebound, abdominal guarding, or the psoas sign, may indicate inflammation involving specific regions of the peritoneum. Nerve fibers that are present may help directly to locate the site of abdominal disease; however, bowel inflammation can present differently. Mucosal damage may not be interpreted as well by the body as a pain presentation.

Pain is often referred to areas that may or may not correlate well with the actual site of disease. Disease processes that involve foregut derivatives such as the stomach and duodenum will present with epigastric pain. Midgut derivatives such as the jejunum may present with pain in the periumbilical region, while hindgut derivatives such as the colon may present with pain in the hypogastrium. The more inflammation that is present involving the peritoneum, the more localized the symptoms tend to be and the more closely the abdominal pain will correlate with a true anatomic location. It is much more difficult in younger children and infants to use these signs, however, and a high index of suspicion should be raised in this situation if there is concern for significant pathology, such as appendicitis.

Use of technology as adjunct to the history and physical examination

With the significant proliferation of technology such as 'smartphones', readily available digital video or pictures may be a helpful adjunct to the physical examination. Transient findings that may not be apparent on examination in the office may be captured for evaluation. An example of this technology is seen in Figure **1.12**. A boy presented to clinic with a chief complaint of rectal prolapse not responsive to measures such as softening the stools with laxative therapy. However, in discussion with the family, his symptoms did not appear to be an exact fit in terms of the typical presentation of rectal prolapse. A smartphone image was obtained by the family of the findings which were not seen in clinic. The child was taken to the endoscopy suite, and a solitary rectal polyp was found instead. The images obtained by the parents made the correct diagnosis easier and led to appropriate intervention. The use of brief videos or pictures by patients and their families may be used to help delineate physical examination findings or specific symptoms not observed in clinic.

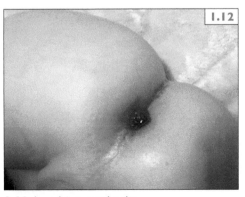

1.12 Low-lying rectal polyp.

CHAPTER 2

Oral Problems Associated with Gastrointestinal Disease

Slava Shapiro

- Introduction
- Benign melanotic macules
- Juvenile periodontitis
- Ankyloglossia
- Labial frenula
- Cleft lip and palate
- Geographic tongue
- Fissured tongue
- Gingival overgrowth

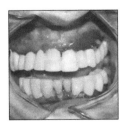
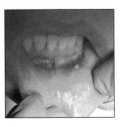
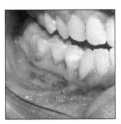
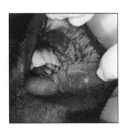

- **Hemangioma**
- **Lymphangioma**
- **Mucocele**
- **Ranula**
- **Fibroma**
- **Parulis**
- **Eruption cyst**
- **Aphthous ulcer**
- **Systemic lupus erythematosus**
- **Bullous pemphigoid**
- **Mucous membrane pemphigoid**
- **Pemphigus vulgaris**
- **Erythema multiforme**
- **Stevens–Johnson syndrome**
- **Coxsackie virus**
- **Rubeola**
- **Rubella**
- **Varicella-zoster virus**
- **Herpes simplex virus**
- **Oropharyngeal candidiasis**

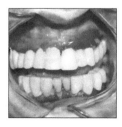
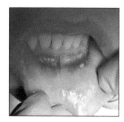
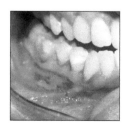
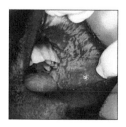

Introduction

The lips and oral cavity are the most antral portion of the gastrointestinal (GI) tract and are most accessible to visual examination by the clinician. A lingual or oral problem can be an independent abnormality or a component of a systemic disease, nutritional deficiency, or a GI disease. Thorough lingual and oral examination including identification of disease is an essential part of a routine physical examination.

Benign melanotic macules

CLINICAL PRESENTATION

Oral melanotic macules occur on the oral mucosa and present with one or more flat brown to black areas, sometimes with irregular borders and mottled pigmentation, on average 2–4 mm in size, but no larger than 1 cm. These macules do not darken when exposed to sunlight.

EPIDEMIOLOGY AND ETIOLOGY

Mucosal melanotic macules, most commonly develop on the vermilion portion of the lower lip and are common in white adolescent girls and young women (**2.1**). The etiology of a single or small number of flat brown to black pigmented areas is unknown and is considered to be idiopathic. Multiple perioral and oral mucosal melanotic macules characterize disorders such as Peutz–Jeghers syndrome, Laugier–Hunziker syndrome, and Addison disease.

DIFFERENTIAL DIAGNOSIS

The most important lesion to distinguish from melanotic macule is early melanoma, although it is very rare. The appearance is also similar to an amalgam tattoo or oral nevus.

DIAGNOSIS

Single lesions should undergo excisional biopsy to rule out early melanoma. With identification of multiple lesions, a screening work-up for Peutz–Jeghers syndrome, Laugier–Hunziker syndrome, and Addison disease is required.

PATHOPHYSIOLOGY

A melanotic macule is a variation of normal mucosal pigmentation. It is not malignant and cannot transform into a melanoma.

TREATMENT

Excisional biopsy of melanotic macule is diagnostic. When there are multiple lesions, it is always important to biopsy the largest, darkest, most raised lesion with irregular borders.

PROGNOSIS

Excision of isolated melanotic macule(s) can be performed for cosmetic reasons without recurrence. However, lesions associated with Peutz–Jeghers syndrome, Laugier–Hunziker syndrome, and Addison disease may recur as new lesions.

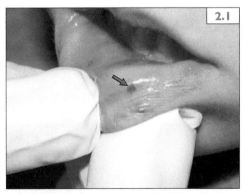

2.1 Benign melonotic macule. Labial melanotic macule of the lower lip (arrow). (Courtesy of Robert D. Kelsch, DMD; Department of Dental Medicine at North Shore Long Island Jewish Health (LIJ) System.)

Juvenile periodontitis

CLINICAL PRESENTATION

Most cases of periodontitis in children are not obvious clinically. Probing for attachment loss, checking for tooth mobility, and obtaining radiographs to assess the bone levels around the teeth helps with the diagnosis. Gingival recession, gingival erythema, and gingival edema typically are not found, except in patients with neutrophil defects. Periodontal disease in a child suggests the need for further investigation of a possible systemic condition.

EPIDEMIOLOGY AND ETIOLOGY

Juvenile periodontitis has three presentations: prepubertal, juvenile, and rapidly progressing periodontitis.

Prepubertal periodontitis can present in a localized form involving minimal inflammation but with deep gingival pockets localized to primary molars, followed by primary incisors. The generalized form shows severe gingival inflammation and deep pockets involving all primary teeth.

Juvenile periodontitis initially involves permanent molars, then incisors in healthy teenagers with associated inflammation, rapid bone loss, and tooth mobility (**2.2**).

Rapidly progressive periodontitis presents similarly to juvenile periodontitis but is more prevalent in young adults.

DIFFERENTIAL DIAGNOSIS

Unexpected bone loss in a child with loose teeth could involve serious diseases, such as Langerhans cell histiocytosis (LCH), Papillon–Lefèvre syndrome, leukocyte adhesion deficiency (LAD), leukemia, neutropenia, hypophosphatasia, chronic granulomatous disease, histocytosis X, diabetes mellitus, Down syndrome, human immunodeficiency virus (HIV), and acquired immunodeficiency syndrome (AIDS).

DIAGNOSIS

Clinical and radiographic data and tissue biopsy as well as tissue specimens should be submitted for culture identification. Pertinent testing for specific immune deficiencies should be considered.

PATHOPHYSIOLOGY

Juvenile periodontitis has been linked to LAD and is also associated with the bacterium *Actinobacillus actinomycetemcomitans*.

TREATMENT

The goal is to extract severely affected teeth as part of periodontal surgery, plaque control, and postsurgical prophylaxis with tetracycline.

PROGNOSIS

In patients with LAD type 1, less than 1% of CD18 surface expression (required for firm adhesion of leukocytes on endothelial cells) predisposes patients to worsening infections and surgical complications.

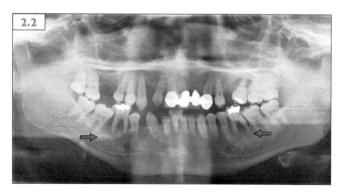

2.2 Juvenile periodontitis. Panoramic film showing bone loss localized to the permanent molars (arrows).

Ankyloglossia

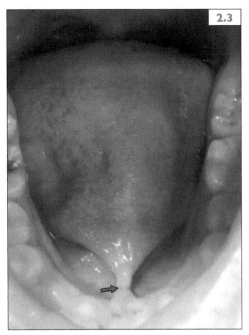

2.3

CLINICAL PRESENTATION
Ankyloglossia, or tongue-tie, is a congenital anomaly with a short lingual frenulum or with a highly attached genioglossus muscle restricting tongue movement (**2.3**).

EPIDEMIOLOGY AND ETIOLOGY
Most cases are sporadic. There is an increased frequency in boys, with a male-to-female ratio of 2:1.

DIAGNOSIS
An abnormally short frenulum, inserting at or near the tip of the tongue, causes difficulty lifting, protruding, or side-to-side movement of the tongue. There is inability to protrude the tongue more than 1–2 mm past the lower central incisors.

PATHOPHYSIOLOGY
Impaired tongue mobility may be associated with breastfeeding difficulty, speech articulation difficulty, and masticatory problems.

2.3 Ankyloglossia, showing a large band of fibrous tissue (arrow) extending from the ventral tongue to the lingual gingiva of the anterior mandible.

TREATMENT
The two most commonly performed procedures for ankyloglossia are frenotomy and frenuloplasty. Frenotomy (also called frenulotomy) is a simple surgical release of the frenulum. This procedure is often performed for infants with breastfeeding difficulty. Frenuloplasty is a release of the frenulum with surgical plastic repair. It is reserved for ankyloglossia that is not relieved by simple division of the frenulum, very thick frenula, or for revision cases.

PROGNOSIS
Definitive treatment requires surgery. Consultation with a lactation specialist may help with feeding problems; speech therapy may help the child improve speech.

Labial frenula

CLINICAL PRESENTATION
Abnormalities of the attachment and hypertrophy of labial frenula may occur in both the upper and lower lips (**2.4**).

PATHOPHYSIOLOGY
The persistence of maxillary attachment during dental eruption may cause widely spaced central incisors (diastema). The extension of the mandibular frenulum to the interdental papilla may produce periodontal disease and bone loss.

TREATMENT
Labial frenulum is typically treated with surgical division.

PROGNOSIS
Prognosis is good with timely diagnosis and surgical management.

Cleft lip and palate

CLINICAL PRESENTATION
In the unilateral cleft lip, there is discontinuity of the orbicularis oris in the region of the cleft. Fibers of the orbicularis oriented in parallel to the cleft margin, insert into the alar base on the lateral side of the cleft and onto the columellar base and septum on the medial side of the cleft. In the complete bilateral cleft of the lip there is a failure of the premaxillary segment to fuse with the lateral maxillary segments. The clefts of both the primary and secondary palate may range from simple notching of the alveolus to clefts that extend through the alveolus or through the hard and soft palate. Clefts of the secondary palate range from simple bifid uvula to complete clefts that may extend anteriorly to the incisive foramen.

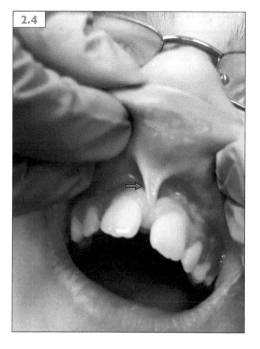

2.4

2.4 Labial frenula showing a hypertrophic, heavy band of mucosa (arrow) attaching to the crest of the alveolar ridge.

EPIDEMIOLOGY AND ETIOLOGY

There is significant racial heterogeneity in the incidence of clefts of the lip and palate. In the Caucasian population, cleft lip and palate occur in approximately 1 in 1000 births, while the incidence in the Asian population is 2 in 1000 births; in African Americans, it is approximately 0.41 per 1000 live births. In contrast, the incidence of clefts of the secondary palate alone is similar for all ethnic groups at 0.5 per 1000 live births. Approximately 60–80% of children born with a cleft of the lip and palate are males; isolated clefts of the secondary palate occur more frequently in females. Distribution of clefts is as follows: 25% of patients present with isolated cleft lip, 50% with cleft lip and palate, and 33% with clefts of the secondary palate alone. Bilateral cleft lip and palate is present in about 20% of patients, and bilateral cleft lip without palate cleft occurs in 5%.

PATHOPHYSIOLOGY

The use of phenytoin during pregnancy has been associated with a 10-fold increase in the incidence of cleft lip. The incidence of cleft lip in infants born to mothers who smoke during pregnancy is twice that of those born to nonsmoking mothers.

Cleft deformities may be syndromic or nonsyndromic in nature. The most common syndromic cleft deformity is seen with Van der Woude syndrome, an autosomal dominant disorder characterized by clefts of the lip or palate and blind sinuses, or pits of the lower lip. Syndromic clefts associated with secondary cleft palate alone include velocardiofacial syndrome, DiGeorge syndrome, and conotruncal anomaly face syndrome, which are all associated with microdeletions of chromosome 22q11.2. Inheritance is autosomal dominant with considerable variability in phenotypic expression, which may include facial dysmorphism, developmental delay, cardiovascular anomalies, immunologic abnormalities, cleft palate, and velopharyngeal dysfunction.

Nonsyndromic palatal clefts with multifactorial inheritance, or from abnormalities at a major single-gene locus may be associated with Stickler syndrome, ectrodactyly-ectodermal clefting (EEC) syndrome, and popliteal pterygium syndrome.

TREATMENT

It is recognized that palatal repairs that denude bone heal with scar formation and result in midfacial growth distortion. This results in a prognathic profile. Correction of maxillary hypoplasia and retrusion usually requires transverse maxillary expansion to correct crossbite deformities. Maxillary advancement with LeFort I osteotomies and rigid fixation is commonly performed to correct for midfacial growth retardation.

PROGNOSIS

The goal of surgical treatment staging is to close the lip and possibly the soft palate at 3 months and to align musculature such as the orbicularis oris, tensor veli palatini, and levator palatine. If the cleft lip is wide, then a lip adhesion procedure is considered. At 18 months of age, speech is of primary concern and closure of the hard palate is required. Closure of the soft palate should be done in conjunction with the lip and not the hard palate. At 7–12 years of age, alveolar cleft repair is advised since 95% of anteroposterior and transverse growth is completed. The procedure can be performed when the permanent cuspid root is at least 60% developed. The procedure includes a four corner flap with autogenous bone grafting.

Geographic tongue

CLINICAL PRESENTATION
Geographic tongue, or benign migratory glossitis, is a chronic condition characterized by red lesions with irregular, elevated, white or yellow borders. The lesions occur predominantly on the dorsum and lateral borders of the anterior two-thirds of the tongue. They are typically asymptomatic (**2.5**).

EPIDEMIOLOGY AND ETIOLOGY
Geographic tongue is more common in girls than boys. The etiology is not known, but it has been associated with childhood allergies.

DIFFERENTIAL DIAGNOSIS
Tongue lesions can resemble oral candidiasis, lichen planus, lupus, and premalignant dysplasia.

DIAGNOSIS
Clinical recognition is important. If symptomatic, biopsy is indicated to rule out other entities.

PATHOPHYSIOLOGY
The lesions are areas of dekeratinization and desquamation of filiform papilla which are continuously changing, creating a migratory appearance.

PROGNOSIS AND TREATMENT
No treatment is indicated in asymptomatic cases. Parental reassurance relieves anxiety associated with this finding.

Fissured tongue

CLINICAL PRESENTATION
Fissured tongue, or lingua plicata, is a developmental anomaly characterized by anterior–posterior fissures from which smaller fissures radiate laterally (**2.6**).

EPIDEMIOLOGY AND ETIOLOGY
Fissured tongue is common in children with Down syndrome. It is seen in Melkersson–Rosenthal syndrome, a rare disorder consisting of recurrent facial and/or lip edema and relapsing facial nerve paralysis.

DIFFERENTIAL DIAGNOSIS
This finding can resemble geographic tongue.

DIAGNOSIS
No biopsy is needed on a fissured tongue because of its characteristic clinical appearance.

PATHOPHYSIOLOGY
The fissures can be shallow or deep. Deep fissures may trap food debris, causing inflammation or secondary fungal infections.

TREATMENT
Patients and parents are advised to brush the surface of the tongue daily.

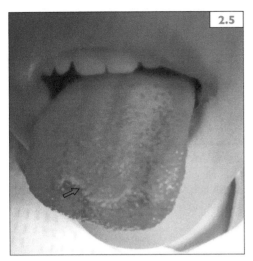

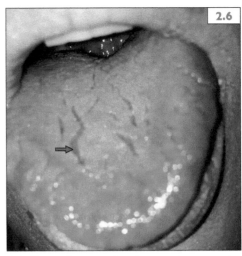

2.5 Geographic tongue showing erythematous patches with a distinctive white rim on the dorsal surface (arrow).

2.6 Fissured tongue showing anterior–posterior fissures on the tongue surface (arrow).

Gingival overgrowth

CLINICAL PRESENTATION AND PATHOPHYSIOLOGY

Gingival overgrowth in children can be hereditary, inflammatory, infiltrative, or an adverse effect of certain medications. In hereditary gingival overgrowth there is a progressive fibrous enlargement of the buccal and lingual gingival surface, with failure or delayed eruption of primary and permanent teeth. Inflammatory gingival overgrowth can result from longstanding gingivitis in young patients, especially when plaque accumulates around orthodontic appliances or in patients who are mouth breathers. It can be localized or generalized, involving interdental papillae and the marginal gingival surface that leads to friable and bleeding mucosa.

The infiltrative type of gingival overgrowth as seen in leukemia can cause gingival enlargement due to infiltration of the gingival tissues with edematous and hemorrhagic features. Drug-induced gingival overgrowth occurs as a side-effect of phenytoin, cyclosporin-A, and nifedipine. This gingival hypertrophy is painless and firm, with little bleeding tendency. Initially gingiva enlarges in the interdental region and then may progress to cover the crowns of the teeth, where it may interfere with occlusion.

DIAGNOSIS

Complete blood count (CBC) count is recommended to rule out anemia or leukemia.

PROGNOSIS AND TREATMENT

With hereditary gingival fibromatosis and inflammatory gingival enlargement, the treatment of choice is gingivectomy. Good oral hygiene is also required to reduce the risk of recurrence.

Patients with leukemic gingival hypertrophy may have difficulty maintaining good oral hygiene because of gingival bleeding. Good oral hygiene and evaluation and management of an underlying systemic disease is necessary. Gingivectomy and discontinuation of medication may be necessary in drug-induced gingival hypertrophy.

Hemangioma

CLINICAL PRESENTATION
Hemangiomas can occur in any soft tissue location and are common on the lip, dorsum of the tongue, gingiva, and buccal mucosa. They are red or bluish-red, slightly raised lesions that are moderately firm to palpation. They are usually painless but can ulcerate or bleed if traumatized (**2.7**).

EPIDEMIOLOGY AND ETIOLOGY
Hemangiomas appear early in life and typically enlarge rapidly during infancy and regress slowly during childhood.

DIFFERENTIAL DIAGNOSIS
Hemangiomas resemble lymphangiomas and hemangiolymphangioma.

DIAGNOSIS
A clinical examination with emphasis on location and size of a lesion with possible mass effect is essential. If a life threatening arteriovenous hemangioma is suspected, further work-up with Doppler imaging, computed tomography (CT), magnetic resonance imaging (MRI), and angiography is recommended.

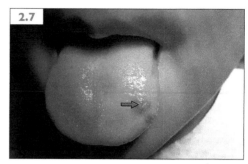

2.7 Hemangioma showing raised, soft, bluish-purple lesion of the dorsal and lateral tongue (arrow).

PATHOPHYSIOLOGY
Hemangiomas are enlarged vascular tumors of mesenchymal origin, characterized by the formation of vascular tubes of endothelial cells.

PROGNOSIS AND TREATMENT
Treatment is indicated if the hemangioma interferes with breathing, eating, or speech, or is grossly deforming.

Lymphangioma

CLINICAL PRESENTATION
Superficial lymphangiomas appear as pink to reddish-blue, soft, compressible lesions, in contrast to a deeper lymphangioma that may not be as apparent. The tongue, lips, and buccal mucosa are the most common sites of lymphangioma occurrence. Large lymphangiomas that involve the floor of the mouth and the neck are called cystic hygromas.

EPIDEMIOLOGY AND ETIOLOGY
Lymphangiomas present at birth or develop later in life.

DIFFERENTIAL DIAGNOSIS
Hemangiomas, hemangiolymphangioma, lipomas, and salivary retention cysts may share similar features with lymphangiomas.

PATHOPHYSIOLOGY
Lymphangiomas are benign tumors of the lymphatic vessels.

PROGNOSIS AND TREATMENT
Surgical resection is the most common treatment, despite a high frequency of recurrences and complications. Image-guided percutaneous chemoablation has shown good surgical outcomes with minimal complications.

Mucocele

CLINICAL PRESENTATION
Mucoceles typically present as painless swellings on the lower lip. They are usually less than 1 cm in diameter, smooth walled, and bluish or translucent. Mucoceles may resolve without intervention or persist, where the surface can become keratinized.

DIFFERENTIAL DIAGNOSIS
Mucoceles can resemble a developing salivary gland tumor, such as a pleomorphic adenoma, basal cell adenoma, or canalicular adenoma.

DIAGNOSIS
Excisional biopsy is diagnostic and serves as a definitive treatment.

PATHOPHYSIOLOGY
Mucoceles are pseudocysts of minor salivary origin. They are formed when salivary gland secretions dissect into the soft tissues surrounding the gland, usually as a result of trauma to a minor salivary gland that causes pooling of mucous in an obstructed and dilated excretory duct (**2.8**).

PROGNOSIS AND TREATMENT
Treatment is excision of the mucocele with removal of the associated minor salivary gland to prevent recurrence.

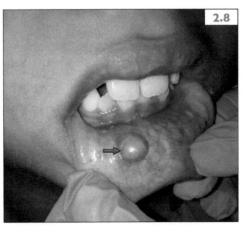

2.8 Mucocele showing tissue swelling of the lower lip composed of pooled mucus (arrow). Lesion is soft and fluctuant on palpation.

Ranula

CLINICAL PRESENTATION

Ranulas appear as blue, fluctuant swellings lateral to the midline in the lower mouth. Large ranulas, or 'plunging' ranulas, can present as neck masses if they extend below the mylohyoid muscle of the floor of the mouth (**2.9**).

EPIDEMIOLOGY AND ETIOLOGY

Ranulas can be congenital, probably from improper drainage of sublingual glands, or acquired after oral trauma.

DIFFERENTIAL DIAGNOSIS

Other lesions should be considered including low-grade mucoepidermoid carcinoma, cavernous hemangioma, lymphangioma, and a venous varix.

DIAGNOSIS

Diagnosis is on clinical examination and CT scan.

PATHOPHYSIOLOGY

Ranulas are pseudocysts associated with the sublingual glands and submandibular ducts.

PROGNOSIS AND TREATMENT

Complete excision with the associated sublingual gland is preferred. Marsupialization and suturing of the pseudocyst wall to the oral mucosa may be effective if complete excision cannot be performed.

Fibroma

CLINICAL PRESENTATION

Fibromas may occur on the palate, tongue, cheek, and lip. Fibromas are usually flesh-colored, sessile or pedunculated, smooth, firm masses less than 1 cm in diameter (**2.10**).

DIFFERENTIAL DIAGNOSIS

This mass can resemble many types of lesions including lipoma, schwannoma, pleomorphic adenoma, basal cell adenoma, and canalicular adenoma.

DIAGNOSIS

Excisional biopsy is the diagnostic and definitive treatment.

PATHOPHYSIOLOGY

Fibromas are lesions that are formed when chronic irritation results in reactive connective tissue hyperplasia.

PROGNOSIS AND TREATMENT

Fibromas can be surgically removed and will not recur if the source of irritation is removed.

Parulis

Parulis is the end of a draining fistulous tract of a necrotic primary tooth. It is a soft, solitary, reddish papule located apical and facial to the abscessed tooth. Purulent drainage may be observed (**2.11**).

Treatment is to extract the abscessed tooth or perform root canal therapy.

Eruption cyst

Eruption cysts are soft tissue lesions associated with erupting primary and permanent teeth. They are caused by fluid accumulation within the follicular space of the erupting tooth. Eruption cysts are called eruption hematomas when the cyst fluid is mixed with blood (**2.12**).

No treatment is needed as these cysts resolve spontaneously as the tooth erupts through the lesion.

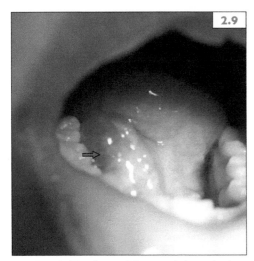

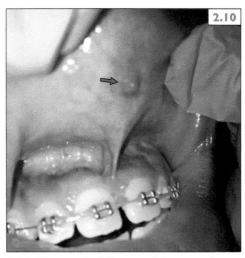

2.9 Ranula. The floor of the mouth has a finely vascularized, distended appearance (arrow), and fluctuant mucus escape phenomenon as a consequence of sublingual gland severance.

2.10 Fibroma. Oral fibroma of the upper lip (arrow) secondary to chronic irritation from orthodontic treatment.

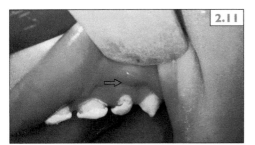

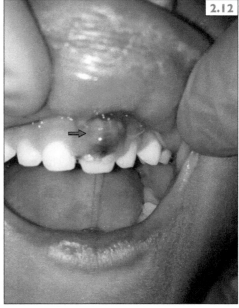

2.11 Parulis. Small nodule is shown (arrow), representing opening of a draining tract on gingiva secondary to dental infection.

2.12 Eruption cyst showing a fluctuant, hemorrhagic swelling of the alveolar ridge (arrow) confined to soft tissues, associated with an erupting tooth.

Aphthous ulcer

CLINICAL PRESENTATION

Aphthous ulcers, also known as canker sores, are painful oral lesions that appear as localized, shallow ulcers of the oral gland-bearing mucosa (**2.13**). Pain is out of proportion to the size of the lesion. Lesions spare attached gingiva, the hard palate, and dorsum of the tongue. The most common presentation of aphthous ulcers is the aphthous minor form while the other forms are aphthous major and herpetiform.

Aphthous minor ulcers are small, painful ulcers that heal spontaneously within 10–14 days without scarring. More severe disease, with larger lesions (aphthous major, characterized as being greater than 5 mm) can last for 6 weeks. Herpetiform ulcers present as multiple small clusters of pinpoint lesions that coalesce to form large irregular ulcers, lasting 7–10 days.

EPIDEMIOLOGY AND ETIOLOGY

Aphthous minor lesions occur episodically with two to four outbreaks per year. Aphthae occur more commonly in childhood and adolescence and become less frequent in adulthood.

DIFFERENTIAL DIAGNOSIS

Traumatic ulcers, caused by mechanical, chemical, or thermal injury are very common causes of oral ulcers in children. The appearance of the lesions varies depending on the intensity of the trauma. These ulcers typically heal within 2 weeks of trauma.

Behçet disease is a neutrophilic inflammatory disorder that presents with recurrent oral and genital ulcerations. It most often presents in young men. Oral aphthae tend to be more extensive and often multiple, healing spontaneously within 1–3 weeks. Genital lesions occur in about 75% of patients with Behçet disease.

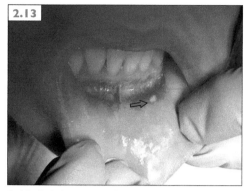

2.13 Aphthous ulcer (arrow). Small, shallow ulcers with a whitish base and erythematous halo of oral mucosa.

PATHOPHYSIOLOGY

Factors that may predispose to the development of aphthous ulcers include familial predisposition, trauma, hormonal factors, food or drug hypersensitivity, immunodeficiency, and emotional stress. Aphthous ulcers may be seen in patients with celiac disease, inflammatory bowel disease, and with use of antimetabolites such as methotrexate.

PROGNOSIS AND TREATMENT

The treatment for aphthous ulcers includes symptomatic relief with topical steroids and topical analgesics.

Systemic lupus erythematosus

CLINICAL PRESENTATION
Systemic lupus erythematosus (SLE) can involve the lips and oral mucosa. Discoid lip lesions are characterized as keratotic papules or plaques with pigment alteratio, and associated photosensitivity. Oral ulcers are red, shallow, and found on the palate and marginal gingiva (**2.14**). Oral ulcers are usually painless.

EPIDEMIOLOGY AND ETIOLOGY
Oral mucus membrane involvement occurs in up to 50% of patients with SLE.

PROGNOSIS AND TREATMENT
Skin biopsy and other features of SLE are used for diagnosis. Treatment of lip lesions includes glucocorticoids as well as antimalarial agents.

Bullous pemphigoid

Bullous pemphigoid is an autoimmune blistering disorder with oral involvement, consisting of intact bullae or erosions occurring in about one-third of adult cases. It rarely presents in children. Skin lesions may consist of bullae or urticarial plaques and typically occur in the flexural areas, groin, and axillae.

The diagnosis is made with immuno-fluorescence testing of lesional and perilesional skin. Therapy is with oral gluco-corticoids.

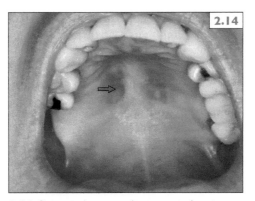

2.14 Systemic lupus erythematosus showing palatal diffuse annular leukoplakic lesions, erythema, and chronic ulcerations (arrow). (Courtesy of Robert D. Kelsch, DMD; Department of Dental Medicine at North Shore Long Island Jewish Health (LIJ) System.)

Mucous membrane pemphigoid

Mucous membrane pemphigoid affects oral, ocular, pharyngeal, laryngeal, genital, or anal mucosa where squamous mucosal involvement predominates. The disease process involves breakdown of adhesive factors that anchor the epithelium to basement membrane and connective tissue. A potential clinical test, though not specific, consists of rubbing the tissue, producing a blister or bulla (Nikolsky sign). Oral lesions include desquamative gingivitis and bullae with a tendency to scar (**2.15**).

The diagnosis is made by immuno-fluorescence testing along with the appropriate clinical findings. Immunosuppressant therapy is needed to control this disease.

Pemphigus vulgaris

CLINICAL PRESENTATION

Pemphigus vulgaris occurs very rarely in children and is characterized by flaccid bullae that typically begin in the oropharynx and then spread to involve the skin of the scalp, face, chest, axillae, and groin. Pemphigus vulgaris can be life threatening. There is a loss of adhesion between cells above the basal cell layer resulting in bullous formation. The bullae rupture easily, so that the patient often presents with only painful erosions and no intact bullae. One specific type, paraneoplastic pemphigus, tends to involve the oral and ocular mucosa (**2.16, 2.17**).

PROGNOSIS AND TREATMENT

The diagnosis of pemphigus vulgaris is made by immunofluorescence testing and serum levels of immunoglobulin G autoantibody to desmoglein III. Standard therapy is with oral glucocorticoids, but relapsing disease can be treated with cyclophosphamide, mycophenolate mofetil, azathioprine, intravenous gamma globulin, and in severe cases, plasmapheresis.

Erythema multiforme

CLINICAL PRESENTATION AND PATHOPHYSIOLOGY

Erythema multiforme is a hypersensitivity reaction that presents with both mucosal and skin lesions. Mucosal involvement is seen in greater than 90% of patients with erythema multiforme. Erythema and edema of the lips along with intraoral bullae may occur. The bullae often rupture, leaving painful raw surfaces and hemorrhagic crusts (**2.18, 2.19**). Oral lesions are very painful.

Erythema multiforme is frequently associated with herpes simplex virus (HSV) infections, medications, or can be idiopathic. Target skin lesions are a characteristic feature of erythema multiforme.

PROGNOSIS AND TREATMENT

Erythema multiforme can be managed with symptomatic therapy alone. For patients with cutaneous disease and/or mild oral mucosal involvement, treatment with topical corticosteroids, oral antihistamines, and/or an anesthetic mouthwash is sufficient. Antiviral therapy often is effective for the prevention of recurrent HSV-associated erythema multiforme.

2.15 Mucous membrane pemphigoid showing gingiva containing patchy areas of erythema and superficial erosions (arrow). (Courtesy of Robert D. Kelsch, DMD; Department of Dental Medicine at North Shore Long Island Jewish Health (LIJ) System.)

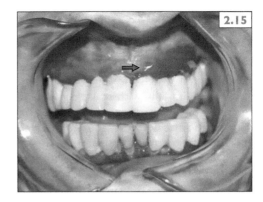

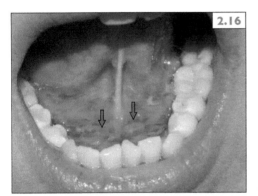

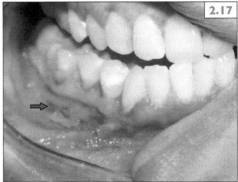

2.16, 2.17 Pemphigus vulgaris showing erosive lesions and blister formation of gingiva (arrows). (Courtesy of Robert D. Kelsch, DMD; Department of Dental Medicine at North Shore Long Island Jewish Health (LIJ) System.)

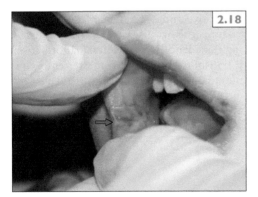

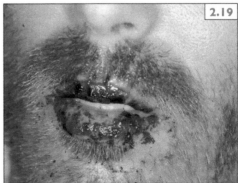

2.18, 2.19 Erythema multiforme showing diffuse areas of superficial sloughing and focal erosions of labial mucosa (arrow). (Courtesy of Robert D. Kelsch, DMD; Department of Dental Medicine at North Shore Long Island Jewish Health (LIJ) System.)

Stevens–Johnson syndrome

CLINICAL PRESENTATION

Stevens–Johnson syndrome is a clinical condition in which the skin is sloughing. It presents initially with malaise and fever, followed by the rapid onset of erythematous or purpuric macules and plaques. Erythematous, purpuric macules and skin detachment may also occur in Stevens–Johnson syndrome. Mucosal membranes are affected in 92–100% of patients, usually at two or more distinct sites, such as the ocular, oral, and genital regions. Stevens–Johnson syndrome is commonly induced by drugs such as nonsteroidal anti-inflammatory drugs, allopurinol, phenytoin, carbamazepine, barbiturates, anticonvulsants, and sulfa antibiotics.

PROGNOSIS AND TREATMENT

Supportive care includes wound care, fluid and electrolyte management, nutritional support, pain control, and treatment of secondary skin infections.

Coxsackie virus

Coxsackie virus infections present as intraoral and palmar or plantar lesions. It is common in children younger than 5 years of age and is often labeled as 'hand, foot, and mouth disease'. The lesions appear as oval shaped, pale papules with a rim of erythema on the palms and soles, and small aphthae intraorally. The intraoral lesions tend to spare the lips and gingiva, unlike HSV. Fever, sore throat, and a malaise often precede the onset of lesions.

Treatment is supportive. Lesions and symptoms disappear within 2 weeks.

Rubeola

Measles, or rubeola, present orally on the buccal mucosa as lesions called Koplik spots. Koplik spots are flat, erythematous macules with 'salt crystal' centers. They appear during the prodrome that precedes the skin rash by 1–2 days. Rubeola is also associated with diffuse pharyngitis and bilateral cervical lymphadenitis.

Measles is self-limiting with a 2 week clinical course. Serious complications, such as acute encephalitis, corneal ulcerations, pneumonia and otitis media, are infrequent in pediatrics and usually seen in nonimmunized adults. Supportive care is important.

Rubella

With increased pediatric immunization practice, rubella, or German measles, is no longer common in children. It manifests as a fine reddish maculopapular rash on the face, progressing down the trunk and extremities. Throat and palate erythema present without Koplik spots. Fever, mild malaise, and involvement of posterior cervical lymph nodes and suboccipital lymphadenopathy are common.

Rubella is a self-limiting viral disease where supportive care is recommended. Worrisome features of this disease are attributed to a high incidence of congenital malformations if transmitted to a first trimester embryo in nonimmunized pregnant women. Diagnosis is made with a fluorescent antibody test.

Varicella-zoster virus

Varicella-zoster virus infection presents as vesicles and erosions seen in patients with varicella (chickenpox). In patients with herpes zoster, grouped vesicles or erosions may be seen unilaterally on the hard palate. Other oral areas that may be involved include the buccal mucosa, tongue, and gingiva.

It is a self-limiting disease in the immunocompetent patient. Supportive care, such as with hydration, analgesics, and antipyretics, is recommended. Lesions may persist for 10–21 days.

Herpes simplex virus

CLINICAL PRESENTATION AND PATHOPHYSIOLOGY

Primary HSV infection occurs in young children approximately 1 week after contact with an infected child or adult. The infection may be subclinical or be associated with symptoms such as fever, malaise, irritability, or sleeplessness. The oral presentation includes red, edematous marginal gingivae that bleed easily, and clusters of small vesicles that become yellow after rupture surrounded by a red halo. The vesicles coalesce to form large, painful ulcers of the oral and perioral tissues. HSV remains latent in the trigeminal ganglion until it is reactivated. Reactivation occurs on the lips as herpes labialis, a vesicular eruption on the skin adjacent to the vermilion border of the lip. The vesicles rupture to form ulcers and crusts and heal without scarring in 1–2 weeks. In the oral cavity HSV presents as herpetic stomatitis and primary reactivation occurs on the hard palate or gingiva.

PROGNOSIS AND TREATMENT

Primary herpetic gingivostomatitis is self-limiting and only supportive care consisting of hydration, nutrition, antipyretics, and antibiotics for secondary infections is recommended. Immunocompromised patients warrant acyclovir therapy.

Oropharyngeal candidiasis

CLINICAL PRESENTATION AND PATHOPHYSIOLOGY

Oropharyngeal candidiasis or 'thrush' is common in young infants, diabetics, patients treated with antibiotics, chemotherapy, radiation therapy, and those with AIDS. Patients receiving inhaled glucocorticoids for asthma or topical glucocorticoids for rhinitis and eosinophilic esophagitis are also prone to this complication.

Oropharyngeal candidiasis can manifest in several ways. The pseudomembranous form is the most common, and is characterized as plaques on the buccal mucosa, palate, tongue, or oropharynx (**2.20**). The atrophic form, which is often found under dentures in adults, presents as erythema without plaques. Candidiasis may also present with a sore beefy red tongue. In addition, *Candida* species can cause angular cheilitis or perlèche, a painful fissuring at the corners of the mouth.

Patients with recurrent or extensive disease need to be tested for HIV or other immune deficiencies. The diagnosis is confirmed by obtaining a potassium hydroxide preparation of the white patches or erosive areas of the mucosa to visualize budding yeasts with or without pseudohyphae.

PROGNOSIS AND TREATMENT

Topical therapy is usually effective with topical nystatin suspension; systemic antifungal treatment can be used if necessary. Candidiasis usually resolves once underlying factors are controlled.

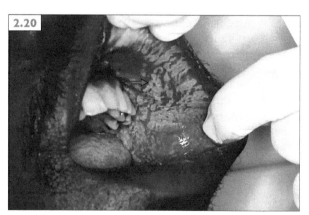

2.20 Oropharyngeal candidiasis. Pseudomembranous candidiasis of the oral cavity (arrow). (Courtesy of Robert D. Kelsch, DMD; Department of Dental Medicine at North Shore Long Island Jewish Health (LIJ) System.)

ESOPHAGUS

CHAPTER 3

Abnormal Anatomy of the Esophagus

Razan Alkhouri, Rafal Kozielski, Daniel Gelfond

- **Congenital esophageal stenosis**
- **Esophageal atresia/tracheoesophageal fistula**
- **Laryngotracheoesophageal cleft**
- **Esophageal diverticula and pouches**
- **Esophageal webs and rings**
- **Esophageal duplication**
- **Esophageal tumors**
- **Hiatal hernia**
- **Persistent embryonic epithelium**
- **Heterotopic gastric mucosa (inlet patch)**

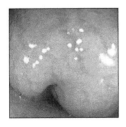
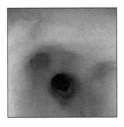
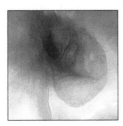
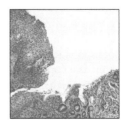

Congenital esophageal stenosis

DEFINITION

Congenital esophageal stenosis is defined as intrinsic stenosis caused by congenital malformation of the esophageal wall. The etiology is represented in three variants:

- Esophageal webs or diaphragms (usually occurs in the proximal and mid esophagus).
- Fibromuscular thickening (middle to lower esophagus).
- Cartilaginous tracheobronchial remnants (TBRs) (distal esophagus or segmental stenosis).

CLINICAL PRESENTATION

Symptoms vary with the location and severity of the stenosis. They often present after 6 months of age when solid food is introduced. Lower lesions present as vomiting, regurgitation of undigested food, aspiration, and recurrent pneumonias. If not diagnosed early, the child can present with growth failure and symptoms of malnutrition. High lesions present with respiratory symptoms.

EPIDEMIOLOGY AND ETIOLOGY

The overall incidence is 1 in 25,000–50,000 live births. 17–33% of cases are associated with other anomalies such as tracheoesophageal fistula, cardiac defects, intestinal atresias, imperforate anus, and chromosomal abnormalities.

DIFFERENTIAL DIAGNOSIS

It is important to differentiate esophageal stenosis from other diseases such as achalasia, stricture from esophageal reflux or eosinophilic esophagitis, and compression from external structures. The majority of esophageal stenosis is acquired and can be seen as a complication of caustic ingestions, postsurgical changes, or inflammatory conditions.

DIAGNOSIS

- Esophagrams reveals stenotic area with a dilated esophagus proximal to the stenotic area.
- Upper endoscopy is diagnostic.
- Esophageal manometry can be done to rule out motor disorders.

PATHOPHYSIOLOGY

- Deformity of TBR is due to an abnormal separation of the foregut into esophagus and trachea, and occurs during the fourth week of gestation. Diaphragms are a form of partial esophageal atresias.

TREATMENT

Treatment of congenital esophageal stenosis typically requires surgical repair. A thin proximal esophageal web and fibromuscular stenosis can be dilated without need of a surgical intervention. Definitive treatment occasionally requires partial resection with electocautery or endoscopic laser ablation followed by dilation. Dilatations are not always successful and there is a risk of esophageal perforation with possible development of Boerhaave syndrome, which carries a high mortality rate.

Esophageal atresia/ tracheoesophageal fistula

DEFINITION

Esophageal atresia (EA) is the lack of communication between the proximal and distal esophagus. Tracheoesophageal fistula (TEF) is an abnormal communication between the trachea and esophagus. Both entities usually occur together. There are five types of TEF (**3.1**), with 85% of patients demonstrating a blind ending upper esophageal pouch with a fistula from the trachea to the distal esophagus.

CLINICAL PRESENTATION

At birth newborns require frequent suctioning for increased secretions. Cough, emesis, and cyanosis are noted with feeding initiation. A distal fistula may produce progressive abdominal air distension.

An H-type fistula (**3.1C**) is often diagnosed late. A patient presents with respiratory distress, recurrent pneumonias, or wheezing.

Premature births occur in approximately one-third of the infants with EA which further increases morbidity.

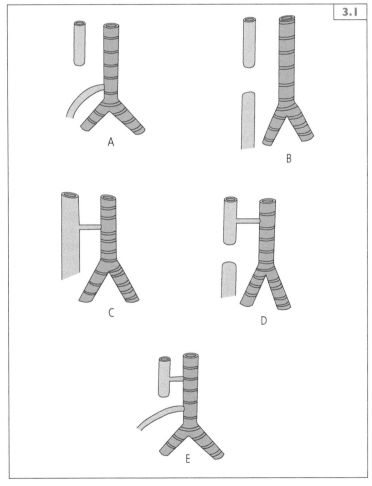

3.1

3.1 Types of tracheoesophageal fistula (TEF). **A**: Esophageal atresia (EA), with distal TEF (85%). Gastric air present on abdominal X-ray; **B**: EA with no TEF (8%). Absent gastric air on abdominal X-ray; **C**: isolated TEF (4%). Gastric air present on abdominal X-ray; **D**: EA with proximal TEF (2%). Absent gastric air on abdominal X-ray; **E**: EA with proximal and distal TEF (<1%). Gastric air present on abdominal X-ray.

EPIDEMIOLOGY AND ETIOLOGY

Incidence is 1/3,000–4,000 live births, highest among Caucasians. There is a 0.5–2% risk of recurrence among siblings of an affected child. The exact etiology remains unknown. Excessive ventral invagination of the ventral pharyngoesophageal fold leading to faulty division of the foregut into tracheal and esophageal channels during the first month of embryonic development is thought to be the underlying mechanism.

DIAGNOSIS

Prenatally, a history of polyhydramnios and an anechoic structure in the fetal neck representing the upper pouch will give suspicion of a TEF and EA. Failure to pass a nasogastric (NG) tube in a newborn can be diagnostic. A NG tube will meet resistance and may potentially coil in the esophagus (**3.2, 3.3**). A communication with trachea is recognized by the presence of intestinal air.

Direct visualization of the fistula by bronchoscopy can localize the fistula. Endoscopy may not be able to visualize the fistula. Introduction of radiographic contrast into the proximal esophagus can lead to aspiration and is typically not warranted unless it is an H-type fistula with no EA. Identification of an H-type TEF requires a special technique to increase detection rate, by withdrawing a NG tube slowly from the esophagus, allowing better visualization of the esophageal mucosa.

Echocardiogram is usually done pre-operatively to assess for associated cardiac defects.

PATHOPHYSIOLOGY

In EA the proximal part is a dilated blind-ended pouch with hypertrophied muscles, while the distal segment is atretic with thin walls. The gastroesophageal sphincter is typically incompetent with defective neural innervations.

Additional congenital anomalies occur in 50% of these infants. Most of the anomalies occur in the midline and have a significant impact on prognosis. Among infants with tracheoesophageal anomalies, 10% will have imperforate anus and 30% will have congenital cardiac defects including ventricular septal defect, patent ductus arteriosus, and tetralogy of Fallot. Multiple malformations are seen with VACTERL (vertebrae, anal, cardiac, tracheoesophageal, radial, renal, and limb anomalies) and VATER (vertebrae, anal, tracheoesophageal, and renal) association.

TREATMENT

Surgical repair is done via standard extra-pleural thoracotomy with division of the fistula and single layer primary anastomosis using polyglycolic acid sutures.

Long gaps between atretic ends might require colonic interposition (**3.4**), lengthening myotomies, or a stomach pull into the chest cavity. If lengthening fails, then ligation of the fistula and gastrostomy tube with delayed repair is considered. Complications include anastomotic leak and strictures, salivary fistula, pneumonitis, and mediastinitis.

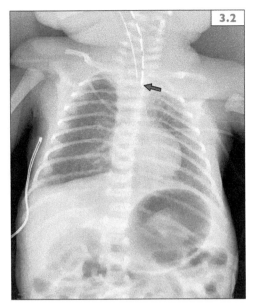

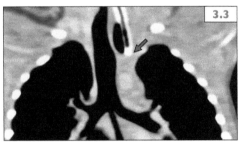

3.2, 3.3 Esophageal atresia. 3.2: The nasogastric tube fails to pass in the esophagus shown on X-ray (arrow); 3.3: CT of nasogastric tube ending above the carina (arrow).

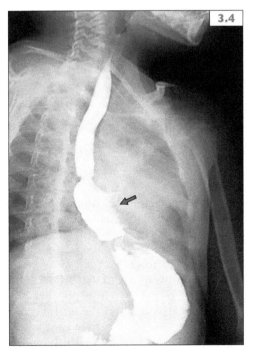

3.4 Esophageal atresia: surgically repaired atretic part with colonic interposition (arrow).

Laryngotracheoesophageal cleft

DEFINITION AND PATHOPHYSIOLOGY

Laryngo–tracheo–esophageal (LTE) cleft (LTEC) is a rare congenital anomaly consisting of midline defect along the posterior portion of the larynx and trachea and the anterior portion of the esophagus, leaving a communication between these structures. LTECs are differentiated by the Ryan classification:

- Type I: cleft above the cricoid.
- Type II: cleft extends beyond the cricoid lamina.
- Type III: cleft extends to the carina.
- Type IV: cleft extends into the main stem bronchi.

CLINICAL PRESENTATION

- Symptoms start after birth and severity depends on length of the cleft.
- Patients present with a weak or absent cry, respiratory distress with feeds, hoarseness, stridor, and aspiration pneumonias.

EPIDEMIOLOGY AND ETIOLOGY

Most cases are sporadic but can be inherited as an autosomal recessive mutation. They are seen with other anomalies including TEF, anal atresia, malrotation, microgastria, bronchobiliary fistula, cardiac anomalies, and Opitz syndrome.

DIAGNOSIS

Chest X-ray might reveal aspiration pneumonia, esophageal air, and distended bowel. Computed tomography (CT) and bronchoscopy are used to evaluate the extension of the cleft. The presence of intact arytenoid fold excludes the diagnosis of a cleft. An esophagram with small contrast volumes shows filling of the esophagus and trachea.

TREATMENT

The main objective in the management of the LTEC is to stabilize the airway. Some patients require intubation and gastric tube placement until the time of repair. Surgical repair is the definitive treatment. It is done with a lateral pharyngotomy approach through a vertical lateral cervical incision. Large clefts frequently require tracheostomy.

Complications include recurrent laryngeal nerve injury, fistulization, granulation tissue at the repair site, esophageal stenosis, aspiration, and esophageal dysmotility.

Esophageal diverticula and pouches

DEFINITION

An esophageal diverticulum or pouch is a pocket of stretched tissue that pushes outwards through the muscular wall and develops anywhere along the esophagus. It is rare and can be congenital or acquired. It is classified according to the location:

- Pharyngeal pouch (Zenker diverticulum) occurs immediately above the cricopharyngeal muscle.
- Midesophageal diverticulum occurs due to dysmotility or due to mediastinal traction.
- Epiphrenic diverticulum is located just above the diaphragm and can be associated with other diseases affecting the esophageal motility.

An esophageal diverticulum can also be classified according to the layers forming the diverticulum, or the cause (traction *versus* pulsion).

CLINICAL PRESENTATION

Large pouches can sometimes be palpated in the neck postprandially. Diverticula do not always cause problems. Some collect food, which can lead to food regurgitation, dysphagia, chest pain, aspiration pneumonia, and feeling a need to clear one's throat. As food collects in the pockets, it promotes bacterial overgrowth in the esophagus, which commonly leads to halitosis.

EPIDEMIOLOGY AND PATHOPHYSIOLOGY

Noncongenital diverticula can develop from pulsion when increased pressure in the oropharynx occurs during swallowing against a closed upper esophageal sphincter (Zenker), or from increased pressure during esophageal propulsive contractions against a closed lower esophageal sphincter (epiphrenic). In contrast, traction diverticula occur as a consequence of pulling forces on the outside of the esophagus from an adjacent inflammatory process (e.g. involvement of inflamed mediastinal lymph nodes in tuberculosis or histoplasmosis). The diverticula can contain all layers of the gastrointestinal (GI) tract, or only the mucosa and submucosa (Zenker diverticulum).

DIAGNOSIS
- Barium swallow can outline mucosal abnormalities (**3.5**).
- Upper endoscopy is used to confirm/ establish visual identification with biopsies and possible dilatation if necessary (**3.6**). The endoscopist should be cautious to avoid advancing into the diverticulum as the risk of perforation increases.

TREATMENT
Asymptomatic patients do not require treatment. Depending on the anatomy and tissue pathology, endoscopic dilatation of a strictured segment and acid suppression might be required.

Surgical management for symptomatic cases is recommended; it includes crico-pharyngeal myotomy with or without diverticulectomy.

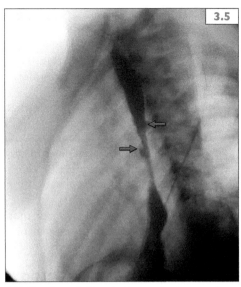

3.5 Esophageal diverticula on a barium swallow (arrows indicate the diverticula).

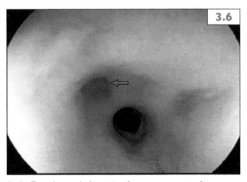

3.6 Esophageal diverticula on upper endoscopy.

PROGNOSIS
Squamous cell carcinoma (SCC) has been reported to develop in patients with a long-term diverticulum, although this is more common in adult patients.

Esophageal webs and rings

DEFINITION

Esophageal rings and webs are thin fragile structures that partially or completely comprise the esophageal lumen.

An esophageal ring is a concentric, smooth, thin extension of normal esophageal tissue consisting of three anatomic layers of mucosa, submucosa, and sometimes include smooth muscle. An esophageal ring can be found anywhere along the esophagus, but is usually found in the distal esophagus.

An esophageal web is a fold of squamous mucosa that protrudes into the lumen at any level of the esophagus.

ETIOLOGY AND PATHOPHYSIOLOGY

Rings and webs may be congenital remnants in which the esophagus fails to recanalize completely during embryogenesis. Schatzki rings arise in response to chronic injury by gastroesophageal reflux. Autoimmune diseases have been associated with esophageal webs and rings. Although webs have been linked to iron deficiency anemia (Plummer–Vinson syndrome), some studies have found no correlation between webs and either overt or latent iron deficiency.

CLINICAL PRESENTATION

Although some patients with esophageal webs are asymptomatic and only get discovered incidentally, most will present with clinical symptoms of dysphagia and esophageal food impaction.

DIAGNOSIS

Barium esophagram or an upper endoscopy is helpful.

TREATMENT

The first line of therapy for webs and rings is endoscopic dilation. Endoscopic laser division can be used for refractory webs along with disruption with biopsy forceps, electrosurgical incision, or steroid injections.

Acid suppression may reduce the risk of recurrence.

Esophageal duplication

DEFINITION

Congenital esophageal duplication is a rare embryologic anomaly of the foregut. It represents either simple epithelial-lined cysts or true esophageal duplications bounded by muscularis mucosae, submucosa, and muscularis externa that can appear as diverticula or as a tubular malformation. Lining of the cystic duplication may include squamous, columnar, or cuboidal epithelium and often will have gastric mucosa.

CLINICAL PRESENTATION

Neonates can present with respiratory distress, while older children usually present with dysphagia owing to the pressure exerted by the cyst. Small duplications can remain asymptomatic. The acid produced from the gastric lining of the duplication can cause erosions and bronchial or GI hemorrhage.

EPIDEMIOLOGY AND ETIOLOGY

The exact incidence of esophageal duplication is not known, but from an autopsy series of nearly 50,000 patients, the incidence of esophageal duplication cysts was estimated to be 1 in 8,200 patients. Congenital duplications occur along any part of the GI tract but most commonly are in the midgut. The foregut accounts for one-third of lesions, and among the foregut duplications, esophageal duplications are the most common.

DIFFERENTIAL DIAGNOSIS

Bronchogenic cyst, enteric cyst of the mediastinum.

DIAGNOSIS

- Chest X-ray and barium esophagram will show a posterior mediastinal mass.
- CT or magnetic resonance imaging (MRI) helps to further identify the lesion.

PATHOPHYSIOLOGY

A cyst or a fistula can form from herniation of the endodermal gut through a split that occurs in the notochord that is present from the 3rd week of gestation. The cyst may interfere with the anterior fusion of the vertebral mesoderm accounting for vertebral anomalies in 50% of the cases.

TREATMENT

Surgical excision.

Esophageal tumors

DEFINITION

Eophageal tumors are rare in children. Small benign mucosal leiomyoma, adenocarcinoma (ACA), and SCC have been reported.

CLINICAL PRESENTATION

Benign esophageal tumors in pediatric patients are usually incidental findings and are often described as small lesions. Larger tumors present with dysphagia, vomiting, anorexia, weight loss, bleeding, recurrent pulmonary symptoms, and pneumonias.

EPIDEMIOLOGY AND ETIOLOGY

In pediatric patients, emphasis is placed on screening and treating conditions that if left untreated will predispose to cancer development in adulthood. A risk factor for ACA is gastroesophageal reflux disease, while risk factors for SCC include achalasia, TEF, chemoradiation, lye ingestion, and other causes of esophagitis. Human papilloma virus has been linked to esophageal papilloma and less certainly to SCC.

DIAGNOSIS

Examination is abnormal only in advanced stages of carcinoma or larger tumors. Lymphadenopathy might be noted; other symptoms may be related to mediastinal spread and superior vena cava obstruction.

Endoscopic ultrasound, CT and MRI help define the depth and degree of tissue involvement. Upper endoscopy and biopsy (or excision for small lesions) are useful.

TREATMENT

Surgical resection. Treatment is tailored to specific lesions, but data on chemotherapy and radiotherapy are not readily available since malignant esophageal tumors are rare in children.

Hiatal hernia

DEFINITION
Hiatal hernia refers to bulging of the stomach through the esophageal hiatus of the diaphragm (**3.7**).

EPIDEMIOLOGY, ETIOLOGY, AND PATHOPHYSIOLOGY
Two types of hiatal hernias are identified: the sliding hernia and the paraesophageal hernia. The sliding hernia occurs when the esophagus and gastroesophageal (GE) junction slides through the hiatus and is the most common, while the paraesophageal hernia occurs when part of the stomach slides adjacent to the esophagus through the hiatus, leaving the esophagus and the GE junction in the abdominal cavity.

CLINICAL PRESENTATION
Patients are usually asymptomatic but may present with symptoms of gastroesophageal reflux and chest pain.

DIAGNOSIS
Hiatal hernia is diagnosed on a barium swallow or during an upper endoscopy.

TREATMENT
Usually no treatment is required for sliding hiatal hernia. Surgical repair is done for paraesophageal hernias that are at risk to strangulate or compromise respiratory status.

Persistent embryonic epithelium

DEFINITION
Persistent superficial patch of columnar epithelium.

CLINICAL PRESENTATION
Persistent embryonic epithelium is an incidental finding on autopsy as microscopic foci. These findings can be found in the proximal or distal esophagus, and have no significant clinical consequence.

EPIDEMIOLOGY, ETIOLOGY, AND PATHOPHYSIOLOGY
The lining of the esophagus changes from ciliated stratified columnar epithelium in an embryo and early infancy to stratified squamous epithelium by week 25 of gestation. Occasionally a patch of superficial columnar epithelium persists at birth, especially in premature infants.

DIAGNOSIS
Physical examination is normal.

TREATMENT
No specific treatment is necessary. The embryonic epithelium is not found after early infancy and is presumed to be replaced by squamous epithelium.

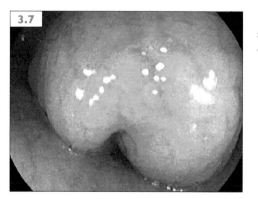
3.7

3.7 Hiatal hernia. Note the bulging of the stomach through the esophageal hiatus of the diaphragm

Heterotopic gastric mucosa (inlet patch)

DEFINITION
Single or multiple patches of gastric mucosa (5–30 mm) in the cervical esophagus (**3.8**).

CLINICAL PRESENTATION
Inlet patch can be an incidental finding, and of little clinical significance. However, some patients present with symptoms of dysphagia/odynophagia, and inlet patch has been found to be associated with gastric *Helicobacter pylori* colonization. Benign complications include esophageal stricture, webs, or stenosis. Exceedingly rare, inlet patch can present with dysplasia and progress to ACA of the esophagus.

In contrast to patients with Barrett esophagus who have intestinal metaplasia, inlet patch is identified by histologic presence of gastric type mucosa (**3.9**).

EPIDEMIOLOGY, ETIOLOGY, AND PATHOPHYSIOLOGY
The incidence in patients undergoing esophagogastroduodenoscopy has been reported to be as high as 3.6%.

TREATMENT
Asymptomatic patients do not require any treatment. Symptomatic patients will benefit from proton pump inhibitors.

Associated strictures can be treated endoscopically with dilatation. Endoscopic biopsy is required to exclude malignant progression.

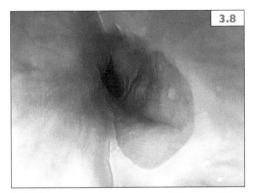

3.8 Heterotopic gastric mucosa (inlet patch) in the cervical esophagus.

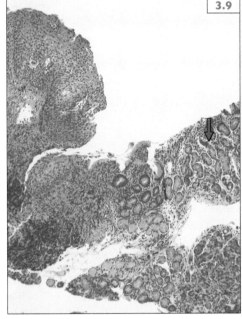

3.9 Inlet patch with gastric mucosa in the esophagus (arrow). (Courtesy of John Pohl, MD; Department of Pediatric Gastroenterology, Primary Children's Hospital, University of Utah, Salt Lake City.)

CHAPTER 4

Gastroesophageal Reflux Disease and Esophagitis

Ricardo A. Caicedo

- **Gastroesophageal reflux**
- **Pill esophagitis**

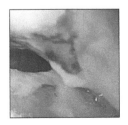
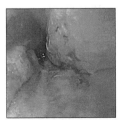
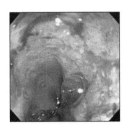
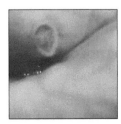

Gastroesophageal reflux

DEFINITION

Gastroesophageal reflux disease (GERD) occurs when the retrograde passage of gastric contents causes recurrent troublesome symptoms or complications. An estimated 2–7% of children report symptoms of GERD, which is the most common cause of esophagitis. Among the general population, the prevalence of reflux esophagitis is about 3–5%. The incidence of esophagitis in patients with GERD ranges between 50% and 80%, based on studies in adults. In a large pediatric study (n = 1788), the prevalence of erosive esophagitis, defined endoscopically, was 12%, and this percentage clearly increased with age. In a United Kingdom primary care study, the incidence of GERD, with or without esophagitis, in children aged 0–18 years was estimated at 0.84 per 1000 person-years. An exact determination of the incidence of reflux esophagitis in children is limited by a paucity of data.

CLINICAL PRESENTATION

Children and adolescents with reflux esophagitis typically present with recurrent pain in the upper abdomen or chest and frequent heartburn. Painful swallowing (odynophagia), difficulty swallowing (dysphagia), and nausea/vomiting are other common manifestations. Infants may regurgitate gastric contents, but clues pointing to reflux esophagitis in this patient population include irritability, posturing (back arching or neck tilting), and Sandifer syndrome (opisthotonus and posturing). Affected infants may also exhibit feeding difficulties or outright feeding refusal, poor weight gain, and, infrequently, hematemesis and/or melena.

ETIOLOGY AND PATHOPHYSIOLOGY

The retrograde passage of stomach contents into the esophagus primarily results from transient lower esophageal sphincter relaxation (TLESR). In infants, increased TLESR leads to physiologic gastroesophageal reflux, often without recurrent symptoms or complications. Other factors, including abnormal esophageal motility, delayed gastric emptying, positioning, meal content, and inflammation also aggravate the process. The net effect is impaired clearance of noxious substances from the esophagus. Repeated exposure of the esophageal mucosa to refluxate composed of hydrochloric acid, pepsin, trypsin, and bile leads to tissue injury and chronic inflammation. GERD is usually mild in children, but over time, it can progress to erosions, ulcerations, and even fibrosis and cellular metaplasia.

GERD and its complications are more commonly seen in children with one or more of the following risk factors: neurologic impairment, obesity, prematurity, chronic lung disease (such as cystic fibrosis), congenital malformations such as esophageal atresia (with or without tracheo-esophageal fistula), hiatal hernia, or a first-degree relative with severe GERD.

DIFFERENTIAL DIAGNOSIS

- GERD.
- Eosinophilic esophagitis.
- Infectious process (candidiasis, cytomegalovirus, herpes simplex virus, human immunodeficiency virus).
- Pill esophagitis.
- Corrosive esophagitis (caustic ingestion).
- Esophageal foreign body.
- Crohn disease.
- Connective tissue disease (scleroderma, polyarteritis nodosa).
- Motility disorder (achalasia).
- Radiation injury.

DIAGNOSIS

Gastroesophageal reflux without complications is usually a clinical diagnosis, but patients with GERD may undergo further diagnostic evaluation. Laboratory tests are of little utility in the diagnosis of GERD. Radiographic studies, such as the upper gastrointestinal (GI) series

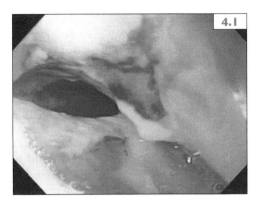

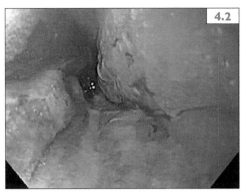

4.1 Severe erosive reflux esophagitis characterized by mucosal breaks, exudate, and bleeding, diagnosed endoscopically in an adolescent with profound neurologic impairment presenting with irritability, hematemesis, melena, and anemia.

4.2 Endoscopic image of eroded esophageal mucosa in a 5-year-old boy with chronic gastroesophageal reflux disease (GERD) and chronic lung disease due to cystic fibrosis. These patients are predisposed to severe GERD.

4.3 Macroscopic appearance of reflux esophagitis in a 6-month-old infant with a history of esophageal atresia repaired in the neonatal period. These patients chronically have abnormal esophageal clearance and are more susceptible to complications of gastroesophageal reflux disease.

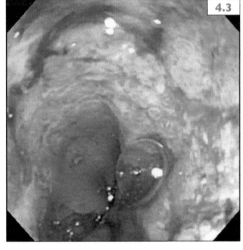

('barium swallow'), should be used to rule out stricture, achalasia, hiatal hernia, or gastric outlet obstruction but should not be used to evaluate for GERD or esophagitis. The most precise diagnostic modality is endoscopy with biopsy in order to detect mucosal breaks, erosions, bleeding and ulcerations (**4.1–4.3**) that, per consensus guidelines, define reflux esophagitis.

Several classification or grading schemes based on endoscopic mucosal findings can be used to determine severity as well as response to therapy. Histologic findings (basal layer hyperplasia, intraepithelial eosinophils) may support a diagnosis of reflux esophagitis, and are important in excluding other diagnoses such as infectious or eosinophilic processes. Esophageal pH (or pH/impedance) probe studies quantify frequency and degree of reflux and attempt to correlate with observed symptoms. These studies may also be useful in determining the efficacy of acid suppression therapy. However, there is not a consistent correlation between abnormal pH probe results and GERD severity or complications. Other adjunctive tests, such as esophageal manometry and scintigraphy scans, have no role in the diagnosis of reflux esophagitis.

TREATMENT

All patients with GERD are likely to benefit from dietary and lifestyle antireflux measures, including caffeine avoidance as well as chocolate and alcohol. Children with reflux esophagitis should be treated with antisecretory (acid suppression) agents. Histamine-2-receptor antagonists (H2RAs, such as ranitidine or famotidine) are better than placebo for healing of esophageal mucosa, but they are more efficacious in mild rather than severe esophagitis. H2RAs are also limited by the development of tachyphylaxis. Conversely, proton pump inhibitors (PPIs, such as omeprazole, lansoprazole, and pantoprazole) are clearly superior to H2RAs in healing esophagitis, without tachyphylaxis. PPIs are the recommended first-line therapy for reflux esophagitis, especially in the higher grade, or erosive esophagitis. The initial treatment duration is typically 12 weeks, with higher dosing or extended duration for refractory cases or patients with GERD-predisposing conditions. Long-term use of PPIs has been associated with an increased risk of *Clostridium difficile* infection, hypomagnesemia, and acute interstitial nephritis in adults. In children, long-term acid suppression may predispose to acquired infections such as gastroenteritis or pneumonia.

Antacid buffering agents, such as magnesium/aluminum hydroxide, may provide symptomatic relief but not mucosal healing. Sucralfate, a surface gel composed of sucrose, sulfate, and aluminum, binds to eroded mucosa and may be effective in treating esophagitis, but usually for a short time only. Long-term sucralfate use may increase the risk of aluminum toxicity. Prokinetic agents, such as metoclopramide or erythromycin, used in the treatment of GERD have no benefit in the treatment of childhood esophagitis. Surgical procedures, such as Nissen fundoplication, should be reserved for children with refractory reflux esophagitis or life-threatening complications of GERD. Postoperative complications often include retching, gagging, and gas bloat, as well as slippage and need for reoperation. In neurologically impaired *versus* nonimpaired children undergoing fundoplication, the complication rate is doubled and the reoperation rate is quadrupled.

PROGNOSIS

Refractory GERD with esophagitis can lead to feeding aversion, poor growth, peptic stricture, and even Barrett esophagus, which is a premalignant lesion of the esophageal mucosa characterized by intestinal metaplasia (columnar rather than squamous epithelium). Barrett esophagitis is very rare in pediatrics (<0.25% prevalence in one population study) but portends an up to 40-fold increased risk of esophageal adenocarcinoma over time. As with GERD in general, the more complicated cases of reflux esophagitis are found in children with neurologic impairment, obesity, and chronic lung disease.

INFANT REFLUX

Infants deserve special mention in this discussion. The prevalence of benign reflux manifesting as recurrent regurgitation is as much as 66% in 4-month-olds, although this percentage decreases to approximately 5% by 12 months. Alternatively, the frequency of GERD in infants is much lower, and complications such as esophagitis are uncommon. In the large study discussed above, the prevalence of reflux esophagitis among infants was less than 5%. The clinical presentation of GERD in infants may include irritability, posturing, feeding refusal, dysphagia, poor growth, and in rare cases, hematemesis. The differential diagnosis includes congenital anomalies, such as an esophageal web or H-type tracheoesophageal fistula, as well as allergic/eosinophilic esophagitis, cow's milk or soy protein hypersensitivity, and metabolic disorders such as galactosemia or urea cycle defects. Diagnosis of esophagitis is best made with endoscopy and histology, but often in infants diagnosis is based on symptoms and response to therapeutic trials of acid suppression and modified feedings (thickened, casein hydrolysate, or amino acid-based formula, smaller volume, positional changes). The natural history of infant GERD is one of gradual resolution, but may be more complicated or even require fundoplication in infants with neurologic impairment, extreme prematurity, complex congenital heart disease, or chronic lung disease.

Pill esophagitis

The incidence and prevalence of pill esophagitis in children are unknown, and this problem is more common in adolescents. The typical patient is a teenager who swallows a large tablet or capsule without sufficient liquid or while lying in a supine position. Typical symptoms include chest pain, odynophagia, dysphagia, and drooling. The most common causative agents are doxycycline and clindamycin (often prescribed for acne); others include nonsteroidal anti-inflammatory drugs, antivirals, beta-blockers, bisphosphonates, and potassium preparations. The pill usually lodges in the midesophagus, leading to inflammation, ulceration, and even necrosis (**4.4**). Diagnosis is usually clinical, but endoscopic examination is helpful to determine severity and to establish etiology of symptoms. Treatment includes analgesics, topical anesthetics, sucralfate, and acid suppression drugs. The prognosis is usually good except in repetitive injury.

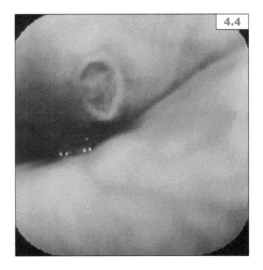

4.4 Endoscopic examination showing a typical example of pill esophagitis. The discrete ulceration in the esophageal mucosa was caused by the impaction of a large tetracycline pill.

CHAPTER 5

Eosinophilic Esophagitis

Raghu U. Varier, Molly A. O'Gorman

DEFINITION

Eosinophilic esophagitis (EoE) is a distinct clinicopathologic diagnosis that involves chronic, antigen-driven, immune-mediated esophageal disease characterized clinically by esophageal dysfunction, and histologically by esophageal eosinophilic infiltration and inflammation. Initially thought to be primarily associated with gastroesophageal reflux disease (GERD), our understanding of the presence of esophageal eosinophils has changed over the past several years. Esophageal biopsies are required to establish the diagnosis of EoE, which is classically defined as 15 or more eosinophils per high-powered field isolated to the esophagus. The related characteristic clinical symptoms are unresponsive to antacid therapy and are typically associated with normal pH monitoring of the distal esophagus.

CLINICAL PRESENTATION

The symptoms of EoE are similar to GERD, although the clinical manifestations of EoE can vary with age. Symptoms include abdominal pain, feeding difficulties, and failure to thrive in younger children. Teenagers and adults also can present with dysphagia and food impactions.

Patients often have a history of atopic disease. Some patients have identifiable food triggers, which have been associated with symptoms and histologic changes that are improved after avoidance of the offending agent. In addition, it has been reported that some patients have seasonal variation in symptoms, implicating an association with aeroallergen exposure.

EPIDEMIOLOGY

EoE has a nearly worldwide distribution and has been reported in various countries in North America, South America, Asia, Europe, and Australia. The incidence of EoE is reported as about 1 in 10,000, with a prevalence of 4.3 per 10,000 people. The overall incidence seems to be increasing, perhaps partially due to a greater recognition of the disease. In children, the disorder is more common in males and is more likely to affect Caucasians. There also seems to be a familial association of EoE in about 10% of patients.

DIFFERENTIAL DIAGNOSIS

The primary differential diagnosis for EoE is GERD, which may be differentiated histologically by changes localized to the distal esophagus, rather than the entire esophagus. It is important to note, however, that eosinophilic inflammation and/or infiltration isolated to the distal esophagus despite high-dose proton pump inhibitor therapy, is consistent with a diagnosis of EoE rather than of GERD. Other considerations include inflammatory bowel disease, celiac disease, and hypereosinophilic syndrome. Esophageal eosinophilia can also be seen with viral esophagitis, parasitic infections, and with drug allergies.

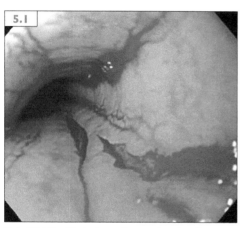

5.1 Middle-third of esophagus showing linear furrows with friable mucosa.

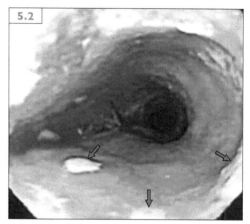

5.2 Middle-third of esophagus with exudate (arrows).

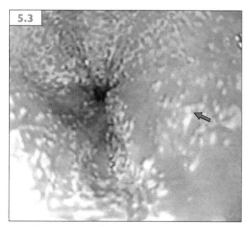

5.3 Middle-third of esophagus with eosinophilic exudate/white plaques (arrow).

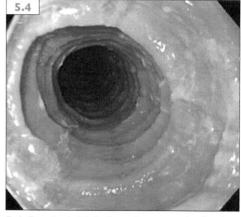

5.4 Proximal-third of esophagus; trachealization. (Courtesy of Richard J. Noel, MD, PhD; Medical College of Wisconsin, Division of Gastroenterology and Nutrition.)

DIAGNOSIS

EoE is a clinicopathologic disorder, as defined above, with symptoms of esophageal dysfunction and an associated isolated esophageal eosinophilia. Endoscopic findings are variable, and can include gross mucosal changes such as linear furrows (**5.1**), exudates (**5.2**), white plaques (**5.3**), decreased caliber of esophageal lumen, esophageal rings, and trachealization (**5.4**) of the esophagus (also known as 'feline esophagus'). Other features include shearing (**5.5, 5.6**) and coarse mucosal texture (**5.7, 5.8**). Tertiary contractions of the esophagus can also be seen. However, EoE has been diagnosed when the appearance of the esophageal mucosa is otherwise grossly normal, further emphasizing the importance of tissue acquisition.

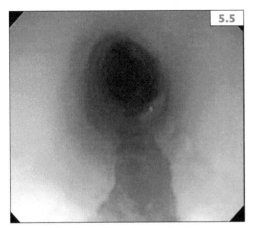

5.5 Middle-third of esophagus; shearing.

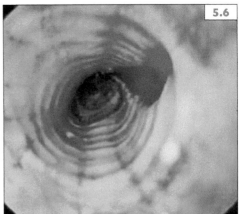

5.6 Middle-third of esophagus; shearing. (Courtesy of Mary P. Bronner, MD; University of Utah, Division of Pathology.)

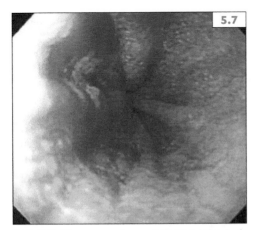

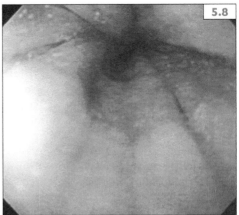

5.7, 5.8 Coarse esophagus. **5.7**: Distal-third of esophagus; **5.8**: middle-third of esophagus.

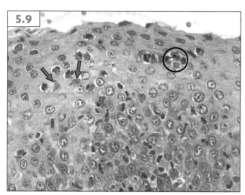

5.9 Proximal esophagus; microabscess (arrows). Single small eosinophilic granules may be remnants of degranulated cells (circle). (Courtesy of Kajsa E. Affolter, MD, Mary P. Bronner, MD; University of Utah, Division of Pathology.)

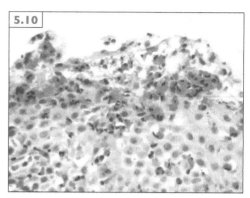

5.10 Distal esophagus; superficial eosinophil layering. (Courtesy of Kajsa E. Affolter, MD, Mary P. Bronner, MD; University of Utah, Division of Pathology.)

Mucosal biopsy specimens should be obtained from the proximal and distal esophagus. The optimal number of specimens from each site to maximize the diagnostic yield is currently being investigated. One study demonstrated a diagnostic sensitivity of 84%, 97%, and 100% for obtaining 2, 3, and 6 biopsy specimens, respectively.

Histologic features of EoE include degranulated eosinophils, superficial eosinophilic microabscesses (>4 eosinophils in a cluster) (**5.9**), eosinophilic surface layering (**5.10**), an increased number of intraepithelial eosinophils (>15 per high-power field [hpf]) [**5.11(A)**]), marked basal cell hyperplasia (**5.11(B)**), elongation of papillae, and lamina propria eosinophilia and fibrosis.

Additional laboratory and radiographic studies may be useful in the work-up of EoE, but have not necessarily been found to be diagnostic of the condition. Because of the high rate of atopic disease in patients with EoE, a complete evaluation for potential aeroallergens and dietary antigens by serum specific immunoglobulin E (IgE), skin prick and/or patch testing should be considered. Currently, there are no data to support the use of total IgE levels as a surrogate marker for disease progression or resolution.

The presence of peripheral blood eosinophilia may provide support for the presence of EoE, but this finding is not diagnostic and disease activity correlation is unknown.

An upper gastrointestinal (GI) contrast study may show an esophageal stricture or decreased esophageal caliber (**5.12**) in patients with dysphagia, or it may rule out anatomic abnormalities is children who present with vomiting. Intraesophageal pH or impedance monitoring may be useful to exclude pathologic gastroesophageal reflux in the presence of esophageal eosinophilia, although having a diagnosis of GERD does not exclude EoE.

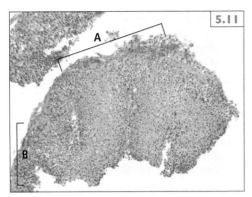

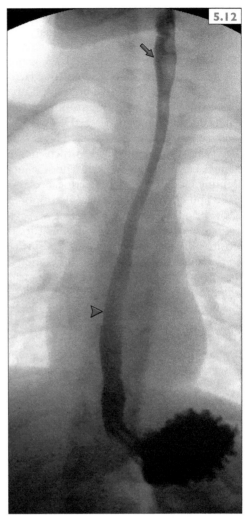

5.11 Esophagus showing increased eosinophils with luminal clustering (A) and basal cell hyperplasia (B). (Courtesy of Kajsa E. Affolter, MD, Mary P. Bronner, MD; University of Utah, Division of Pathology.)

5.12 Upper gastrointestinal contrast study. Examination of the esophagus demonstrates a small caliber esophagus relatively diffusely. There is mild relative increase in the caliber of the esophagus at the level of the distal cervical esophagus (arrow) and the distal thoracic esophagus (arrowhead) when compared with the remainder of the thoracic esophagus.

PATHOPHYSIOLOGY

The pathogenesis of EoE is not completely understood; however, there is growing evidence that the disease is a disorder of immune dysregulation influenced by genetic and environmental factors.

Though not normally found in the esophagus, eosinophils establish themselves as permanent residents of the remainder of the GI tract during early embryonic development, a process regulated by the peptide eotaxin, which also appears to have a central role in antigen-mediated eosinophil recruitment. The recruitment of eosinophils in the GI tract is observed in a variety of infectious or inflammatory conditions including parasitic infections, inflammatory bowel disease, gastroesophageal reflux, and exposure to food allergens. In patients with EoE, an association with allergies is common, suggesting that eosinophil recruitment in these patients may be a response to environmental antigens.

Numerous inflammatory mediators have been implicated in regulating eosinophil migration, adhesion and accumulation. Mediators such as interleukin (IL)-3, granulocyte macrophage-colony stimulating factor (GM-CSF), and IL-5 have been implicated in eosinophil development, migration, and effector function. IL-1, IL-4, IL-13, and tumor necrosis factor (TNF) have been shown to be involved with eosinophil trafficking and adhesion to the endothelium. Murine models support the critical roles of IL-5 and eotaxin in esophageal eosinophil growth and recruitment, respectively.

The recognition of key modulators of eosinophil recruitment and function has important clinical implications. In addition to being potential targets for drug development, these mediators may also have a future role in the diagnosis and monitoring of the disease.

TREATMENT

Dietary therapy with specific food antigen restriction or with changing to a strict diet using amino acid-based formula has been shown to promote symptomatic improvement and mucosal healing with reduced numbers of esophageal eosinophils in children with EoE. Dietary therapy is often guided by allergy testing to identify potential dietary triggers. However, dietary restriction may be based on elimination of common food antigens, such as cow's milk, soy, wheat, egg, peanuts/tree nuts, and seafood, without performing specific allergy testing, after which foods can be gradually reintroduced one by one in a serial fashion while proving tolerance by endoscopic examination. Although studies have shown similar clinical and histologic responses between these dietary therapies, it appears that using an elemental diet is the most effective therapy in patients with food allergy.

Topical and systemic corticosteroids have been proven to resolve clinicopathologic features of EoE. Topical steroids, including liquid budesonide and swallowed fluticasone, have been shown to be effective in inducing EoE remission. Several studies have reported safety with the use of topical steroids, with the exception of localized fungal infections. Swallowed fluticasone propionate, preferably administered with a metered-dose inhaler without a spacer, has been studied in children with EoE, with promising results. Though numerous studies have used varying doses of fluticasone, a general consensus is to use 440–880 µg per day for children and 880–1760 µg per day for adolescents/adults, in split daily doses for a minimum of 6–8 weeks before follow-up. Further studies on pharmacokinetics and long-term effects of fluticasone need to be conducted. Systemic corticosteroid use generally is reserved for emergent situations such as severe dysphagia or severe dehydration secondary to swallowing dysfunction. Because of the potential for significant side-effects, long-term use of systemic corticosteroids is generally not recommended.

Though acid suppression should not be used as the primary treatment for patients with EoE, it should be utilized as cotherapy for patients with associated GERD, as well as to help differentiate between GERD and EoE.

Leukotriene receptor antagonists and mast cell stabilizers have not been shown to have therapeutic benefit in EoE.

Esophageal dilatation can be performed for patients who have symptomatic esophageal strictures; however, use of this procedure carries a risk of mucosal laceration and perforation. It is generally recommended that diagnostic endoscopy with biopsy be performed, followed by medical therapy, prior to esophageal dilatation in patients with EoE.

Emerging data support a potential role of IL-5 biologic agents, such as reslizumab or mepolizumab, in the treatment of EoE. Spergel *et al*. (2011) showed in a large multi-center double-blind, randomized, placebo-controlled study, reslizumab significantly reduced intraepithelial esophageal eosinophil counts in children and adolescents with EoE when compared to placebo. However, improvements in symptoms were observed in all treatment groups including placebo. To date, no biologic agent is approved for this disorder.

PROGNOSIS

Patients with EoE should improve with appropriate medical therapy. However, the natural history of EoE has not been extensively studied. It is thought that progressive esophageal scarring, stricture, and dysfunction can develop if EoE is left untreated. There also appears to be an increased risk for the development of other eosinophilic gastrointestinal disorders, such as eosinophilic gastritis and eosinophilic duodenitis, in patients with EoE.

CHAPTER 6

Esophageal Motility: Measures and Disorders of Esophageal Motor Function

Anil Darbari

- **Esophagus: anatomy and physiology**
- **Disorders of swallowing**
- **Measures of esophageal motility**
- **Achalasia**
- **Isolated LES dysfunction**
- **Nutcracker esophagus**

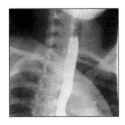
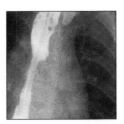
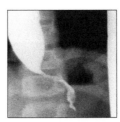
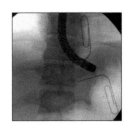

Esophagus: anatomy and physiology

The esophagus is the conduit for food bolus passage from the mouth to the stomach. While the passage of food via the esophagus is typically short, the esophagus serves the following main functions:

- Moving food forward (away from the mouth).
- Preventing food from moving backward (towards the mouth).
- Preventing injury to the organs, such as esophageal mucosa and the airways.

Complex mechanisms are utilized to serve these functions. Deglutition or swallowing is the act of passage of food from the mouth to the stomach. Since the initial phases of swallowing are voluntary and involve complex interaction with breathing, to understand better its physiology, swallowing is traditionally divided into three phases:

- Oral phase.
- Pharyngeal phase.
- Esophageal phase.

ORAL PHASE

This phase is mostly designed to prepare the food for its passage to the stomach. It is entirely voluntary and is controlled by the temporal lobes and the limbic system, with contributions from the motor cortex and other cortical areas. The food is chewed and moistened into a smooth soft bolus, utilizing movements of the lips, tongue, jaws, palate, and oropharynx. At the end of the oral phase, the food is now prepared and is propelled back into the pharynx, mostly by tongue movements.

PHARYNGEAL PHASE

The main function of the pharyngeal phase is to ensure its passage into the esophagus safely and without spillage into the airways. The pharynx utilizes a series of contractions, often called pharyngeal peristalsis, while the bolus is compressed against the posterior pharyngeal wall by the tongue, thereby creating a pressure gradient moving the food bolus forward. The pharyngeal phase is mostly involuntary, although some components, such as stopping the breath, are under voluntary control. To prevent spillage into the airway, several maneuvers are undertaken including the inhibition of breathing, the approximation of the larynx to the pharynx by its elevation, the closing of the epiglottis over the larynx, and the closure of the vocal cords. A partial brief breach is often labeled 'penetration', while a more robust passage of food into the airways is called 'aspiration' in clinical settings.

ESOPHAGEAL PHASE

This phase begins as food, enters the pharynx and the pressure gradient and waves are created in the pharynx. The esophageal phase is entirely involuntary. Using neural mechanisms, a relaxation of the upper esophageal sphincter is achieved, allowing for a quick, smooth passage of the bolus from pharynx to the esophagus. For a more complete understanding of the esophageal phase of swallowing, this phase is further divided into three areas, mostly based on their functions:

- Upper esophageal sphincter (UES).
- Body of the esophagus (body).
- Lower esophageal sphincter (LES).

While initiation of the swallowing in oral phase is under voluntary control, the subsequent phases in pharynx and esophagus are mostly involuntary. The complex neurologic coordination is achieved using sensory information from these structures and is under the control of the brainstem. The nerves mostly involved in the swallowing include cranial nerves V, IX, and X for the sensory portion and cranial nerves V, VIII, IX, X, and XII for the motor control. Once started, the esophageal phase continues without input from the central nervous system.

In the clinical setting, the oral and pharyngeal phases of swallowing are typically evaluated and managed by speech and language pathologists or occupational therapists and, in some instances, by pulmonologists or otorhinolaryngologists. The esophageal swallowing is evaluated and managed by gastroenterologists. For the purposes of this chapter, the subsequent passage will focus on the esophageal motility and its implications in (the esophageal phase of) swallowing.

Disorders of swallowing

Difficulty in swallowing or dysphagia is the usual presentation of disorders affecting swallowing. To understand them better, swallowing disorders can be classified into two types of disorders:

- Anatomic or structural disorders:
  - Stenosis/stricture of the lumen.
  - Congenital anomalies.
  - Esophageal diverticulum.
- Motor disorders of swallowing.
  - Dysfunction of esophageal sphincters.
  - Motor abnormalities of peristalsis:
    Paresis/weakness.
    Spasticity.
  - Achalasia.

Measures of esophageal motility

History and physical examination provide important information towards underlying causes, especially for causes secondary to underlying systemic conditions or a past history of esophageal injury or surgery. Most children however, will present with dysphagia or with vomiting. In most cases no specific physical finding is noted. Tests to evaluate disorders of swallowing can be differentiated into:

- Indirect tests:
  - Barium swallow (**6.1–6.3**).
  - Modified barium swallow (MBS).
  - Esophageal scintigraphy/transit time.
- Direct tests:
  - Esophageal manometry.
  - pH impedance study.
  - Combined impedance manometry study.

BARIUM SWALLOW

The barium swallow is also known as esophagram (**6.1–6.3,** overleaf). This is often the first step in evaluation of a child presenting with a suspected swallowing disorder. The barium swallow allows for evaluation of all the phases of swallowing. It provides objective assessment of the structure and function of oral, pharyngeal, and the esophageal portions of swallowing. It also helps distinguish anatomic or structural causes from functional disorders of swallowing (*Table 6.1*).

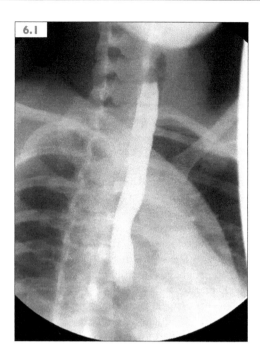

6.1–6.3 Barium swallow studies.
6.1 Normal esophagus.

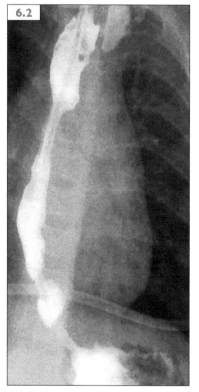

6.2 Eophageal stricture.

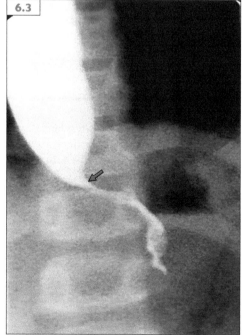

6.3 Achalasia with bird beak appearance (arrow).

Table 6.1 Usefulness and limitations of esophageal motility tests

	Usefulness	Limitations
Barium swallow	Evaluate oral, pharyngeal, and esophageal areas	Does not indicate causes of disorders of swallowing function
	Able to distinguish anatomic causes from disorders of function	It is a one-time study, so caution should be used to apply it in clinical settings
	Can be performed in most radiologic settings	Radiation exposure
MBS	Evaluate oropharyngeal swallow	Dependent on the skill level of the therapist and radiologist
	Various consistencies of food are tested	It is a one-time study, so caution should be used to apply it in clinical settings
	Can determine the presence of laryngeal penetration and/or aspiration	Normal values for pediatrics are not very well established
Esophageal scintigraphy	Noninvasive	Dependent on the experience of the nuclear medicine staff
	Various consistencies of food can be tested	Does not indicate cause of the underlying disorder
	May be useful to detect esophageal clearance after dilatation therapy of lower sphincter	Normal values for pediatrics are not very well established
Esophageal manometry	Definitive evaluation of dysphagia	Requires patient co-operation to allow catheter placement via nostril into the esophagus
	Various consistencies of food can be tested	Performed at specialized centers with physicians and staff specially trained to perform and analyse the study
	Establish the diagnosis of underlying esophageal motility disorder	Normal values for pediatrics are not very well established

MBS: modified barium swallow.

MODIFIED BARIUM SWALLOW

The MBS is typically performed to evaluate the oral and pharyngeal phases of swallowing. In most institutions, this study is performed using fluoroscopy. The patient is given age and skill level appropriate food of different consistencies, mixed with a radiologic contrast. A skilled speech pathologist or occupational therapist with special training in performing and evaluating these studies with an experienced radiologist monitors the passage of the contrast-laden food through the oral and pharyngeal swallow. The test is often useful to determine the presence of laryngeal penetration or frank aspiration (*Table 6.1*). It also helps guide the management by allowing the therapist to recommend the volume and consistency of food that the patient is able to tolerate.

ESOPHAGEAL SCINTIGRAPHY/ TRANSIT TIME

A small amount of radioactive material such as technetium 99 isotope is mixed with age appropriate food that the patient ingests. The use of esophageal scintigraphy is limited in clinical practice in pediatrics (*Table 6.1*). Most institutions commonly substitute the test with a fluoroscopic evaluation of the swallow.

MANOMETRY

Esophageal manometry evaluates the pressure changes in the esophagus during the act of swallowing (**6.4**). The test is performed by inserting a soft catheter via the nostril into the esophagus and measuring esophageal pressure with various swallows. Accurately recording pressure along the entire length of the esophagus is challenged by several physiologic features:

- The pharynx, UES and proximal esophagus contract much more briskly than do the distal esophagus and LES.
- Both sphincters exhibit marked radial asymmetry attributable to a unique anatomy in the case of the UES and to the superimposed crural diaphragm in the case of the LES.
- The esophagus moves during the swallowing both because of the elevation of the UES by the pharyngeal musculature and because of contraction of the longitudinal muscle during peristalsis.

The manometric parameters usually considered in the analysis of a standard esophageal manometry include the analysis of body for peristalsis, the lower esophageal sphincter

---

Table 6.2 Parameters utilized in the analysis of esophageal manometry studies

Body

Amplitude	High	Normal	Low
Co-ordination	Normal	Intermittently abnormal	Persistently abnormal

LES

Resting LES pressure	High	Normal	Low
Relaxation	Normal	Intermittently incomplete	Persistently incomplete

LES: lower esophageal sphincter

for its resting pressure, and percent relaxation noted with swallows (*Table 6.2*):

- Esophageal body:
  - Esophageal pressure waves >10 (mmHg):
    High amplitude.
    Normal amplitude.
    Low amplitude.
  - Esophageal pressure waves peristaltic:
    Normal.
    Intermittently abnormal.
    Persistently abnormal.
- LES:
  - Detectable LES pressure >5 mmHg (resting LES pressure):
    High resting LES pressure.
    Normal resting LES pressure.
    Low resting LES pressure.
  - LES relaxation with swallows:
    Complete relaxation.
    Intermittently incomplete relaxation.
    Persistently incomplete relaxation.

Several configurations of the catheter and manometry systems became commercially available, making this a required test in evaluation of all children with dysphagia (*Table 6.3*). It is also used to determine the location of the LES prior to reflux analysis using pH impedance study.

Conventional esophageal manometry *vs.* high-resolution manometry

The concept of high-resolution manometry (HRM) is to overcome the limitations of conventional manometric systems with advanced technologies. First and foremost, this involved vastly increasing the number of pressure sensors on the HRM catheter. Since the sensors are placed very close to each other, the measured intraluminal pressure becomes a spatial continuum. Also, the sensors are circumferentially sensitive and record in high fidelity, overcoming the fidelity and directionality limitations noted in conventional water perfused systems. With improved software and computerization capabilities, the large digital dataset is plotted in algorithms to display them as colored pressure topography plots rather than a series of line tracings (**6.4–6.6**, overleaf). These advances permit the accurate and dynamic imaging of esophageal pressure along the length of the esophagus. The pressure magnitude along this continuum is depicted in spectral color scale.

Table 6.3 Esophageal manometry systems and catheters

Systems	Perfusion manometry
	Solid state manometry
	High-resolution manometry
	High-resolution impedance manometry
	Video manometry (manometry combined with video-fluoroscopic swallow study)
Catheters	3–4 channels located at the end of the catheter
	Long channel (called sleeve) with one or two pressure transducers
	High-resolution catheters

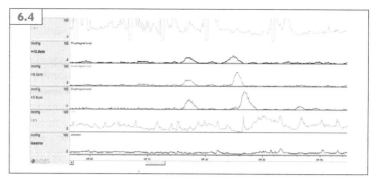

6.4 Conventional esophageal manometry study demonstrating normal swallow from pharynx to stomach. This study is performed using high-resolution impedance manometry perfusion catheter.

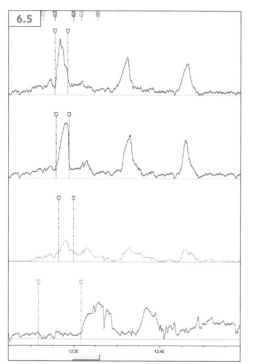

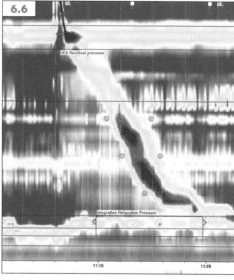

6.5, 6.6 High-resolution manometry (HRM). An example of a normal esophageal response to a water swallow displayed as a conventional line plot on the left, and as a colored topographical HRM plot on the right.

High resolution impedance manometry (HRIM)

A further advancement in technology has been combining the manometry sensors on the catheter with impedance sensors, thereby providing simultaneous information of bolus transit, in addition to high-resolution manometry data (**6.7**).

Silny first described the use of intraluminal impedance to monitor the bolus movement within the gastrointestinal tract in 1991. While manometry provides measurement of pressure gradient, it still does not measure bolus transit. The relationship between peristalsis as measured by manometry and bolus transit can be achieved by combining manometry with either a) video fluoroscopy, or b) intraluminal impedance monitoring (**6.8**).

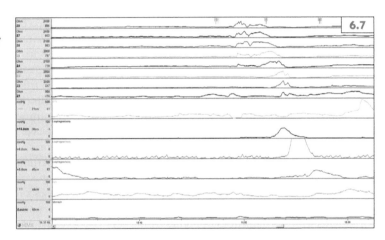

6.7 High-resolution impedance manometry line plot showing combined information about bolus transit in the impedance channels and esophageal pressures in the manometry channels.

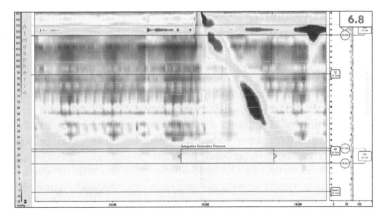

6.8 High-resolution impedance manometry contour plot combining high-resolution manometry with impedance channels.

Disorders of esophageal motor function: achalasia

DEFINITION

Achalasia is a rare esophageal motor disease caused by the absence of peristalsis in the esophagus and defective LES relaxation. The incidence is described as 1:100,000 per year and a lifetime prevalence of 1:10,000. The typical age of onset is in adults between 25 and 60 years, although the pediatric age group including infants can be affected.

It is mostly an isolated condition; however, it can occur together with other abnormalities. The most common syndrome is called triple-A syndrome; an autosomal recessive disease characterized by achalasia, alacrimia, and Addison disease. The gene responsible, AAAS, is located on chromosome 12q13. In children with this syndrome, neurologic and dermatologic disorders are also observed in addition to facial dysmorphism.

Achalasia occurs with equal frequency in men and women, with no racial predilection. Even if it is an uncommon disease, it occurs frequently enough to be encountered at least yearly by most gastroenterologists. Esophageal and motility specialists may see 10 or more cases a year. The overall life expectancy of patients with achalasia does not differ from those of the general population.

CLINICAL PRESENTATION

Symptoms of achalasia primarily include dysphagia or difficulty in swallowing. The symptoms are often gradual, developing slowly over several weeks to years and increase as the disease progresses. The diagnosis of achalasia should be suspected in any patients complaining of dysphagia for solids and liquids with regurgitation of bland food and saliva. Initially the dysphagia may be primarily for solids; however, by the time of clinical presentation, nearly all patients complain of dysphagia for solids and liquids while eating and drinking, especially cold beverages.

Various maneuvers, including 'power swallows' and carbonated beverages, both of which increase intraesophageal pressure, may be used to improve esophageal emptying. As the disease progresses, the increasing contraction of the LES on swallowing leads to regurgitation of food that has not entered the stomach and to retrosternal pain, particularly when there is extreme dilatation of the esophagus. Restricted movement of food and avoidance of food may lead to weight loss. This process can occur swiftly, but typically takes place over a longer period lasting several months or years.

DIAGNOSIS

In cases of suspected achalasia, the diagnostic procedure is aimed mostly at the main symptoms. Endoscopy is the first step in diagnosing the cause of dysphagia. It can also be used to rule out secondary causes of achalasia in adults (for example, inflammation, stenosis, or tumors) and to obtain tissue biopsies. However, if there are grounds in the patient's medical history for suspecting a stricture, a barium swallow and radiograph of the esophagus are recommended first, as endoscopy poses a higher risk of perforation. Once secondary achalasia has been ruled out endoscopically, an esophageal manometry and/or barium swallow and X-ray of the esophagus are performed.

Esophagogastroscopy together with barium swallow or esophagram and esophageal manometry are part of standard diagnostic studies for suspected achalasia. Endoscopically, diagnosis can only be established in approximately one-third of all achalasia patients, and this depends on the stage the disease has reached. In these cases resistance is typically noted at the gastroesophageal junction but can still be overcome relatively easily by the endoscope. In advanced stages with esophageal dilatation, food is typically noted in the esophagus.

On a barium swallow, the esophagus often appears dilated. In a video fluoroscopic swallow study, an astute radiologist will often note a lack of peristalsis, and a tapered, thread- like area of contrast in the cardiac region, often called a 'bird beak appearance' (**6.3**). In many patients, the barium swallow could present with a classic appearance, but esophageal manometry is still considered necessary for making the diagnosis of achalasia. The radiologic findings are nonspecific and make the diagnosis in two-thirds of the cases. Some centers perform modified techniques called a timed barium swallow, where the test is individualized for each patient and primarily assesses esophageal emptying of barium in the upright position over 5 minutes. Swallow studies can be repeated after therapy to evaluate esophageal emptying and correlate with the patients' symptoms.

Esophageal manometry is the gold standard and is required to establish the diagnosis of achalasia. It must be done in any patient where invasive treatments such as pneumatic dilation or surgical myotomy are planned. It can successfully diagnose over 90% of all cases. The cardinal esophageal manometry features noted in achalasia are:

- Failure of LES relaxation.
- Absence of peristalsis.
- High resting LES pressure.
- Simultaneous contractions of esophageal body.

The first two features are consistently noted in achalasia patients, and other features such as a hypertensive LES may be either not present, or not noted consistently in all swallows.

HRM and Clouse contour plots introduced in 2000 for the clinical evaluation of esophageal motility are utilized for esophageal pressure topography (EPT). The Chicago Classification utilizes key EPT-specific metrics and criteria optimized for clinical studies (**6.9**).

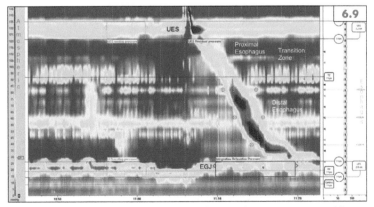

6.9 Normal swallow illustrating a normal peristaltic contraction and key landmarks used in the Chicago classification of esophageal motility.

Based on this classification, achalasia is divided into three distinct types of achalasia (*Table 6.4*, **6.10–6.12**). This classification only applies to primary esophageal motility disorders and is not intended to include postsurgical studies, for example after fundoplication or Heller myotomy.

HRM can be used to predict the outcome of each type of achalasia. This was tested in a logistic regression model in which clinical outcome was the dependent variable and achalasia subtype was the independent categorical variable while controlling for age, sex, presence or absence of dilatation on index endoscopy, and esophagogastric junction (EGJ) basal and relaxation pressure (4 second integrated relaxation pressure [IRP]) on HRM. Achalasia subtype I was considered the control for calculating the odds ratio (OR) since this represents the classic achalasia. Achalasia subtype II was much more likely to respond to therapy compared with subtype I (OR 11.2). In contrast, achalasia subtype III was much less likely to respond to therapy than subtype I (OR 0.24).

PATHOPHYSIOLOGY

Achalasia involves the selective loss of inhibitory neurons in the myenteric plexus, leading to the production of vasoactive intestinal polypeptide (VIP), nitric oxide (NO) and inflammatory infiltrate responsible for abnormal esophageal function. An unopposed excitation of the LES causes its dysfunction or failure to relax in response to swallowing. Even though the mechanisms responsible for selective loss of inhibitory neurons in the myenteric plexus that produces VIP, NO, and inflammatory infiltrates responsible for abnormal LES dysfunction are still not well understood, the most acceptable hypothesis suggests that achalasia may be caused by viral and autoimmune factors leading to the inflammatory changes and damage to the myenteric plexus.

Table 6.4 Chicago classification of achalasia, based on high-resolution manometry and esophageal pressure topography

Type I achalasia	Classic achalasia	100% failed peristalsis Mean IRP > upper limit of normal
Type II achalasia	Achalasia with esophageal compression	No normal peristalsis Mean IRP > upper limit of normal Panesophageal pressurization with >20% of swallows
Type III achalasia	Peristaltic fragments or Spastic esophagus	No normal peristalsis Mean IRP > upper limit of normal Preserved fragments of distal peristalsis or premature (spastic) contractions with >20% of swallows

IRP: integrated relaxation pressure in mmHg referenced to gastric pressure. It is the mean esophagogastric junction pressure measured with an electronic equivalent of a sleeve sensor for 4 contiguous or noncontiguous seconds of relaxation in the 10 second window following deglutive upper esophageal sphincter relaxation.

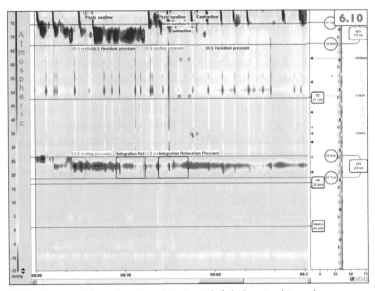

6.10 Type I achalasia. Classic achalasia with failed peristalsis and impaired esophagogastric junction relaxation as noted in high-resolution manometry image.

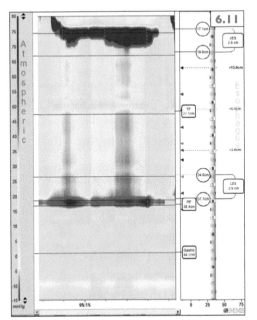

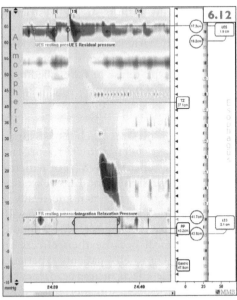

6.11 Type II achalasia. In achalasia with esophageal compression, no lumen obliterating contraction occurs but the esophagus empties by a global contraction in conjunction with some degree of shortening.

6.12 Type III achalasia. In spastic achalasia there is a lumen obliterating spastic contraction shown here in high-resolution impedance manometry image; this is often viewed radiographically as a 'corkscrew' esophagus.

TREATMENT

The goal of therapy is to improve symptoms and esophageal clearance, and to prevent continued dilatation of the esophagus (*Table 6.5*). The muscular activity to the denervated esophagus cannot be restrored. The lack of peristalsis and impaired function of LES are not reversed by any therapy. Medical management is therefore directed towards decreasing the gradient across the LES by using muscle relaxants. Management of achalasia with medications is rarely used anymore in clinical practice because of the side-effects of medications, and poor long-term outcomes.

Pharmacologic therapy

More commonly used pharmacologic agents include calcium-channel blockers and long-acting nitrates. Other agents used sometimes include anticholinergics such as atropine, cimetroprium and dicyclomine, beta-agonists such as terbutaline, and theophylline. Many authors suggest restricting the use of pharmacologic agents in patients who are very early in the disease process, as an adjunct to other forms of therapy, or for patients who refuse or have failed more invasive forms of therapy.

Nitroglycerine

Long-acting nitrates such as isosorbid dinitrate have been shown to provide symptomatic relief in 53–87% of patients. Nitrates cause significant LES relaxation that can be confirmed manometrically as well as on radionuclide studies. Usually nitrates are taken sublingually 15–30 minutes prior to a meal because their effects are short lived. Up to 50% patients experience significant side-effects such as headaches and hypotension, especially in appropriate doses of the medication, or develop resistance. The use of these agents is therefore limited in clinical practice. Their long-term efficacy is not established.

Nifedipine

When indicated, nifedipine, a calcium-channel blocker is the pharmacologic agent of choice. It lowers the LES pressure and the amplitdue of esophageal contractions in doses of 10–20 mg in adults. Its experience in children is limited, however; in adolescents it has been documented to cause a significant fall in LES pressure and provides good clinical response. Some studies have shown excellent long-term effects in up to 65% of patients with rare side-effects.

Nonpharmacologic therapy
Pneumatic dilatation

Pneumatic dilatation (PD) is accomplished by placing a dilating device at the level of LES, and inflating it to stretch the esophageal muscle and LES. Proper placement of the balloon depends upon an endoscopically placed guidewire, and fluoroscopy. The most commonly used technique utilizes a rigid endoscopic balloon inserted over

---

Table 6.5 Aim of treatment of achalasia

Relief of the functional LES obstruction

Relief of symptoms

Prevention of progressive esophageal dilatation

Nutritional rehabilitation:

  Oral *vs.* gastric/transpyloric tube feeding

  Volume of tube feeds

Prevention of gastroesophageal reflux:

  Elevation of head of the bed:

    Improves esophageal emptying

    Decreases nocturnal regurgitation

an endoscopically placed guidewire at the level of the LES. These noncompliant balloons are available in 3.0 cm, 3.5 cm, and 4.0 cm diameters. Under fluoroscopic guidance, the balloon is inflated to disrupt the LES (**6.13–6.15**).

PD should preferentially start with a 3.0 cm balloon to lower the risk of perforation. Using a graded distension protocol with increasing balloon diameter, success rates of 70–80% are reached, further increasing to >90% when redilation is allowed in the case of recurrent

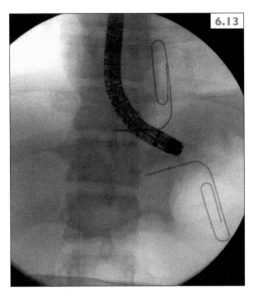

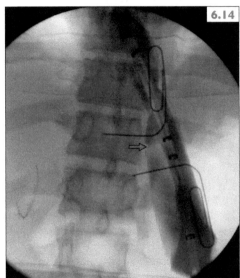

6.13–6.15 Radiograph showing endoscopic balloon dilatation. **6.13**: First a radio-opaque marker is placed externally, when the area of narrowing is noted endoscopically and fluoroscopically; **6.14**: radiograph shows the area of narrowing by indentation in the balloon (arrow); **6.15**: the balloon after dilatation is completed.

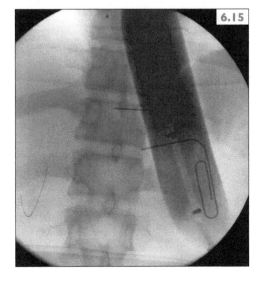

symptoms. The need for further dilatations is determined by the presence of symptoms, often correlated with esophageal emptying studies at 4–6 week intervals after treatment. PD and laparascopic Heller myotomy are the most commonly used nonpharmacologic treatments.

Botulinum toxin therapy

Botulinum toxin is a potent inhibitor of acetylcholine release that binds to presynaptic cholinergic terminals causing inhibition of acetylcholine release at the neuromuscular junction. It reduces LES pressures in achalasia by decreasing the excitatory cholinergic innervations to the sphincter. Temporary paralysis of the innervated muscles occurs. On average, botulinum toxin injections decrease LES pressure by 50%, while partially improving esophageal emptying. A total of 100 units is endoscopically injected into the LES in multiple aliquots in a ring around the sphincter. Based on many studies, some placebo controlled, botulinum toxin markedly improves symptoms in approximately 75% of achalasia patients. About 50% patients relapse within 6 months probably due to regeneration of the affected receptors. Serial injections are required for sustained relief, and comparison studies show long-term efficacy is lower than PD or myotomy.

Surgical therapy

The first successful surgery for achalasia was performed in 1913 by the German surgeon Ernest Heller. The most popular operation now is a minimally invasive single anterior myotomy introduced by Pellegrini and coworkers in 1992. The overall success of the laparascopic operation through the abdomen is superior to the thoracoscopic approach. In a laparascopic Heller myotomy (LHM), the EGJ is laparascopically retrieved/approached and both muscle layers of the LES are cleaved with an extension of the incision 2–3 cm over the proximal stomach, usually combined with an antireflux procedure such as a fundoplication. Retrospective single-center studies reported very high success rates ranging between 89% and100%, resulting in an increasing enthusiasm in favor of the surgical approach. However, more recent prospective multicenter trials with well-defined criteria for therapeutic success, failed to show superior therapeutic success compared to PD as primary treatment for achalasia, after a mean follow-up of up to 43 months. Additionally, no difference in the level of esophageal stasis and quality of life was observed.

Per oral endoscopic myotomy

In this recently developed endoscopic treatment technique, a submucosal tunnel is created to dissect the circular muscle fibers over a 7 cm esophageal and 2 cm gastric length. The procedure is only performed in adults so far, and follow-up after a clear reduction of symptoms and a significant reduction in LES pressure is short (mean 5 months).

PROGNOSIS

Since most treatment techniques do not cure the motor abnormalities of achalasia, recurrences after any form of treatment will occur with longer follow-up periods. In patients treated with PD, treatment failure is more often observed in younger and male patients. Therefore, LHM is the preferred treatment option for males below the age of 40 years. Also, as noted above, HRM and high-resolution EPT can be used to predict successful therapy. Since stasis induces chronic inflammation, persistent stasis should be avoided as this could lead to dysplasia and eventually squamous cell carcinoma. Patients with persistent stasis are also more likely to need additional treatments compared to patients with complete empty-ing. Timed barium esophagrams to determine stasis and a screening program for patients with longstanding achalasia for early detection of dysplasia are therefore recommended.

Isolated LES dysfunction

These patients typically have abnormal LES relaxation with preserved peristaltic activity in the body of the esophagus. Because they have some peristalsis, they fail to meet the criteria for a diagnosis of achalasia (*Table 6.6*).

HRM is useful in such patients as the findings noted are similar to those seen in patients who have established causes of mechanical obstruction of the EGJ, such as fundoplication. These patients typically respond poorly to balloon dilation or botulinum toxin injection, but they may have better response to myotomy.

Table 6.6 Manometry parameters in lower esophageal sphincter (LES) dysfunction

Body	
Amplitude	Normal
Co-ordination	Normal
LES	
Resting LES pressure	High to normal
Relaxation	Normal to persistently incomplete

Nutcracker esophagus

The finding of elevated wave amplitude has been a consistent feature in the diagnostic criteria for 'nutcracker esophagus' (*Table 6.7*). Such a finding could however be sometimes seen in the absence of symptoms, and therefore the presence of dysphagia and chest pain is essential in establishing the diagnosis.

Using HRM, the nutcracker esophagus is defined as a hypercontractile disorder based on mean distal contractile integral (DCI). Subsequently, however, it was further subclassified into patients who had a mean DCI of 5000–8000 mg/s per cm (hypertensive peristalsis, or nutcracker esophagus) and those with a mean DCI >8000 mg/s per cm (spastic nutcracker). The distinction is suggested because patients with spastic nutcracker are almost always symptomatic.

Table 6.7 Manometry parameters in nutcracker esophagus

Body	
Amplitude	High (>180 mmHg)
Co-ordination	Normal to mildly abnormal
Lower esophageal sphincter (LES)	
Resting LES pressure	Normal
Relaxation	Normal to intermittently incomplete

CONCLUSION

Technological advances have led to the development of new methodology for assessing esophageal motility in health and disease. Techniques that integrate HRM with pressure topography plotting and with measures of bolus transit, such as HRIM, are replacing rather than complementing conventional manometry in motility centers. Subcategorization of achalasia and better understanding of esophageal motility have been shown to correlate with responsiveness to treatment. There is no evidence of superior outcomes with myotomy as compared to endoscopic therapy for achalasia.

ACKNOWLEDGMENTS

The author would like to acknowledge Lindsay Clarke, PA, Co-ordinator for the Comprehensive GI Motility Center, Children's National Medical Center, for critical review of the manuscript and contribution in selection of manometry studies for illustration. Thanks are also due to John Desbiens, senior motility technician for manometry studies and image selection.

CHAPTER 7

Esophageal Varices

Cathy Sampert, Kyle Jensen

DEFINITION
Esophageal varices are dilated intraesophageal veins resulting from portal hypertension. If variceal bleeding occurs, this is considered a life-threatening emergency.

CLINICAL PRESENTATION
Patients most often present with signs or symptoms of chronic liver disease and cirrhosis, but they may also be asymptomatic until the initial gastrointestinal (GI) bleed occurs, manifesting as hematemesis, melena, hematochezia, or pallor and fatigue.

DIFFERENTIAL DIAGNOSIS
The different conditions which result in esophageal variceal bleeding vary depending on the level of the impeded blood flow:

- Prehepatic causes occur with portal vein obstruction (thrombosis most commonly), which represents approximately 30% of children with bleeding varices.
- Intrahepatic causes include those which affect the parenchyma, such as cirrhosis and hepatic fibrosis, but vascular complications may also result (e.g. veno-occlusive disease or schistosomiasis).
- Posthepatic causes include Budd–Chiari syndrome or constrictive pericarditis.

Additional causes of portal-hypertensive bleeding include gastric varices, portal gastropathy, and possibly gastric antral vascular ectasia.

Nonvariceal causes of GI bleeding such as peptic ulcer disease, Mallory Weiss tears, or vascular lesions also should be considered, as management differs from a variceal bleed (outlined below).

DIAGNOSIS
The most common findings are those seen in cirrhosis (i.e. ascites, muscle wasting, possible jaundice), but the most specific finding suggestive of esophageal varices in children is splenomegaly. Additional findings may include bruising or petechiae, and less commonly, dilated abdominal veins (caput medusa). Internal hemorrhoids due to increased venous pressure are an uncommon finding in children.

A complete blood count should be obtained, which often shows leukopenia and thrombocytopenia, with a variable decline in the hemoglobin from low-grade bleeding. Coagulation markers (prothrombin time (PT)/international normalized ratio (INR)) also may be elevated, indicating variable degrees of synthetic dysfunction. Values of standard 'liver function tests' such as alanine aminotransferase (ALT), bilirubin, or albumin also will vary based on the underlying etiology for portal hypertension, and may even be normal in the setting of portal vein thrombosis.

Varices or other signs of portal hyper-tension (i.e. splenomegaly or abnormal portal venous flow) can be identified with radiologic procedures including ultrasound, computed tomography, or magnetic resonance imaging. These modalities are noninvasive and allow for evaluation of the portal venous system and liver parenchyma. Upper endoscopy is the preferred approach, however, as grading of the lesions and therapeutic interventions for acute bleeding or bleeding prophylaxis may be performed simultaneously. Varices are graded based on size during endoscopic evaluation. These are generally graded as small, medium, or large, where 'small' varices are straight dilated esophageal veins, 'medium' varices (7.1) are enlarged, tortuous esophageal varices occupying less than one-third of the lumen, and 'large' (7.2) are coil-shaped esophageal varices occupying more than one-third of the lumen. A four-point scale also is used with grade I representing dilated veins less than 5 mm in diameter that are compressed with insufflation. Grade II are still straight, but protrude into the lumen without obstructing the endoscopic view. Grade III are large, tor-tuous, and obstruct the esophageal lumen. Grade IV varices obstruct the lumen with red spots (7.3) suggesting impending hemorrhage.

PATHOPHYSIOLOGY

Portal hypertension occurs when the portal venous pressure increases as a result of 1) increased resistance within the liver, or 2) increased blood flow. As portal blood flow increases, more blood is transported through other routes to return to the systemic circulation. This increased blood flow leads to the dilatation of esophageal veins and varices result.

TREATMENT
Prophylaxis

Two forms of prophylaxis exist: primary prophylaxis interventions performed prior to the first episode of variceal hemorrhage, and secondary prophylaxis interventions performed after the initial episode of variceal hemorrhage, to prevent rebleeding.

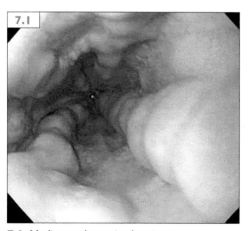

7.1 Medium to large sized varices.

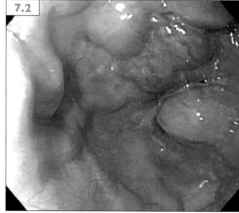

7.2 Large varices in the distal esophagus.

Medical

The most common medications used to prevent variceal bleeding are nonselective beta-blockers. Although commonly used in adults with medium to large esophageal varices, there are little data regarding this practice in children with esophageal varices. The avoidance of medical prophylaxis in children is because children rely almost exclusively on tachycardia to maintain cardiac output when bleeding occurs, as stroke volume is relatively fixed. This is contrasted with adults, who maintain cardiac output by increasing stroke volume through increased peripheral vascular resistance improving preload, as well as tachycardia. This difference in compensatory physiology increases concern for decreased survival of variceal hemorrhage in children on beta-blockers. Determining the appropriate response in children can also be challenging as the hepatic vein–portal gradient is not frequently measured.

Endoscopic

Endoscopic variceal ligation (EVL) and sclerotherapy are invasive approaches for primary or secondary prophylaxis of esophageal varices. EVL involves attaching a banding device to the videoendoscope, passing it into the esophagus, identifying a varix at increased risk for bleeding, suctioning the mucosa, and deploying a small elastic band to ligate the varix (**7.4**).

In smaller children, especially those under 2 years old, the banding device is difficult to pass through the oropharynx, and sclerotherapy is typically the only endoscopic alternative. This requires passing a needle through the biopsy channel of the videoendoscope and injecting the varix with a sclerosant such as ethanolamine or sodium morrhuate. Large adult and smaller pediatric studies suggest sclerotherapy is less effective than EVL and is associated with a higher complication rate; thus, sclerotherapy should be considered only in those patients for whom EVL is not feasible.

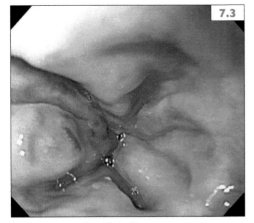

7.3 Varices with red spots.

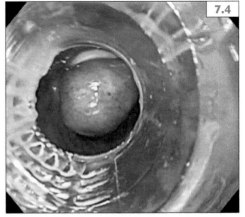

7.4 Varix post banding, as seen via banding apparatus.

Acute management
Medical

Fluid resuscitation and transfusion to maintain hemoglobin levels of 8–10 g/dl (80–100 g/l) are the first steps of stabilization. Correction of coagulopathy with Vitamin K, fresh frozen plasma, or other blood products also is used to reduce hemorrhage.

Octreotide is used to decrease GI bleeding through vasoconstriction of the splanchnic circulation. Patients should not be fed while on this medication as vasoconstriction increases the risk of bowel ischemia during feeding. Additional side-effects include hypoglycemia, cholelithiasis, nausea, vomiting, and rarely arrhythmias. Octreotide is typically continued for a short time after EVL to minimize the risk of rebleeding, which is greatest in the first 3–5 days after intervention.

Vasopressin is the most potent splanchnic vasoconstrictor, decreasing portal flow and pressure, but in contrast to octreotide, it has a more significant side-effect profile including peripheral, mesenteric, and cardiac ischemia, hypertension, arrhythmias, and cerebrovascular accidents. It is typically not considered safe to continue vasopressin at high doses for more than 24 hours, favoring use of octreotide.

Proton pump inhibitors are useful in the acute management of bleeding esophageal varices as these patients often have portal hypertensive gastropathy and gastric protection is beneficial, as is reduction of gastric acid to minimize further esophageal injury from reflux.

Antibiotics are typically given immediately before and for a minimum of 7 days after esophageal variceal hemorrhage, because cirrhotic patients with upper GI hemorrhage have a high risk of developing serious bacterial infections.

Endoscopic

EVL or sclerotherapy are acute treatment options for bleeding esophageal varices. Depending on the severity of the bleeding varices, medical therapy may be utilized to slow bleeding and allow visualization of the targeted varix to perform either procedure. In cases of severe hemorrhage, the patient cannot wait for effective medical therapy and urgently needs endoscopic intervention while continuing medical therapy. Adult guidelines recommend EVL within 12 hours of presentation with an acute variceal bleed.

Occlusion tubes

If bleeding persists and endoscopic intervention cannot be performed to control the bleeding, balloon tamponade with a Sengstaken–Blakemore tube should be considered. This procedure is rarely performed in children and contains significant risks including aspiration, perforation/necrosis, and migration. These tubes should not remain inflated more than 12 hours consecutively, necessitating close monitoring. Variceal tamponade is a temporizing measure but may allow time for endoscopic management and allow more time for efficacy of medical therapy.

Surgical/interventional

Transplantation: ultimately, esophageal varices are the result of portal hypertension, and when due to cirrhosis will only be cured with liver transplantation. Multiple or severe esophageal variceal hemorrhage in patients with chronic liver disease warrants evaluation for liver transplantation. In those patients with chronic liver disease who are listed for transplantation, exception points (used to raise the Pediatric End-Stage Liver Disease or PELD score) are available to prioritize transplantation. If synthetic dysfunction does not exist, surgical shunts should be considered.

Surgical shunts: portosystemic shunts are another option for resolving portal hypertension. Shunts should be considered in patients with normal synthetic function, without cirrhosis. Risks include worsened encephalopathy, rebleeding, and relatively high surgical complication and shunt malfunction rates. Although shunts in children are uncommon, the most frequently used selective shunt is a distal splenorenal shunt, which decompresses varices at the gastroesophageal junction and spleen, decreases bleeding risk for the majority of patients, and has a lower risk of encephalopathy than systemic shunts.

An additional shunt is the 'Rex-shunt' which can be helpful in the setting of presinusoidal portal hypertension with normal hepatic parenchyma. This form of portal hypertension most commonly results from portal vein thrombosis. In this group of patients, the thrombosed portion of the portal vein can be bypassed, and first-pass hepatic metabolism is maintained which decreases the risk of encephalopathy.

Adults suffering variceal hemorrhage are sometimes triaged to urgent transjugular intrahepatic portosystemic shunt (TIPS) after failing endoscopic and medical therapy. This intervention is not a standard practice in children, as smaller vessel size makes this technique more challenging. Ultimately, TIPS serves as a temporizing measure for those patients with decompensated cirrhosis while awaiting transplantation. Hepatic encephalopathy may also increase after TIPS.

Suguira procedure: the Sugiura procedure is a devascularizing procedure used for refractory variceal hemorrhage. There are limited pediatric data, but a case series demonstrated good results of this technique in 12 children with variceal hemorrhage refractory to conservative management.

PORTAL HYPERTENSIVE GASTRIC LESIONS

The management of gastric lesions resulting from portal hypertenson is less well defined in children. In adults, portal hypertensive gastropathy (**7.5**) is managed with beta blockade and iron supplementation and with TIPS if the patient becomes transfusion-dependent. Gastric antral vascular ectasia is often treated similarly, although some

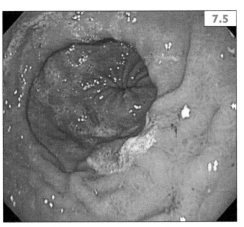

7.5 Portal hypertensive gastropathy with mosaic appearance to the mucosa.

providers advocate the use of argon plasma coagulation when iron supplementation is not effective, or medical management by maintaining adequate platelet count and appropriate INR.

PROGNOSIS

Children with esophageal varices are at variable risk for hemorrhage depending on the extent and etiology of their portal hypertension. Fifty percent of children with biliary atresia who survive more than 10 years without transplantation will experience variceal hemorrhage, as will half of children with portal vein thrombosis by age 16 years. The mortality rate of an episode of GI bleeding in children with portal hypertension also is variable, with reported ranges of 2.5–20%. Because of the somewhat unpredictable risk of death with variceal hemorrhage, careful monitoring and prevention are key in these patients.

CHAPTER 8

Esophageal Infections

Niraj Patel

DEFINITION

'Esophagitis' is a general term for inflammation, irritation, or swelling of the esophagus. Infectious esophagitis is caused by fungi or yeast, most commonly *Candida albicans*, viruses such as herpes simplex virus (HSV) or cytomegalovirus (CMV), and less commonly bacteria.

Infectious esophagitis is a rare finding in previously healthy individuals, and is usually an indicator of a primary or secondary immunodeficiency. The exact incidence is unknown, and several risk factors increase the risk for esophagitis including chemotherapy for hematologic malignancies, solid organ or hematopoietic stem cell transplantation, primary immunodeficiencies, diabetes, prolonged corticosteroid therapy, and infection with human immunodeficiency virus (HIV).

CLINICAL PRESENTATION

Dysphagia and odynophagia are the most common complaints of esophagitis, although these symptoms may escape detection in very small children. Fever is caused by systemic infections such as disseminated CMV disease or tuberculosis. Nausea and vomiting are more commonly associated with CMV esophagitis. Hematemesis can be a common initial symptom of fungal esophagitis. Oral lesions suggest infection with *Candida* species, HSV, or HIV, and less commonly with CMV infection and tuberculosis. Oral thrush in the setting of esophagitis is most commonly seen in infants and immunocompromised hosts. Other signs and symptoms of infectious esophagitis include abdominal pain, diarrhea, cough, and rash.

ETIOLOGY AND PATHOPHYSIOLOGY

Several mechanisms exist that protect the esophagus from microbes. These include motility from the oropharynx to the stomach with flow of luminal contents that decrease the esophageal colonization of pathogens, mucosal lining of stratified squamous epithelium which protects from invasion, and innate and adaptive immune responses. Factors that disrupt these protective mechanisms, such as chemotherapy, prolonged corticosteroid therapy, immunosuppression, and malignancy, increase the risk for fungal and viral infections. Dysmotility of the esophagus is a risk factor for infectious esophagitis in immunocompetent children. The majority of esophageal infections are predominantly

8.1 *Candida* spp. esophagitis showing diffuse white plaques.

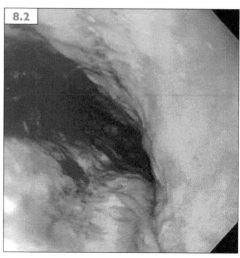

8.2 Ulcerative lesions associated with herpes simplex virus esophagitis.

fungal or viral. The most common etiologies include *Candida* spp. (especially *Candida albicans*), HSV, and CMV. Other etiologies have been reported and include *Pneumocystis*, *Aspergillus* spp., *Histoplasma* spp., varicella-zoster virus (VZV), papillomavirus, Epstein–Barr virus (EBV), HIV, *Cryptosporidium*, and *Leishmania donovani*. Bacterial infections make up only 10–16% of esophageal infections.

DIFFERENTIAL DIAGNOSIS

- Pathologic gastroesophageal reflux.
- Eosinophilic esophagitis.
- Chagas disease.
- Achalasia.
- Diffuse esophageal spasm.
- Foreign body impaction.
- Mediastinal or retropharyngeal abscesses.

DIAGNOSIS

Although a clinical history, barium esophagram, and appearance by esophagoscopy can provide clues to the etiology of esophagitis, histopathology, cultures, and immunohistochemistry are essential in confirming the pathogens. Serology for HSV, CMV, or EBV may be helpful for acute infection, and deoxyribonucleic acid (DNA) detection methods can be useful for tissue and serum.

Barium esophagraphy details the mucosal lining, but an esophagram is not as sensitive as endoscopy for detailing infectious esophagitis. Lesions of HSV and CMV are usually limited to the mid and distal esophagus, whereas *Candida* spp. esophagitis may be more diffuse and appear as white longitudinal plaques or tiny nodular lesions with a granular appearance (**8.1**). Discrete stellate ulcers in the mid esophagus is typical of HSV (**8.2**), whereas elongated or oval large ulcers are characteristic of CMV.

The macroscopic appearance of infectious lesions can overlap. Diffuse lesions suggest *Candida* spp. infection, but lesions of the distal esophagus are more common with HSV and CMV. White plaques adhering to mucosa is associated with *Candida* spp. infection. In HSV esophagitis, ulcers may appear

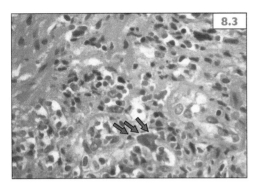

8.3 Hematoxylin and eosin stain of cytomegalovirus (arrows). (Courtesy of Lisa Dixon, MD; Department of Pathology, University of Florida.)

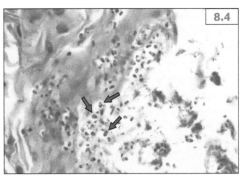

8.4 Hematoxylin and eosin stain of *Candida* spp. (arrows). (Courtesy of Lisa Dixon, MD; Department of Pathology, University of Florida.)

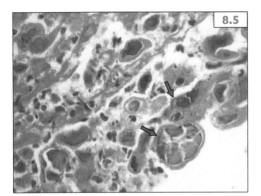

8.5 Hematoxylin and eosin stain of herpes simplex virus (arrows). (Courtesy of Lisa Dixon, MD; Department of Pathology, University of Florida.)

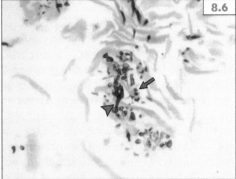

8.6 Grocott's methenamine silver stain for *Candida* spp., budding yeast (arrow) and elongated pseudohyphae (arrowhead). (Courtesy of Lisa Dixon, MD; Department of Pathology, University of Florida.)

as 1–3 mm vesicles, or more commonly as ulcers with a raised edge and necrotic center. If disease progresses, these ulcers can coalesce and have a similar appearance to candidal esophagitis. CMV esophagitis may reveal multiple shallow or large elongated ulcers in the distal esophagus. Ulcers caused by *Mycobacterium tuberculosis* can vary in size and generally demonstrate a shallow, necrotic base.

Biopsy specimens are best obtained from the edge and base of the lesions and analyzed by a pathologist. Hematoxylin and eosin stain (**8.3–8.5**), Gram stain and culture, viral culture, and special stains for fungi and mycobacterium should be considered (**8.6**).

Immunohistochemical staining and DNA hybridization may also aid in the diagnosis (**8.7, 8.8**).

TREATMENT
Fungal esophagitis

Candida spp. esophagitis requires systemic therapy and the preferred agents are oral fluconazole, intraconazole, or voriconazole. The duration of therapy is 14–21 days. For patients with severe dysphagia, intravenous formulations of azole medications may be needed initially. Although resistance to azoles of various species of *Candida* exist, data regarding pediatrics are sparse. An alternative to azole therapy is intravenous therapy with an echinocandin such as caspofungin, anidulafungin, or micafungin. Intravenous amphotericin B deoxycholate is another alternative for refractory disease; however, nephrotoxicity is a major side-effect. Lipid formulations of amphotericin B have reduced toxicity and low-dose therapy of 7–14 days is generally sufficient. Therapy is similar for other causes of fungal esophagitis including *Aspergillus*, *Mucor*, and *Cryptococcus* spp., and should be guided by antimicrobial susceptibility. Echinocandin should not be used for *Cryptococcus* spp. given its lack of activity against this agent.

Viral esophagitis

Intravenous acyclovir is used to treat HSV esophagitis. Alternatives include valacyclovir and famciclovir because of their bioavailability and clinical efficacy. VZV esophagitis is also treated with intravenous acyclovir. Therapy for CMV esophagitis is intravenous ganciclovir. Patients with HSV, VZV, or CMV esophagitis unresponsive to the above therapy can be treated with intravenous foscarnet. Duration of therapy is 14–21 days.

Bacterial esophagitis

Broad spectrum antibiotics should be used as empiric therapy for *Staphylococcus aureus*, gram-negative organisms, and viridans streptococci. When infection due to *Mycobacterium tuberculosis* is suspected, therapy directed at systemic disease associated with this pathogen is appropriate.

PROGNOSIS

Complications from viral esophagitis include hemorrhage, fistula formation, dissemination, and superinfection. Late complications include esophageal narrowing with stricture formation and necrosis. Fungal esophagitis in the presence of acquired human immunodeficiency syndrome (AIDS) generally carries a survival rate of approximately 1 year in untreated HIV patients. Sequelae from untreated or improperly treated fungal esophagitis include esophageal strictures, fistulas, obstruction, and perforation.

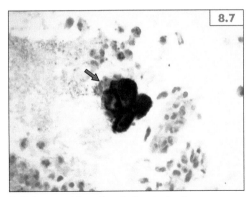

8.7 Immunohistochemical stain for herpes simplex virus (arrow). (Courtesy of Lisa Dixon, MD; Department of Pathology, University of Florida.)

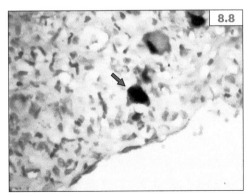

8.8 Immunohistochemical stain for cytomegalovirus (arrow). (Courtesy of Lisa Dixon, MD; Department of Pathology, University of Florida.)

CHAPTER 9

Esophageal Foreign Bodies

David Brumbaugh

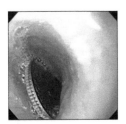
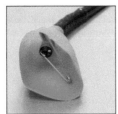
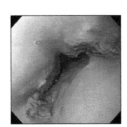
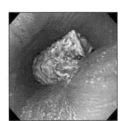

Introduction

The accidental ingestion of foreign bodies is largely a pediatric problem. These items are frequently swallowed by children, leading to significant anxiety for caregivers and health care providers alike. Older children with developmental delay or pervasive developmental disorders may be at higher risk of foreign body ingestion. Adolescents with psychiatric disease may intentionally swallow objects in an attempt at self-harm. Coins are the most commonly ingested foreign body by children (**9.1**). Fortunately, the large majority (80–90%) of swallowed foreign bodies are able to traverse the gastrointestinal (GI) tract without complication. However, in certain circumstances, such as the ingestion of a button battery, an acute pediatric emergency exists where timely care is critical.

ANATOMY

A swallowed foreign body must first clear the esophagus. This hollow tube is comprised of two muscular layers, an inner circular layer and outer longitudinal layer, which are designed to propel the food bolus in an anterograde fashion. Unique to the esophagus within the digestive tract is the transition from striated muscle to smooth muscle from proximal to distal esophagus, mirrored in the change from voluntary control of swallowing to involuntary control of GI tract motility distal to the mid esophagus. Critical structures adjacent to the esophagus (**9.2**) include the trachea, which lies just anterior to the esophagus in the neck and upper thorax, the carotid arteries, the aortic arch, and descending aorta, which descends to the left of the esophagus in the lower thoracic cavity.

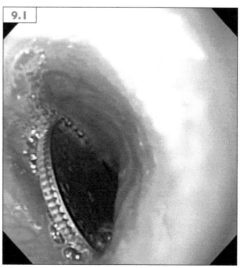

9.1 Endoscopic view of a coin lodged in the esophagus.

There are at least three anatomic points within the esophagus that represent common sites for entrapment of foreign bodies (**9.3**). The first anatomic point is the upper esophageal sphincter (UES), where approximately two-thirds of retained esophageal foreign bodies will be located. The UES represents the anatomic transition from the posterior pharynx to the esophagus. The cricopharyngeus muscle is the dominant muscle of the UES and is under voluntary control. Relaxation of the cricopharyngeus is an important component of a normal swallowing mechanism. The second anatomic narrowing is in the mid esophagus where the aortic arch crosses to the left. The intimate anatomic relationship between the aortic arch and esophagus is very familiar to the endoscopist, who on every examination of the upper intestinal tract visualizes the pulsations of the adjacent aorta. The third anatomic narrowing is the lower esophageal sphincter (LES), which is the anatomic junction of the esophagus and stomach. Unlike the UES, which is composed of striated fibers, the LES is a ring of smooth muscle that relaxes in co-ordination with esophageal peristalsis to allow for the movement of a swallowed food bolus into the stomach.

Children with a history of previous esophageal surgery or with known esophageal stricture are at increased risk of esophageal foreign body impaction. The most frequent example of this phenomenon is the child with a previous surgical repair of esophageal atresia or tracheoesophageal fistula. These children may have narrowing of the esophagus at the site of the surgical anastamosis and invariably have distal esophageal dysmotility that may increase the risk of foreign body impaction. Vascular rings and slings can lead to extrinsic esophageal compression that may lead to

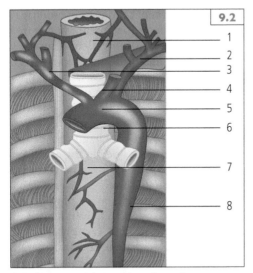

9.2 Anatomic relationships of esophagus to adjacent vascular and respiratory structures. 1: Proximal esophagus; 2: left subclavian artery; 3: brachiocephalic artery; 4: left common carotid artery; 5: aortic arch; 6: trachea; 7: middle esophagus; 8: descending aorta.

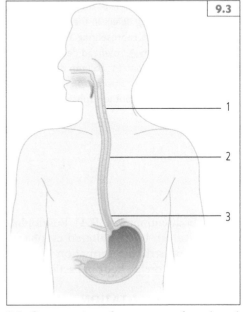

9.3 Common sites of entrapment of esophageal foreign bodies. 1: Upper esophageal sphincter; 2: aortic arch; 3: lower esophageal sphincter.

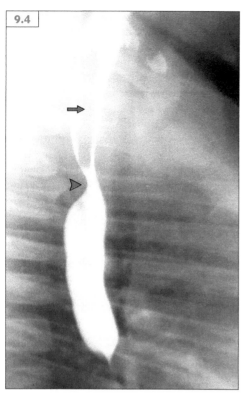

9.4 Contrast radiography of the esophagus. Arrow shows a filling defect in the column of esophageal contrast, representing a nonradio-opaque foreign body. Arrowhead demonstrates indentation of the contrast column due to external posterior compression of the esophagus by an aberrant left subclavian artery.

foreign body entrapment (**9.4**). Eosinophilic esophagitis can lead to altered esophageal motility and stricture formation and thus predispose to foreign body impaction

CLINICAL PRESENTATION

In the pediatric population, it has been estimated that up to 30% of children with an esophageal foreign body will be asymptomatic and are brought to medical care only because the ingestion was witnessed by a caregiver. Acute symptoms of an esophageal foreign body include throat or chest pain, dysphagia, vomiting/regurgitation, odynophagia, choking, and drooling. Respiratory symptoms such as cough, dyspnea, stridor, and wheezing can be present with acute foreign body ingestion, but interestingly, several retrospective studies have shown that respiratory symptoms will predominate when the foreign body ingestion is unwitnessed and the foreign body has been entrapped in the esophagus for greater than 1 week. Fever can also be present in the setting of a chronic esophageal foreign body. Thus, a high index of suspicion must be maintained for esophageal foreign body when a toddler presents with fever and respiratory symptoms. There are multiple reports of acute upper GI tract bleeding in the setting of a chronic esophageal foreign body, especially button batteries, which are discussed in depth later in this chapter.

Complications

Fortunately, complications from esophageal foreign body ingestion are rare in children. Acutely, a foreign body that completely obstructs the lumen of the esophagus can lead to the inability to swallow oral secretions, placing the younger child at particular risk of aspiration. Most complications, however, result from either (1) the presence of a sharp foreign body in the esophagus, or (2) the presence of a foreign body in the esophagus for greater than 24 hours. Sharp foreign bodies can migrate through the esophageal wall, leading to development of infectious complications such as mediastinitis or abscess, or hemorrhagic complications by penetration of an adjacent vascular structure. It is theorized that the chronically impacted esophageal foreign body mechanically exerts pressure on the esophageal wall, leading to compromise of local esophageal vascular supply. Pressure necrosis can then lead to esophageal perforation or the development of fistula to vascular structures or the trachea.

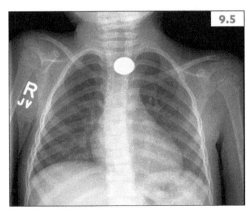

9.5 Posterior–anterior radiograph of the chest demonstrates the classic appearance of an esophageal coin.

DIAGNOSIS AND TREATMENT

In any pediatric foreign body ingestion, the initial diagnostic strategy is radiographic. The X-ray series should include adequate visualization of the cervical esophagus and abdomen in order to determine precisely the location of the object. If the exact nature of the foreign body is uncertain, a lateral projection is mandatory because it allows for discrimination between a coin and button battery. Coins are easily visualized by radiograph and lie almost always in the coronal plane (**9.5**). Metal detectors have been advocated by some as a mechanism for determining the location of an ingested coin within the digestive tract without the cost and radiation exposure associated with radiography.

Many types of foreign bodies, such as nonmetallic toys, are not radio-opaque and thus cannot be visualized on simple X-ray. When a foreign body is not radio-opaque but the clinical suspicion for esophageal foreign body impaction is high, as in the patient who is drooling and complaining of chest discomfort, it is reasonable to proceed to procedural removal. However, where symptoms are more subtle or absent but ingestion is suspected, contrast radiography can be very helpful. Swallowed barium may reveal the foreign body as a filling defect within the usual column of esophageal contrast (**9.4**).

As a general rule, esophageal foreign bodies should be removed within 24 hours of ingestion. This time frame is derived principally from retrospective reviews of pediatric patients, where complications of impacted esophageal foreign bodies have been seen with duration of impaction as short as 24 hours.

The first steps in management are determined by (1) the type of foreign body, (2) severity of patient symptoms, (3) the location of the foreign body, and (4) the age of the patient. Sharp foreign bodies and button batteries should be removed immediately because of the risk of severe injury to the esophagus and adjacent structures. Patients who are very uncomfortable or unable to swallow oral secretions should proceed to emergent foreign body removal. Data from children who have ingested coins suggest that location within the distal esophagus and older age are predictors of spontaneous foreign body passage. Thus, in the previously healthy older toddler/school-aged child with a distal esophageal foreign body that is neither sharp nor a button battery, and who has minimal symptoms, a period of observation of 12–24 hours is a reasonable approach. In randomized clinical trials, the use of glucagon to encourage spontaneous passage of a foreign body has not been shown to be an effective strategy in the pediatric population.

There are multiple procedural strategies for the removal of esophageal foreign bodies. In principle, esophagoscopy (rigid or flexible) allows for direct visualization of the foreign body and surrounding esophageal mucosa. Thus, esophagoscopy is the gold-standard approach for esophageal foreign body removal. However, in the case of esophageal coin impaction, there are several alternative approaches to removal, discussed below, that are likely just as safe and effective as esophagoscopy.

Techniques for foreign body removal

Nonendoscopic techniques for esophageal foreign body removal are reserved for patients who have no known anatomic abnormality of the esophagus, whose witnessed ingestion is <24 hours prior, who are clinically stable, and where the foreign body is blunt and round (typically a coin).

One nonendoscopic technique involves a balloon-tipped catheter (commonly a Foley catheter) introduced into the esophagus under fluoroscopic guidance with minimal sedation. The balloon is then inflated within the esophagus distal to the foreign body. The entire catheter is then pulled back, dislodging the object into the oropharynx. The procedure is carried out in the Trendelenburg position to help keep the dislodged foreign body from causing airway compromise. Esophageal bougienage has

been reported in a small number of pediatric patients with an esophageal coin. With this strategy, a rubber semi-rigid esophageal bougie is introduced into the esophagus without sedation. The bougie is advanced, thus pushing the ingested coin into the stomach.

Both rigid and flexible endoscopic techniques have been employed for removal of esophageal foreign bodies. Choice of endoscopic technique is typically training-specific, with otolaryngologists and pediatric surgeons most commonly utilizing the rigid endoscope and gastroenterologists preferring the flexible endoscope. Limited data suggest that both endoscopic devices are equally efficacious in the removal of esophageal foreign bodies, although rigid endoscopy may be associated with a higher risk of esophageal perforation and postprocedural dysphagia. The rigid endoscope, by dilating the esophagus proximal to the foreign body, may allow for better visualization of the esophagus, particularly in the proximal esophagus just beyond the UES. In cases of chronic foreign body impaction, where there is significant edema of the surrounding tissue, the enhanced visualization afforded by rigid endoscopy may be of benefit.

There are multiple catheter-deployed devices, introduced through the working channel of the endoscope, which can be utilized for foreign body removal. The most commonly used device is the forceps, which grasps the edge of the foreign body prior to removal (**9.6, 9.7**). Endoscopically deployed nets (**9.8, 9.9**) can be used for blunt objects with no graspable edge, and snares (**9.10, 9.11**) are used to lasso a protruding surface that cannot be adequately grasped with forceps.

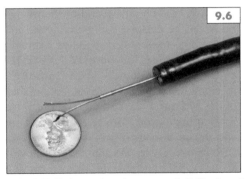
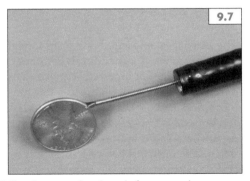

9.6, 9.7 Endoscopic coin grasper. **9.6**: Deployed; **9.7**: coin grasped and ready for removal.

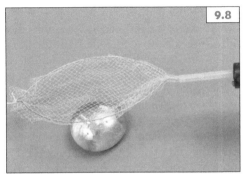
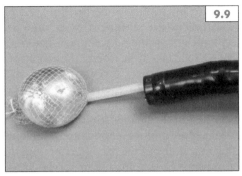

9.8, 9.9 Endoscopic Roth net foreign body retriever. **9.8**: Net is opened over a glass marble; **9.9**: Roth net secured around the marble, ready for removal.

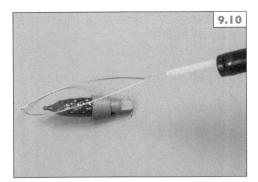
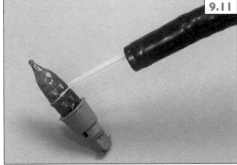

9.10, 9.11 Endoscopic snare. **9.10**: Snare prepares to grasp a tree light; **9.11**: snare is secured around the light, ready for removal.

Sharp objects

The esophageal impaction of a sharp foreign body presents a procedural challenge. Among commonly ingested types of sharp objects are pins, including open safety pins, toothpicks, needles, jewelry, broken glass, and bones. Fish bones are more common in Asia, where fish is a more common dietary staple. The principal risk of a sharp foreign body is perforation of the esophageal wall, which can lead to infectious or hemorrhagic complications. On plain radiograph of the chest, the presence of a linear stripe of air along the border of the esophagus can indicate an esophageal perforation (**9.12**). Toothpicks are noteworthy as they are typically not visible on plain radiograph yet have a tendency to perforate the esophagus and migrate into surrounding tissue. Moreover, due to their porous nature, toothpicks may then spread bacteria and lead to mediastinal contamination.

There are multiple endoscopic techniques that may decrease the risk of perforating the esophagus in the process of foreign body removal. Endoscopic overtubes are hollow tubes that fit over the shaft of the endoscope (**9.13, 9.14**). The sharp end of the foreign body can be grasped using a conventional endoscopic tool, and the hollow overtube is then advanced beyond the end of the endoscope, allowing the sharp end of the foreign body to rest within the hollow shaft of the overtube. This technique protects the walls of the esophagus when the endoscope and grasped sharp object are pulled back and removed. A second approach, deploying a rubber foreign body hood, can only be utilized if the foreign body is advanced first to the stomach. Advancement of a sharp object into the stomach first requires control of the sharp end of the object using graspers, bringing the sharp end of the object as close to the end of the endoscope as possible, then effecting a slow, controlled advance that maintains the endoscope in the middle of the esophageal lumen. This technique can be very challenging if the sharp end is oriented distally. Once in the stomach, the endoscope is withdrawn through the gastroesophageal junction, thus flipping the foreign body hood over the end of the endoscope (**9.15–9.17**) and protecting surrounding tissue from injury.

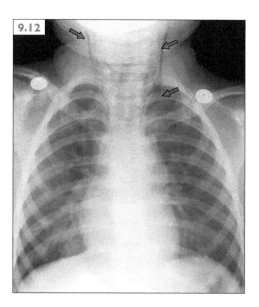

9.12 Posterior–anterior radiograph of the chest. Arrows demonstrate mediastinal free air due to esophageal perforation.

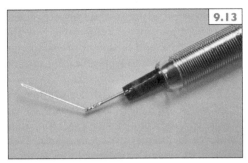

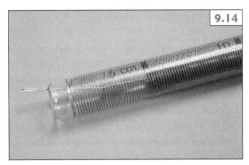

9.13, 9.14 Endoscopic overtube used for removal of a sharp foreign body. **9.13:** An endoscopically deployed device is used to grasp the sharp end of a sewing needle; **9.14:** the endoscope is pulled back into the overtube, protecting surrounding mucosa while the endoscope is withdrawn.

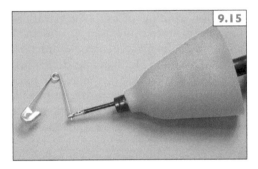

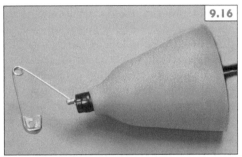

9.15–9.17 Use of a foreign body hood for removal of a sharp foreign body. **9.15:** With the foreign body hood in place at the end of the endoscope, a rubber-tipped device is used to grasp the sharp end of a safety pin; **9.16:** the grasping device is pulled back to the tip of the endoscope; **9.17:** when the endoscope is withdrawn through the gastroesophageal junction, the foreign body hood is flipped over the end of the endoscope, protecting surrounding tissue from injury.

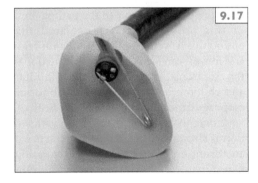

Food impactions

Food impactions represent the most common type of esophageal foreign body in adults. In pediatrics, food impactions are most common in older school-aged and adolescent children. However, certain children may present at any age with a food impaction, in particular those with a previous history of esophageal surgery (such as correction of esophageal atresia), known esophageal stricture, or history of an antireflux surgery procedure. The most commonly impacted foods in the esophagus are meats such as chicken, beef, and hot dogs (**9.18**).

In the child with a food impaction but without a history of esophageal surgery, the clinician must be highly suspicious for the diagnosis of eosinophilic esophagitis (EoE). Multiple recent single-institution reviews have demonstrated a high incidence of EoE amongst biopsied pediatric patients with food impactions. Some investigators have reported a seasonal variation in the frequency of esophageal food impactions, with relatively more food impactions in the summer and fall months, suggesting that aeroallergen exposure may play a role in the pathogenesis of this problem. It is postulated that eosinophil-driven esophageal inflammation and fibrosis can lead to motor dysfunction of the esophagus, and multiple studies in adults and children have demonstrated abnormal esophageal motility in patients with EoE.

A diagnosis of esophageal food impaction is strongly suggested by the history of an abrupt onset of symptoms after eating. Chest pain and drooling are common. The food bolus is unlikely to be seen on simple radiograph, but a contrast study may show a filling defect within the esophagus or complete obstruction of the esophagus (**9.19**). Radiologic confirmation of an esophageal food impaction is not necessary before proceeding to endoscopy. If the patient history supports food impaction and the patient remains uncomfortable with the persistent sensation of an esophageal foreign body, endoscopy can be both diagnostic and therapeutic.

Endoscopic removal of an esophageal food impaction can be tedious as the food bolus typically falls apart with manipulation. Multiple techniques exist for removal. Nets can be deployed through the esophagus to secure the entirety of the food bolus for removal. Grasping devices can be used to remove the bolus or to shred the food bolus into smaller pieces that can then be advanced without obstruction into the stomach. Banding devices, more commonly used for banding of esophageal varices, have been successfully used in adults and children for management of esophageal food impaction. The banding device may provide a 'suction cap' that more effectively attaches the food bolus to the end of the endoscope. Because of the tendency for food boluses to disintegrate, the food bolus frequently is removed in multiple pieces. To accomplish this, the esophagus must be endoscopically intubated multiple times during the procedure, increasing the risk for esophageal perforation and postprocedure discomfort. In a patient of sufficient size, an endoscopic overtube can be utilized to diminish these risks as the endoscope can be withdrawn through the tube without causing injury to the posterior pharynx and upper esophageal sphincter. Endoscopes with two working channels are available for adolescents and adults, which can allow for more efficient shredding of the food bolus prior to advancement of the food into the stomach.

Because of the high likelihood of discovering EoE in pediatric food impaction, it is essential for the endoscopist to obtain mucosal biopsies from the proximal and distal esophagus during the procedure.

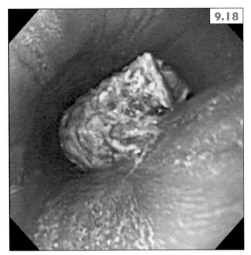

9.18 Endoscopic view of a meat impaction in the distal esophagus. Note linear ridging and white exudates along the esophageal mucosa, endoscopic features of eosinophilic esophagitis.

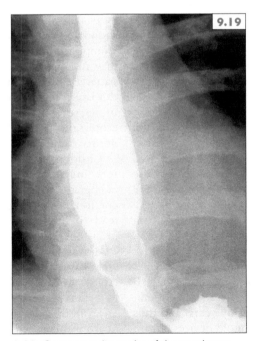

9.19 Contrast radiography of the esophagus demonstrating a filling defect in the distal esophagus due to a food impaction. There is dilatation of the esophagus proximal to the food impaction.

Button batteries

Impaction of a button battery within the esophagus must be considered a pediatric emergency as life threatening injury has been sustained within 2 hours of ingestion. The button battery (**9.20**), also known as a watch battery or disk battery, must be removed immediately from the esophagus to limit the extent of tissue damage.

The mechanism of esophageal injury due to battery ingestion has been worked out by careful experiments in animal models. The cathode and anode of a button battery sit in close proximity, and within the lumen of the esophagus mucosa collapses around the battery and bridges the cathode and anode, completing a circuit that allows for the flow of current through tissue (**9.21**). The flow of current then leads to a rapid change of pH, first in esophageal tissue, and with time, in adjacent tissue such as trachea or vascular endothelium. A simple experiment depicted in Figure **9.22** demonstrates the rapidity with which the pH changes in fluid making contact with a button battery. A severely basic pH is toxic to human cells, leading to individual cell death, and with time, tissue necrosis.

Button batteries were first introduced in the 1950s for use in hearing aids. Their use in consumer electronics and toys has increased exponentially in the last decade with the development of batteries with lithium as the principal metal component of the battery anode. Whereas traditional alkaline button batteries carried a maximum voltage of 1.5 V, newer lithium button batteries are 3 V, thereby increasing current flow to devices or, in the case of ingestion, esophageal tissue. Lithium button batteries can retain their capacitance for many years, and thus discarded batteries from old devices remain potentially dangerous to the curious toddler. Increased voltage and capacitance, which make lithium button batteries more injurious to humans, have also made them desirable for incorporation in electronic devices. An abbreviated list of devices that include lithium batteries includes wristwatches, remote controls, key fobs, greeting cards, and toys. Several types of lithium batteries are large (>2 cm) and thereby are more likely to become stuck within the esophagus.

Data collected by the National Poison Data System, which tracks cases reported to United States poison control centers, has shown an alarming increase over the last decade in the percentage of battery ingestions with severe outcomes, including death. This increase has mirrored the shift in the battery industry towards production of 3 V lithium button batteries. The most common fatal complication of button battery ingestion is hemorrhage, typically due to the development of a fistula between the esophagus and the aorta. Additional severe complications include the development of a secondary tracheoesophageal fistula, esophageal stricture, esophageal perforation, spondylodiscitis, and vocal cord paralysis. Complications of button battery ingestion may not be seen for days to weeks after battery removal. In the case of fistulization, this late complication may reflect the depth of necrotic injury emanating from the esophagus, leading to the destruction of normal tissue planes.

Children with witnessed button battery ingestion should have immediate radiographs to assess for battery location. The confirmation of esophageal location should lead to immediate endoscopic removal in an operating room with surgeons and cardiovascular surgeons on standby. If the child has recently ingested food or liquids, rapid-sequence intubation should be used to secure the patient airway prior to removal. Delay in the administration of anesthesia is unacceptable as time is likely a critical factor in determining the severity of battery-induced esophageal injury.

When a foreign body ingestion is unwitnessed, or where the nature of the swallowed

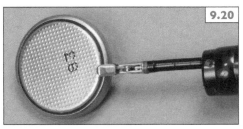

9.20 Lithium button battery.

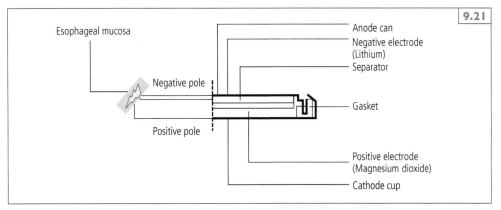

9.21 Cross-sectional schematic of a lithium button battery. The cathode and anode of the battery lie in close proximity. When esophageal tissue lies across the rubber gasket of the battery, bridging the negative and positive electrodes, a circuit is created and current flows through esophageal tissue.

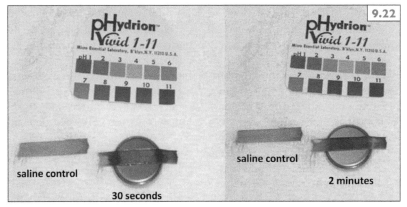

9.22 In this experiment, pH paper is laid across the surface of a 3 V lithium button battery and a drop of saline is applied. Basic pH changes are seen within 30 seconds at the edge of the battery, which is where the positive and negative electrodes lie in close proximity. Within 2 minutes the entire surface of the battery has changed to a pH >11. Such basic changes in pH are injurious to cells.

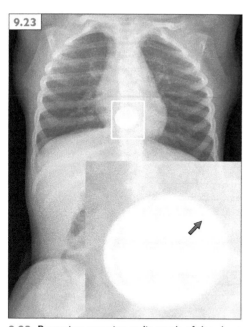

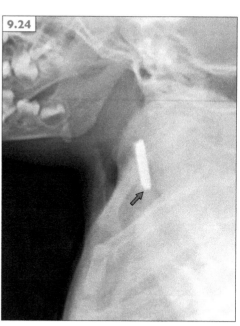

9.23 Posterior–anterior radiograph of the chest demonstrating an esophageal button battery. Inset is a higher magnification of the button battery. The arrow shows the visible ring around the circumference of the battery, a hallmark radiographic feature of a button battery.

9.24 Higher magnification of lateral radiograph of the neck demonstrating a button battery in the cervical esophagus. The arrow points to the step-off from posterior to anterior, a second hallmark radiographic feature of a button battery.

object is in doubt, a frequent source of confusion is the distinction between an esophageal button battery and an esophageal coin. Because the urgency of removal is very different for these two objects, radiographic discrimination is critical. A coin and a button battery can appear very similar on a posterior–anterior radiograph, but a hallmark radiographic feature of a button battery is a distinct rim along the edge of the battery (**9.23**). A lateral view will reveal the 'step off' between the anode and cathode that is an additional classic radiographic feature of a button battery (**9.24**).

At endoscopic battery removal, there will frequently be extensive mucosal ulceration at the site of esophageal impaction (**9.25**). When the injury is severe, placement of a nasogastric tube will allow for delivery of nutrition while maintaining the patient NPO. A contrast esophagram using a water-soluble agent should be performed after battery removal to assess for esophageal perforation. Any radiographic evidence of perforation or patient fever should prompt the administration of intravenous antibiotics.

Proper follow-up of children with moderate-severe battery-induced esophageal injury is unclear. However, considering the well-documented risk of late fistulizing complications of these injuries, surveillance should be strongly considered. Follow-up endoscopic and cross-sectional imaging evaluation may be considered for the purposes of (1) visualizing mucosal healing, and (2) understanding the anatomic structures at risk. Magnetic resonance imaging (MRI) with contrast administration may demonstrate the depth of tissue injury without radiation exposure (**9.26, 9.27**).

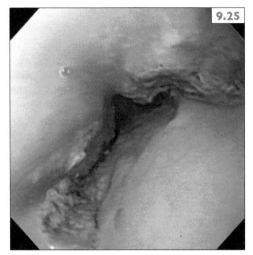

9.25 Endoscopic view of esophageal mucosal ulcerations due to button battery impaction.

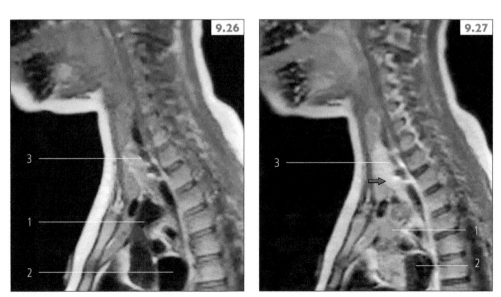

9.26, 9.27 MRI of the chest 4 days after esophageal button battery impaction. **9.26**: Sagittal T1 image of the chest showing irregularity of the esophageal mucosa at the site of battery impaction and the close relationship of this area to the ascending aorta; **9.27**: T1 image with contrast agent gadolinium. Arrow shows the anterior extent of contrast enhancement due to inflammation. 1: aorta; 2: left atrium; 3: esophagus.

Any evidence of esophageal bleeding in association with battery ingestion should prompt the clinician to consider the possibility of an esophageal fistula to an adjacent vascular structure. The 'herald bleed' of an aortoesophageal fistula, whether presenting as hematemesis or melena, is a well-described clinical event that precedes a fatal hemorrhage event by minutes or hours.

Conclusion

Esophageal foreign bodies are common in pediatrics. Respiratory symptoms may be prominent when a foreign body is chronically impacted in the esophagus. Most esophageal foreign bodies can be safely removed within 24 hours with the prominent exception of sharp foreign bodies and button batteries, which are associated with higher risk of complications that necessitates immediate removal.

ACKNOWLEDGMENTS
The author acknowledges Robert E. Kramer, MD for his careful reading of the manuscript and contribution of illustrations.

CHAPTER 10

Esophageal Burns

Mitchell Shub

- **Introduction**
- **Caustic ingestions with acids and alkalis**
- **Button (disk) battery ingestion**
- **Pill-induced esophagitis**

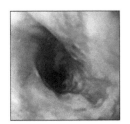
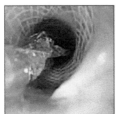
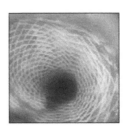
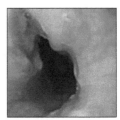

Introduction

Esophageal burn injury remains a significant medical problem in children despite efforts to reduce exposure to caustic household products. Most of these injuries are the result of accidental ingestion of caustic agents and occur in children less than 6 years of age. Teenagers are also at risk, but in many of these instances the ingestion was purposeful with the motive being self-harm. The likelihood that an agent will result in a serious burn is dependent on several factors including pH, concentration, amount consumed, whether the substance can generate an external electrical current, and length of time that it is in contact with the mucosa. Depending on the type of ingestion, the event may result in a medical emergency with the child requiring immediate intervention.

Caustic ingestions with acids and alkalis

MECHANISM OF TISSUE INJURY

Acids (pH 2–6) and alkalis (pH 7–12) produce different types of tissue injury. Acids cause coagulation necrosis with eschar formation that can limit depth of penetration. Conversely, alkalis cause a liquefactive necrosis and saponification injury with potential for deeper tissue damage. In general, alkaline substances tend to be more palatable than acidic products, which often results in the ingestion of larger quantities and a higher risk of serious injury.

The most common caustic substances ingested by children are those that are readily available within households. These include household bleach and oven cleaners. Others include drain cleaners, herbicides, rust removers, swimming pool chemicals, toilet bowl cleaners, and liquid battery acid. Often, these events occur when the caustic agent is stored in a nonchild-proof container that is easily accessible.

Table 10.1 Classification of caustic injury

Grade	Esophageal mucosal appearance
Grade 0	Normal examination
Grade 1	Edema (loss of vascular pattern) and hyperemia of the mucosa
Grade 2a	Friability, hemorrhage, erosions, blisters, white membranes, exudate, and superficial ulcers
Grade 2b	Deep discrete or circumferential ulceration in addition to Grade 2a findings
Grade 3a	Small scattered areas of necrosis (identified by brown-black or grayish discoloration)
Grade 3b	Extensive necrosis

(From Zargar *et al.*, 1991. The role of fiberoptic endoscopy in the management of corrosive ingestion and modified endoscopic classification of burns. *Gastrointest Endosc* **37**:165–169.)

CLINICAL PRESENTATION

Several studies have shown that the presence or absence of symptoms is not an accurate predictor of whether a caustic ingestion has taken place or if a serious esophageal injury has occurred. In addition, the presence or absence of an oral tissue injury is a poor indicator of an esophageal burn. Common symptoms following a caustic ingestion include drooling, dysphagia, feeding refusal, chest pain, abdominal pain, and vomiting. An increased number of symptoms tend to correlate with a significant injury although absence or minimal symptoms do not exclude the possibility of a serious burn. Airway symptoms are not common, but dyspnea is usually a sign of a substantial injury. Severe symptoms following a caustic ingestion can result from perforation of a hollow viscus with mediastinitis, peritonitis, shock, and death.

DIAGNOSIS

The most important step in assessing an esophageal burn is to identify accurately the location, extent, and severity of the injury. Studies have shown that clinical and radiologic evaluations alone are not adequate to predict the type and severity of the injury. Endoscopic evaluation has become a mainstay in assessing burn injuries and is typically performed 12–48 hours after the ingestion. Early endoscopy prior to 12 hours could miss evolving lesions, and late endoscopy beyond 48 hours may increase the risk of perforation. If there is a strong degree of suspicion that a perforation exists then imaging studies such as a plain upright radiograph of the chest and abdomen, water-soluble oral esophagram, or computed tomography with oral contrast should be performed before proceeding with endoscopy. Esophageal injury is graded at the time of endoscopy. A grading system developed by Zargar (*Table 10.1*), classifies caustic injuries from Grade 0 (no visible damage) to Grade 3b (extensive necrotic tissue). The degree of esophageal injury closely correlates with morbidity and mortality. Grade 1 injury, seen in the majority of caustic ingestions, consists of edema and erythema. These children can be fed normally and discharged home. Patients with Grade 2a lesions (superficial and noncircumferential ulcers) rarely progress to esophageal stenosis and usually have an uncomplicated course. Grade 2b injury (circumferential ulceration) is associated with increased risk of stricture formation. These patients will require careful observation as the diet is advanced, and a barium contrast esophogram will need to be performed after 3 weeks to look for stricture formation. Grade 3a (scattered area of necrosis) or Grade 3b injury results in a high degree of stricture formation (**10.1**).

10.1 Extensive esophageal injury with necrosis (Grade 3a) after alkaline ingestion.

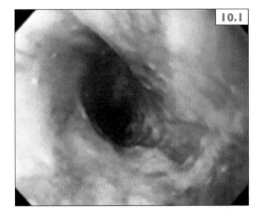

10.1

TREATMENT
Initial management
If endoscopic evaluation reveals a burn injury of 2b or greater, children are hospitalized, intravenous fluids are given, and oral feeds are initially withheld. Often, a nasogastric tube is placed under direct endoscopic vision or over a guide wire. This tube can provide a route for feeding and can also act as a stent if a stricture occurs. As children recover and the edema in the esophagus diminishes, oral feedings can be initiated. If oral or enteral feeds are not tolerated then total parenteral nutrition will be required. Corticosteroids have not been shown to reduce the incidence of stricture formation and are not generally advocated. There is not sufficient data to support the universal use of antibiotics; however, they are warranted in patients at high risk for perforation (Grade 3 injury). Acid reflux has been shown to impair the healing process, therefore treatment to reduce acid production should be considered in children with Grade 2b or greater injuries. Proton pump inhibitor (PPI) therapy can be given until tissue injury has healed, usually in 2–3 weeks. Long-term treatment with PPI therapy may be needed in patients with extensive esophageal injury, due to impaired esophageal motility leading to slow clearance of acid reflux.

Long-term management
Children with Grade 2b and Grade 3 injuries need to be closely monitored for signs of dysphagia as an indication of esophageal stricture formation. Diagnostic testing is usually performed 2–3 weeks after the injury. A barium esophagram can outline a stricture (**10.2**) and determine the extent of stricture formation. Endoscopy can identify the degree of mucosal healing, the location of a stricture, and can be used to initiate esophageal dilatation with bougies or balloons of graduated size (**10.3–10.5**). Strictures may require serial dilations over several months or years. Esophageal perforation can occur as a complication of dilation therapy, especially with severely fibrotic lesions.

10.2 Radiograph taken 4 weeks after a Grade 3a caustic injury demonstrating a long esophageal stricture.

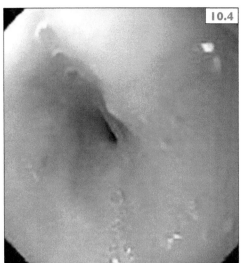

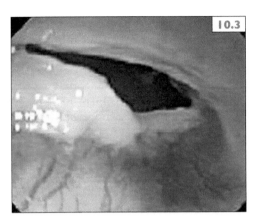

10.3 Circumferential esophageal burn injury with ulcer and white exudate at 12 hours after caustic ingestion.

10.4 Esophageal stricture formation at 6 weeks following the injury.

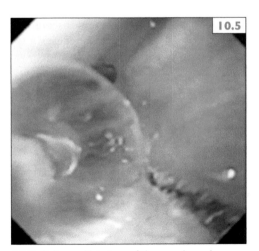

10.5 Balloon dilatation of the esophageal stricture.

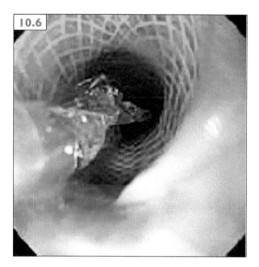

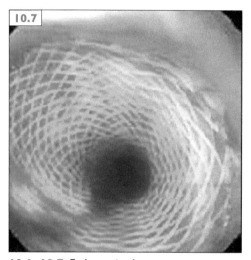

There is observational evidence that the application of mitomycin C solution to the fibrotic area immediately after dilation may slow down the regeneration of scar tissue. Other therapies that have been used include steroid injection at the stricture site following dilation, placement of a self-expanding esophageal stent (**10.6, 10.7**), or prolonged use of a nasogastric tube. Strictures that are refractory to management may require partial esophageal resection with reversed gastric tube esophagoplasty or colonic interposition.

There is an increased risk for developing esophageal carcinoma in all patients with an esophageal stricture following caustic ingestion. Most patients develop esophageal dysmotility with delayed clearance of gastric refluxate following severe caustic burn injury. It is thought that the combination of caustic injury and chronic peptic esophagitis increase the risks of developing both adenocarcinoma and squamous carcinoma. It is recommended that endoscopic surveillance begins 15–20 years after caustic stricture injury, with endoscopy performed every 1–3 years thereafter.

10.6, 10.7 Endoscopic placement of a self-expanding esophageal stent.
10.6: Placement following balloon dilation;
10.7: self-expanding stent after deployment.

Button (disk) battery ingestion

DEFINITION AND PATHOPHYSIOLOGY

Foreign body ingestion in children is a common problem and usually involves objects that pass through the gastrointestinal tract without causing serious injury. However, ingestion of a button battery, which becomes lodged within the esophagus, has emerged as a serious and potentially life-threatening problem. A severe burn injury can result from a charged button battery retained in the esophagus. This type of ingestion has become an increasingly common problem because of the ready availability of these types of batteries. The most dangerous battery is the 20 mm diameter lithium cell battery that is used to power electronic toys and other common devices found in the household. These batteries are large enough to become lodged in the esophagus of a small child and powerful enough to cause severe burn injuries.

Button cell batteries generate an external electrolytic current that hydrolyzes tissue fluids. Lithium 20 mm batteries are 3 V cells and generate sufficient current to produce deep tissue injuries. Even discharged cells, which are unable to power a product, have enough residual voltage to produce damage. The most serious injury occurs in the area adjacent to the negative battery pole where the external electrolytic current is generated. The negative pole is the narrower side of the disc when viewed laterally on a radiograph. Tissue injury can progress for days to weeks after the battery has been removed.

CLINICAL PRESENTATION

Most children will present with nonspecific symptoms that can be seen with other types of foreign body ingestions. The initial symptoms might include dysphagia, drooling, cough, chest pain, fussiness, feeding refusal, and vomiting. Also, fever and signs of shock can be seen in cases where a perforation has occurred. Some children will have minimal or no symptoms. In children where the ingestion was not witnessed, the correct diagnosis may be missed for hours or days, resulting in a serious outcome or fatality.

DIAGNOSIS

An urgent radiograph of the chest and abdomen is usually performed to determine if a foreign body is present within the esophagus. In cases where the ingestion was witnessed, the radiograph can rapidly establish whether the battery is lodged in the esophagus. Unfortunately, in unwitnessed ingestions, it may be difficult to differentiate between a coin and a battery. Certain features, such as a 'double rim' or 'double disk' sign on an anterior–posterior film (**10.8**) or tapered contour on a lateral film may help correctly identify a battery. Even an experienced radiologist will incorrectly identify a battery as a coin about 20% of the time. In situations where a missed diagnosis occurs, there can be a prolonged delay, which can lead to significant morbidity and mortality. When in doubt, repeat X-rays at different angles may help make the correct diagnosis.

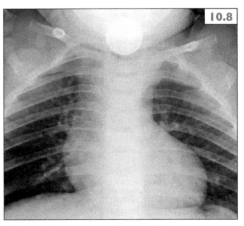

10.8 Radiograph of a 20 mm disk battery in the esophagus of a 1-year-old showing a 'double rim' sign.

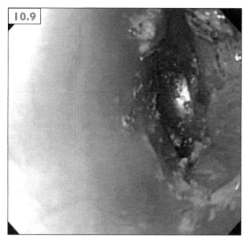
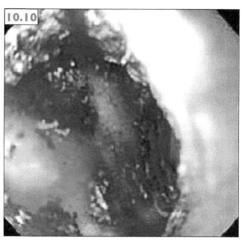

10.9, 10.10 Button battery ingestion. **10.9**: Button battery impacted in the esophagus with burn injury. (Courtesy of Robert Kramer, MD; Children's Hospital of Colorado, Denver.) **10.10**: necrotic injury observed after disk battery removal.

TREATMENT
Initial management
Urgent endoscopic removal of the battery from the esophagus after ingestion is the recommended treatment choice (**10.9, 10.10**). Serious burn injury can occur as soon as 2 hours after ingestion. Endoscopy should not be delayed if a child has recently eaten as this could lead to prolonged mucosal exposure and higher risk for deep burn injury. Endoscopic removal is preferred over other forms of extraction as it allows direct visualization of tissue injury and the direction the negative pole of the battery is facing. If mucosal injury is present, children should be monitored for delayed complications.

Long-term management
If severe mucosal injury is initially documented, then delayed complications should be anticipated including: esophageal perfor-ation, mediastinitis, esophageal stricture, tracheoesophageal fistula, tracheal stenosis, empyema, pneumothorax, or exsanguination from perforation into a large vessel. Specific complications can be anticipated based on battery orientation (direction of negative pole) and location of esophageal injury. Patients at risk of perforation into vessels should be monitored in the hospital with serial radiologic imaging.

Early intervention may prevent a catastrophic bleeding event. Patients should also be monitored for signs of respiratory symptoms, especially those associated with swallowing, as this could indicate development of a tracheoesophageal fistula. Development of dysphagia can indicate presence of an esophageal stricture. It is critical to know that perforations, fistulas, and severe bleeding events may occur up to 18 days after battery removal and esophageal or tracheal strictures may be delayed for weeks to months.

Pill-induced esophagitis

Pill induced esophageal burn injury 'pill esophagitis' is an under-reported problem and seems to occur most commonly in young women including adolescents. Over a hundred different medications have been implicated with the most common being nonsteroidal anti-inflammatory drugs, acne medicine (tetra- or doxycyclines), and potassium chloride tablets. Esophageal injury occurs when a caustic medicinal pill becomes lodged in the esophagus and releases a concentrated amount of irritant content. Risk factors for developing this injury include taking a pill with little or no fluid, reclining while ingesting a medication, underlying anatomic abnormalities (i.e. esophageal stricture, atrial enlargement), and esophageal motility abnormalities. Patients will usually present with odynophagia with or without dysphagia. A localized, circular area of ulceration characterizes a typical injury (**10.11**) and most often involves the junction of the proximal and middle esophagus. Diffuse erythema may surround the ulcer(s) with normal appearance of the mucosa in the rest of esophagus. Usually the injury heals without sequela but rare cases of mediastinitis and penetration of the great vessels have been reported.

Treatment consists of withdrawal of the offending medication with resolution of symptoms within a few days to a few weeks. No treatment regimen has been adequately studied; however, topical anesthetics, acid suppression, and sucralfate are commonly used.

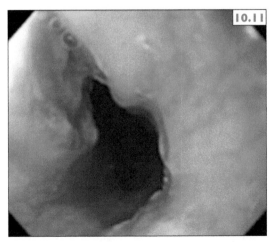

10.11 Ulceration from 'pill esophagitis' in a 14-year-old taking a nonsteroidal anti-inflammatory drug.

STOMACH AND DUODENUM

CHAPTER 11

Gastritis and Gastric Ulcers

Ian Kang

DEFINITION

'Gastritis' is the microscopic evidence of inflammation of the gastric mucosa, indicating histologic evaluation of biopsy samples. 'Gastropathy' indicates epithelial cell damage without inflammation. Both are best diagnosed by endoscopy. There is no universally accepted histologic grading system in pediatrics. 'Ulcers' are mucosal lesions that disrupt the muscularis mucosa. A recent publication estimated the incidence of bleeding from a peptic ulcer to be 0.5–0.9 and 4.4/100,000 individuals.

The overall incidence of gastritis is not well known. Incidence of *Helicobacter pylori* is low in western Europe, the United States, and Canada. The prevalence of *H. pylori* at 10 years of age in developed countries is approximately 10% and increases with age, while the prevalence of this infection is much higher in Asia, Africa, South America, Mexico, and southern and eastern Europe with rates up to 90%. Infection is usually acquired by 5 years of age. Risk factors include low socioeconomic status, bed-sharing, and a large number of siblings. There are conflicting data on the effects of breastfeeding and daycare attendance. Reinfection rates are considered to be low after successful treatment but are more likely in young children.

CLINICAL PRESENTATION

Presentation is variable as there may be multiple causes and varying ages of patients. Common symptoms are as follows: abdominal pain (variable location, but particularly epigastric), irritability, vomiting, and poor appetite. Additional symptoms may include nocturnal awakening, early satiety, and weight loss. Hemorrhagic gastritis (**11.1**) may be associated with hematemesis, anemia, melena, and occult blood in stool.

ETIOLOGY AND PATHOPHYSIOLOGY
Infectious gastritis

H. pylori is a gram-negative bacterium responsible for nodular gastritis (**11.2**) in humans and is the most common cause of gastritis worldwide. Transmission is not understood but considered to be by person-to-person contact based on familial clustering. It survives stomach acid by producing urease to buffer acid and by colonizing the mucous layer. Other bacterial-related gastropathies include *Helicobacter heilmannii* which is uncommon and is associated with gastric carcinoma/mucosa-associated lymphoid tissue (MALT) lymphoma. It is approximately twice the size of *H. pylori*, and its treatment is similar to that of *H. pylori*.

Viral infections related to gastritis include cytomegalovirus (CMV see below), Epstein–Barr Virus (EBV), human herpes virus-7, influenza, and herpes simplex virus (HSV). These causes of gastritis are relatively rare. HSV is most commonly seen in immunocompromised patients.

Parasitic infections include *Anisakis* from sushi/sashimi/ceviche ingestion, and parasites are notable for causing eosinophilia and worms visible on endoscopy. Treatment may involve endoscopic removal of the worms. *Giardia* is a rare cause of gastritis and seems to affect those with abnormal gastric acid secretion.

Fungal infections of the stomach are most common in neonates, malnourished patients, and immunocompromised children. Notable organisms include *Candida*, *Aspergillus*, *Histoplasma*, and *Mucorales* spp.

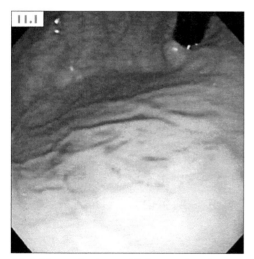

11.1 Hemorrhagic gastritis in retroflex view.

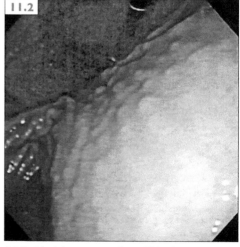

11.2 Nodular gastritis from *Helicobacter pylori*.

Reactive gastropathy

Stress ulcers are related to physiologic stress such as critical illness (shock, acidosis, sepsis, burns, surgery, head injury) and associated mucosal hypoperfusion.

Uremic gastropathy is exacerbated by steroid usage and liver disease. In chronic renal failure, patients have increased parietal, chief and gastrin–producing cells but normal gastric pH, which may be from neutralization secondary to increased ammonia.

Long distance runners may suffer from an erosive or nonerosive gastropathy related to hypoperfusion and dysmotility. The lesions may be visualized anywhere in the stomach.

Neonatal gastropathy

Neonatal gastropathies are usually related to prematurity, sepsis, or prolonged ventilation. This disorder also may be seen with use of indomethacin or dexamethasone. Prostaglandin E usage to maintain patency of the ductus arteriosus can lead to mucosal thickening and gastric outlet obstruction.

Medication-induced gastritis

Nonsteroidal anti-inflammatory drug (NSAID)-related gastritis is secondary to topical irritation and inhibition of cyclo-oxygenase, and can occur after the first dose. Aspirin, unique among NSAIDs, also inhibits thromboxane production in platelets. Other medications associated with gastritis include corticosteroids, potassium chloride, and iron preparations. Proton pump inhibitors (PPIs) may cause parietal cell hyperplasia and endoscopic visualization of gastric pseudopolyps. These pseudopolyps are not true polyps, have not been shown to be dysplastic, and usually resolve after stopping therapy.

Traumatic gastropathy

Traumatic gastropathies may occur from repeated retching (prolapse gastropathy), or may be related to foreign bodies in the stomach such as nasogastric tubes, gastrostomy tubes, or coins.

Radiation gastropathy

Currently, gastric tolerance to radiation is unknown. Acid suppression is not protective. Radiation damage may lead to stricture formation.

Corrosive gastritis

Corrosive gastropathy occurs from ingestion of acid or alkaline products. Acid ingestion causes coagulation necrosis, and induces pylorospasm, which may lead to gastric outlet obstruction. Alkali ingestion causes liquefaction necrosis and also may cause gastric outlet obstruction. Button batteries may lead to gastric ulceration within minutes to hours but are usually most dangerous in the esophagus.

Bile gastropathy

In adults, bile gastropathy is known to occur after gastric surgery. Bile may be found in the stomach at the time of endoscopy and may not have clinical significance. Bile reflux is usually seen in teenagers and does not respond to acid suppression. The usual endoscopic findings include erythema, but histologically there is usually venous congestion with inflammation.

Granulomatous gastritis

The most common cause of granulomatous disease in the stomach is Crohn disease (**11.3**). Gastritis in patients with ulcerative colitis is not uncommon, but is usually mild and not granulomatous. Unless granulomas are visualized, it may be difficult to differentiate between the two entities. Other causes of granulomatous gastritis include lymphoma, sarcoid, chronic granulomatous disease (CGD), and rarely Wegener granulomatosis.

Allergic and eosinophilic gastritis

Allergic gastropathy is usually related to milk protein intolerance in infancy and typically resolves with allergen avoidance, with shellfish and nuts as notable exceptions. Eosinophilic gastropathy may involve all layers of the gastrointestinal (GI) tract. This disorder may improve with allergen avoidance if a specific antigen can be identified. Signs and symptoms may include diarrhea, anemia, hypoproteinemia, and peripheral eosinophilia. Endoscopically, it is common to see erosions or pseudopolyps associated with eosinophilic gastropathy (**11.4**).

Lymphocytic gastritis

Lymphocytic infiltrates are seen in celiac disease, CMV infection, and Ménétrier disease. In celiac disease, these infiltrates regress with the institution of a gluten-free diet. CMV gastritis is almost always in immunosuppressed patients. Ménétrier disease usually presents around 4 years of age and is associated with giant gastric folds and a protein-losing gastropathy. Although dramatic in appearance, Ménétrier disease is usually benign and self-limited.

Hyperplastic gastropathy

If not from a previously noted cause, investigation should consider polyposis syndromes such as Peutz–Jegher syndrome.

Portal hypertensive gastropathy

Portal hypertensive gastropathy is variable in appearance, from small erythematous patches to cherry-red spots or a hemorrhagic appearance. The mucosa may have a mosaic or 'snake skin' appearance (**11.5**). The most common cause is cirrhosis, and there may be other evidence of portal hypertension seen on endoscopy such as gastric varices (**11.6, 11.7**).

Graft versus host disease

While chronic graft versus host disease (GvHD) (>100 days post-transplant) rarely involves the stomach, acute GvHD in the GI tract is more common. Symptoms include abdominal pain, nausea, vomiting, anorexia, weight loss, and diarrhea. Histologic findings include epithelial cell apoptosis, crypt loss, and lymphocytic infiltration.

Collagenous gastritis

Collagenous gastritis is rare, and may occur alone or be associated with another disorder such as celiac disease, collagenous colitis, or lymphocytic colitis. Histology is notable for subepithelial fibrosis.

Hypersecretory gastritis

Zollinger–Ellison syndrome (ZES) is rare in children. ZES results from gastrinomas that are either sporadic or related to multiple endocrine neoplasia type 1 (MEN1). The gastrinomas cause increased gastrin release and lead to excess acid. Diagnosis is made by laboratory and radiographic testing. The common laboratory finding of ZES is an elevated fasting gastrin level (>100 pg/ml), and this can also be seen in patients receiving chronic PPI therapy. An elevated serum gastrin (>1000 pg/ml) is considered diagnostic, and secretin or calcium stimulation tests have also been used. Computed tomography and magnetic resonance imaging have excellent specificity but poor sensitivity. Nuclear imaging, particularly somatostatin receptor scintigraphy, can also be helpful.

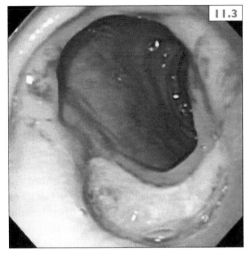

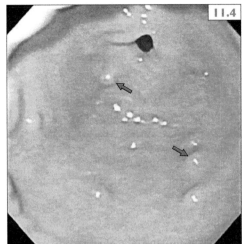

11.3 Crohn gastritis with ulceration.

11.4 Eosinophilic gastritis with pseudopolyps (arrows).

11.5 Mosaic or 'snake skin' appearance of portal hypertensive gastropathy.

11.6, 11.7 Gastric varices due to portal hypertension.

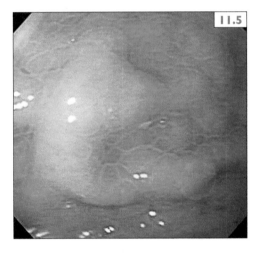

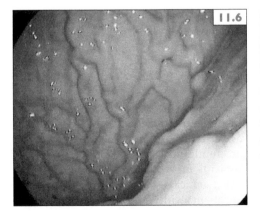

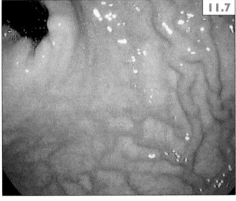

Short bowel syndrome has been linked to gastritis due to the lack of a negative feedback loop inhibiting gastrin secretion. Hypercalcemia from hyperparathyroidism may lead to elevated gastric acid secretion.

DIFFERENTIAL DIAGNOSIS OF ABDOMINAL PAIN NOT INCLUDING GASTRITIS

- Gastrointestinal:
  - Constipation.
  - Gastroesophageal reflux/reflux esophagitis.
  - Nonulcer dyspepsia.
  - Cholecystitis.
  - Inflammatory bowel disease.
  - Pancreatitis.
- Genitourinary:
  - Urinary tract infection.
  - Sexually transmitted disease.
- Functional bowel disorders:
  - Recurrent abdominal pain of childhood.
  - Irritable bowel syndrome.
- Trauma.
- Musculoskeletal.
- Neurologic:
  - Central nervous system neoplasm.
  - Pseudotumor cerebri.

DIAGNOSIS

The diagnosis of gastritis is histologic. There may be poor correlation of scoring between endoscopy and histology unless there are ulcers present. Multiple biopsy samples should be obtained from several different areas of the stomach.

Histologic diagnosis is the gold standard for *H. pylori*. Urea breath testing has excellent specificity and sensitivity. Sensitivity is decreased in urea breath testing if the patient takes medications such as antibiotics, PPI, or bismuth-containing compounds. Patient co-operation may be a limiting factor in breath testing. Stool antigen testing has good positive and negative predictive values. Antibody testing from blood, urine, and saliva is of little value as there is poor sensitivity.

Also, antibody tests may remain positive for years postexposure, and there is no benefit in testing for eradication of infection.

TREATMENT

The mainstay of treatment of gastritis is acid suppression. There are two primary types of medications: histamine H2 receptor antagonists (H2-blockers) and PPIs. H2-blockers reversibly inhibit parietal cell H2 receptors. They have a rapid onset of action and may be taken anytime throughout the day. There are oral and intravenous (IV) forms available. Patients may develop tolerance to H2-blockers which may limit long-term use. Cimetidine blocks cytochrome P450, and it may lead to drug interactions with anticoagulants, phenytoin, propranolol, and tricyclic antidepressants. Cimetidine has also been linked to gynecomastia which reverses upon cessation of the medication.

PPIs are more potent and have a longer half-life. PPIs irreversibly bind to the hydrogen/potassium adenosine triphosphate enzyme system (H+/K+ ATPase), or the proton pump in the gastric parietal cell. The half-life of the H+/K+ ATPase is approximately 48 hours in adults. PPIs are most effective if administered 30 minutes prior to meals; they have a delayed onset of action in the oral form, and may act rapidly if given IV. PPI use in critically ill patients has been associated with increased risk of pneumonia in adults. There is recent literature suggesting an increased risk of *Clostridium difficile* colitis in patients receiving a PPI. Long-term use of PPIs is associated with hypomagnesemia.

Antacids chemically neutralize gastric acid with bicarbonate salts and aluminum or magnesium. These medications have rapid onset but short duration of action. Antacids should not be given to toddlers because of toxicity risk from the sodium or aluminum content. Magnesium-based antacids may cause diarrhea. Aluminum-based antacids must be given with caution in patients with renal disease. Antacids may chelate and interfere with the absorption of other medications such as H2-blockers and antibiotics.

Sucralfate is a local mucosal barrier agent which increases release of prostaglandins. Sucralfate works best in an acidic environment and should be taken separately from antacids, acid suppression agents, and meals. Because it also contains aluminum salts, sucralfate should be given with care in patients with renal failure or prematurity. Sucralfate may also inhibit absorption of multiple medications as with antacids noted above.

Misoprostol is a synthetic prostaglandin E analog that prevents gastric acid secretion and is approved for prevention of NSAID-induced ulcers. Because of its other side-effects (uterine rupture, induced labor, and abortion of pregnancy), it must not be used in women of childbearing age (pregnancy category X). The most common side-effects include abdominal pain and dose-related diarrhea.

Treatment of *H. pylori* infection is recommended only if the patient has the infection with associated gastritis or ulcers. There is no evidence that patients with abdominal pain without ulcers have improvement of their pain after treatment. There are several first-line regimens with 70–90% eradication rates. Three-drug regimens consist of a PPI plus two of three antibiotics (amoxicillin, clarithromycin, or metronidazole), or bismuth salts with amoxicillin and metronidazole. Four-drug regimens include a PPI or H2-blocker, bismuth salts, metronidazole, and one of three other antibiotics (amoxicillin, clarithromycin, or tetracycline). Alternatively, a sequential therapy example may include PPI and amoxicillin for 5 days; then PPI, clarithromycin and tinidazole for an additional 5 days.

Portal hypertensive gastropathy may be treated with beta-blockers to decrease portal pressure or somatostatin analogs (octreotide).

Eosinophilic gastropathy/gastritis is treated by identification/avoidance of allergens, corticosteroids, acid suppression, and may also improve with the use of mast cell stabilizers. Celiac disease-related gastropathy resolves with a gluten-free diet. ZES is treated by acid suppression followed by surgical removal of the gastrinoma(s), although total gastrectomy is rarely required with current medical therapy.

GvHD gastropathy is treated with a variety of immune suppression medication including corticosteroids, cyclosporine, FK506 (tacrolimus), mycopholate mofitil, and acid suppression. Collagenous gastritis may improve with steroids and acid suppression, and radiation gastropathy may improve with argon plasma coagulation, or possibly surgical resection.

CHAPTER 12

Abnormal Anatomy of the Stomach and Duodenum

Rafal Kozielski, Sonal Desai, Daniel Gelfond

- **Introduction**
- **Congenital and acquired anomalies of the stomach**
- **Congenital and acquired anomalies of the duodenum**

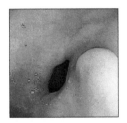 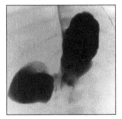 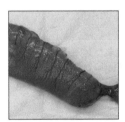 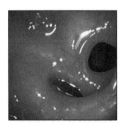

Introduction

In the majority of infants born with congenital malformations of the stomach or the duodenum, clinical symptoms become evident during the first few weeks of life, coinciding with feeding and leading to intolerance, vomiting, abdominal distention, and irritability. Some of the malformations are asymptomatic or may not warrant early investigation and present in later childhood or adulthood. Emphasis is placed on more critical clinical presentations requiring early endoscopic or surgical intervention.

Congenital and acquired anomalies of the stomach

Microgastria

Microgastria is a rare disorder characterized by a congenitally small stomach that is often accompanied by other anomalies such as malrotation, asplenia, tracheoesophageal fistula and other intestinal anomalies. Infants present with postprandial vomiting, reflux often associated with recurrent pulmonary infections, and increased gastric emptying that can present as diarrhea. Diagnosis is made radiologically with an upper gastrointestinal (UGI) series outlining a small stomach (**12.1**). Treatment is based on adequate nutrition, often consisting of continuous enteral nutrition and prevention of aspiration to minimize pulmonary exacerbation. Surgical correction with a double lumen Roux-en-Y jejunal reservoir (Hunt–Lawrence pouch) has been used in severe cases.

Gastric atresia

Gastric atresia is a rare form of intestinal atresia with an incidence of 1:100,000. Depending on the degree of gastric lumen occlusion, this finding can have either partial or complete obstruction, and usually is seen in the area of pylorus or antrum. It is often seen along with other intestinal atresias and associated with genetic syndromes such as trisomy 21.

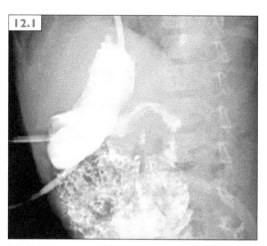

12.1 Microgastria. (Courtesy of John Pohl, MD; Department of Pediatric Gastroenterology, Primary Children's Hospital, University of Utah.)

Atresias with membranous or diaphragm occlusion can be congenital or seen in association with junctional epidermolysis bullosa. Onset and degree of clinical symptoms correlate with the type of atresia. Infants with complete atresia develop early nonbilious vomiting and hypochloremic hypokalemic acidosis. Diagnosis is made with radiologic images showing no air in the intestine, UGI barium studies, and endoscopic evaluation. Treatment is endoscopic transection of the membrane or web or surgical repair.

Gastric duplication

Gastric duplication is a rare embryologic anomaly of the foregut described as a cystic structure most commonly on the greater curvature of the stomach that does not communicate with the gastric lumen. The mucosal lining is usually gastric or intestinal with some reports of respiratory-type epithelium and occasional pancreatic tissue inclusions. Most will present during infancy with nonbilious vomiting, abdominal distention, and failure to thrive. Depending on the type of mucosa lining, ulceration with bleeding and gastrointestinal (GI) hemorrhage or fistula formation with perforation can be observed. An abdominal mass may be appreciated with the enlargement of the duplication. Diagnosis is confirmed radiologically with ultrasonography, computed tomography (CT), or magnetic resonance imaging (MRI). This finding is typically not visualized with UGI study as contrast material fails to enter the cyst lumen. More recent techniques of endoscopic ultrasound have also been used in older children and adults. Management is excision of the cystic structure as there are reports of neoplastic transformation arising from the duplication cysts.

Gastric volvulus

Gastric volvulus is an abnormal rotation of one part of the stomach around another, with obstruction of the lumen and compression of vessels that can result in tissue ischemia and necrosis. Defective fixation of the stomach can lead to three different types of abnormal rotation: organoaxial, mesenteroaxial, or a combination of the two. Most of the congenital gastric volvuli are seen in infants with diaphragmatic defects (congenital diaphragmatic hernia) and absence or excessive laxity of gastric ligaments. Clinically, 70% of infants present with a classic Borchardt triad: pain, retching (with little vomiting), and inability to pass a nasogastric tube. Radiographic studies with plain radiographs and UGI barium series will outline an abnormal contour and position of the stomach as well as abnormal position of pylorus in relation to gastroesophageal junction. Timely recognition is essential to facilitate urgent surgical intervention with reduction of the volvulus and gastric fixation.

Gastric diverticulum

Gastric diverticulum is a rare finding in a pediatric age group. Congenital gastric diverticulum is an outpouching comprising all layers of the gastric wall usually seen in the antrum, pylorus, or posterior wall. Gastric diverticulum has been described in children with hiatal hernia, and pyloric or duodenal obstruction. Occasional presence of pancreatic tissue in the gastric diverticulum supports an embryologic origin of this malformation. In the pediatric population, most of the gastric diverticula are asymptomatic and are identified as an incidental finding. Clinical symptoms of abdominal pain, emesis, and gastroesophageal reflux are usually seen in adults. Bleeding and perforation is a rare manifestation of gastric diverticulum. If symptomatic, surgical resection or invagination with fixation can be therapeutic.

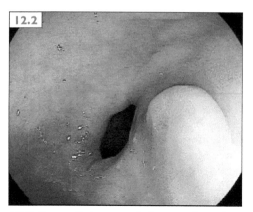

12.2 Pancreatic heterotopia (pancreatic rest).

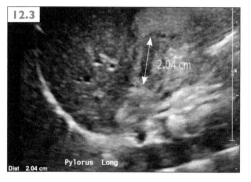

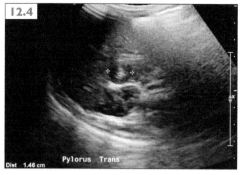

12.3, 12.4 Abdominal ultrasound of hypertrophic pyloric stenosis. Width of pyloric muscle >4 mm (12.4); elongated length of the pyloric channel >16 mm (12.3).

Pancreatic heterotopia

Pancreatic heterotopia is an uncommon and usually benign finding identified during endoscopy often referred to as a 'pancreatic rest'. This extrapancreatic tissue can be found throughout the GI tract and is frequently described as a raised protrusion in the antrum or pylorus that is covered with a gastric mucosa, with a classic central umbilication that corresponds to a draining duct (12.2). Because of its benign nature, no intervention is required. Biopsy might be warranted as they do differentiate from neoplastic lesions or confirm histology. Endoscopic or surgical resection can be done in rare symptomatic cases.

Hypertrophic pyloric stenosis

Hypertrophic pyloric stenosis is defined as a hypertrophied pyloric muscle that results in a narrow pyloric channel with a well recognized clinical presentation of projectile nonbilious vomiting in an infant. Persistence of vomiting can lead to dehydration and metabolic alkalosis. This disorder is not congenital and often presents in the first few weeks of life. Incidence is 6–8/1000 live births with higher incidence among males, in particular first-born males. Diagnosis is confirmed with radiologic studies (UGI barium series or ultrasound) outlining thickened pyloric muscle (>4 mm) with a narrow and elongated channel (>16 mm) (12.3, 12.4). Treatment consists of a surgical pyloromyotomy.

Congenital and acquired anomalies of the duodenum

Duodenal atresia

Duodenal atresia is an intrinsic obstruction in the duodenum most commonly in the second portion of the duodenum at the level of the ampulla of Vater. This abnormal development of the intestine typically occurs *in utero* after the seventh week of gestation. The incidence is 1:2,500–1:40,000 live births. Pathophysiology is presumed to be secondary to failure of vacuolization or inadequate endodermal proliferation. Vascular compromise with ischemia has also been entertained as a possible mechanism of injury. Duodenal atresia can be classified into three anatomic types (**12.5**):

- Type 1: (most common) complete occlusion by a mucosal membrane preserving an intact muscularis layer and serosa with normal continuity.
- Type 2: discontinuous segments connected by a fibrous cord.
- Type 3: complete separation of segments.

Infants present with bilious vomiting shortly after birth. In contrast to a duodenal stenosis, where type 1 duodenal atresia has a communicating lumen, onset of symptoms can be delayed. A duodenal web (diaphragm) (**12.6**) is a mild form of duodenal atresia, often with an opening allowing some luminal contents and air to advance to the distal bowel. On examination, a scaphoid abdomen

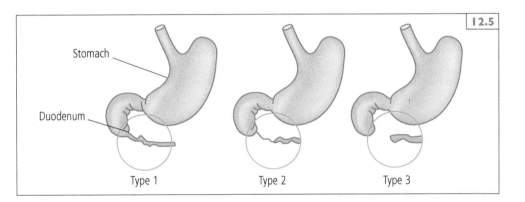

Stomach

Duodenum

Type 1   Type 2   Type 3

12.5

12.5 Diagram of duodenal atresia.

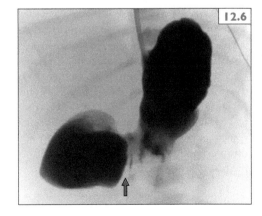

12.6

12.6 Duodenal web (arrow). (Courtesy of Kaveh Vali, MD; Department of Surgery, Women & Children's Hospital of Buffalo.)

is often appreciated in infants with duodenal atresia. Index of suspicion can be raised during a prenatal ultrasound identifying polyhydramnios and a fluid-filled 'double bubble' sign which is pathognomonic for duodenal atresia (**12.7**). Duodenal atresia is strongly associated with Down syndrome (Trisomy 21) as well as GI, cardiac, genitourinary, and vertebral anomalies.

Treatment consists of initial fluid resuscitation followed by surgical repair consisting of resection of the atresia (**12.8**) with side-to-side or end-to-side duodenuodeonostomy or duodenojejunostomy. Resection of the obstructing membrane or duodenal web is controversial, as it can damage pancreatic or biliary ducts. Successful endoscopic techniques of duodenal web resection have been recognized and published.

Duodenal duplication

Duodenal duplication is embryologically similar to the gastric duplication described above and tends to occur on the mesenteric border of the first or second part of the duodenum. Although most of the duplications do not communicate with the intestinal lumen, rare forms of communicating duplications can be observed during endoscopy (**12.9**). Gastric epithelial differentiation is most frequently found within the lumen of the duplication cysts. Symptoms of duodenal or biliary obstruction consist of vomiting and abdominal pain. Elevation of the transaminases along with amylase and lipase can be observed, with enlargement of the duplication cyst obstructing biliary and pancreatic drainage. Ulcer formation along with hemorrhage within the cyst and pancreatitis may also occur. Imaging with ultrasound, CT, or MRI is used to characterize the lesion further. Surgical resection is warranted, although surgery is often complicated by its close proximity to the biliary and pancreatic tree.

Intestinal malrotation

Intestinal malrotation is a congenital defect that occurs at approximately 10 weeks of embryonic life. Estimated incidence of anomalous intestinal rotation is approximately 1 in 500 live births. The overall incidence of malrotation is not known because some patients do not present until later in life or remain asymptomatic. Malrotation is more prevalent in trisomy 9, 13, 18, and 21 and is frequently associated with heterotaxia. Malformation results from failure of the intestine to undergo a normal 270 degree rotation during reduction of the midgut loop back into the abdomen following the temporary, physiologic herniation into the umbilical stalk.

The development of the intestinal tract is often described as the process of bowel rotation and fixation occurring in three stages:

- Stage 1 – period of umbilical cord herniation (week 5 to week 10).
- Stage 2 – period of reduction of the midgut loop back into the abdomen (weeks 10–11).
- Stage 3 – period of fixation and lasts from the end of stage 2 until shortly after birth.

The arrest of intestinal rotation may be complete (nonrotation), or can take place at any stage following the initial counterclockwise 180 degree movement. Nonrotation is an example of early failure of rotation and is considered a misnomer as the initial 90 degree rotation is completed. However, without further rotation, the small bowel is located on the right side while the colon occupies the left side of the abdomen (**12.10**). In addition, there are rare variants of nonrotation affecting only the duodenum and small bowel. Incomplete rotation (malrotation) is more common and may present during the neonatal period. Midgut

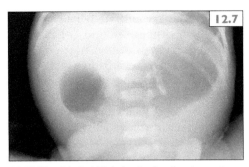

12.7 'Double bubble' sign in duodenal atresia.

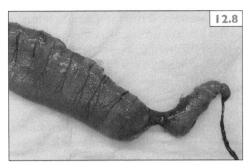

12.8 Surgical resection of the intestinal atresia.

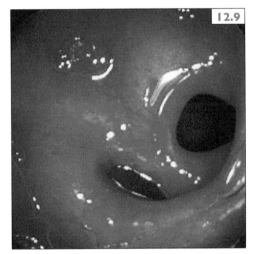

12.9 Endoscopic view of the communicating duplication cyst. (Courtesy of John Pohl, MD; Department of Pediatric Gastroenterology, Primary Children's Hospital, University of Utah.)

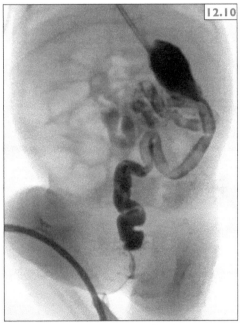

12.10 Barium enema intestinal malrotation with colon (microcolon) on the left side of the abdomen.

volvulus is a frequent complication of malrotation occurring *in utero* or postnatally. Abnormally rotated bowel does not develop a normal mesenteric attachment, rendering the intestine excessively mobile and at a high risk for volvulus leading to bowel ischemia. Peritoneal bands (Ladd's bands) form due to disordered fixation of the malpositioned bowel associated with incomplete cecal descent. Ladd's bands are often found anterior to the duodenum causing extrinsic compression and bowel obstruction.

Infants can present with bilious vomiting, abdominal distention, and colicky pain. Radiologic studies demonstrate an abnormal gas pattern, and a barium study (UGI or barium enema) outlining the abnormal anatomy and an obstruction can be diagnostic. Surgical evaluation to assess bowel anatomy and tissue viability is performed in the operative setting along with a Ladd's procedure to secure bowel in the proper orientation. Depending on the degree and extent of tissue injury, necrotic bowel may need to be resected.

CHAPTER 13

Eosinophilic Gastroenteritis

James P. Franciosi

DEFINITION

Eosinophilic gastroenteritis (EGE) is an inflammatory condition of the stomach and small intestine, in which eosinophils are the predominant cell type, that may affect all layers of the gastrointestinal (GI) tract wall. Unlike eosinophilic esophagitis (EoE), histopathologic criteria have been proposed for EGE but are not currently widely accepted.

CLINICAL PRESENTATION

Although abdominal pain is the most common GI symptom, clinical presentations vary widely and may include bloating, dyspepsia, nausea, vomiting, GI bleeding, iron deficiency anemia, protein-losing enteropathy (with hypoalbuminemia), ascites, abdominal distention, bowel obstruction or perforation, growth failure, and diarrhea. It is important to consider eosinophilic gastritis (with or without mucosal involvement) in the differential diagnosis of hypertrophic pyloric stenosis. A typical presentation may include progressive vomiting, dehydration, electrolyte abnormalities, a thickening of the gastric outlet, atopic symptoms, and an elevated peripheral eosinophil count. At endoscopy, EGE findings may include prominent antral lymphonodularity (often in a radial pattern) (**13.1–13.3**), ulceration, a mass-like appearance, patchy erythema (**13.4, 13.5**), or may be normal.

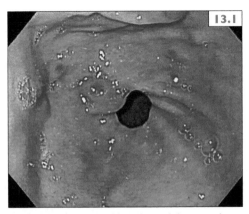

13.1 Scattered antral lymphonodularity and erythema.

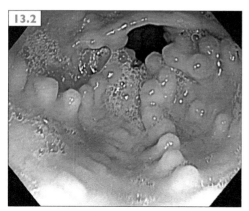

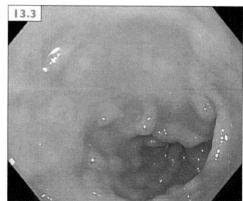

13.2, 13.3 Prominent antral lymphonodularity in a radial pattern.

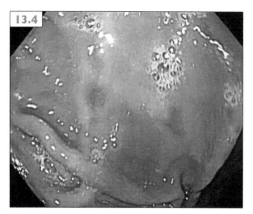

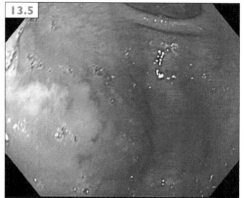

13.4, 13.5 Patchy foci of erythema.

DIAGNOSIS

Physical examination should be directed towards identifying stigmata of atopic disease, infectious etiologies, celiac disease, inflammatory bowel disease, and connective tissue diseases/vasculitis.

In contrast to EoE, peripheral eosinophilia or an elevated immunoglobulin (Ig) E level frequently occur with EGE. Esophagogastroduodenoscopy with biopsies remains the principal diagnostic and disease assessment tool. For isolated eosinophilic gastritis, testing for *Helicobacter pylori* should be performed on all patients. Viral and genetic testing should be considered based on the clinical context. For food antigen driven disease, a combination of skin prick testing and atopy patch testing can be utilized to identify respective IgE-based and non-IgE-based causative food allergens. For EoE, another successful approach is to remove empirically the six most common food groups (milk, soy, wheat, eggs, nuts, and fish/shellfish) without associated allergy testing. Clinical experience suggests that either allergy test directed or empiric food antigen elimination is less effective for EGE as compared to EoE. For patients that also have small intestinal involvement, an additional work-up is warranted.

A colonoscopy with biopsies and terminal ileal intubation should be considered in all patients with significant EGE. Additional investigations for celiac disease, inflammatory bowel disease, and parasitic infections are indicated. Depending on the clinical presentation (e.g. hypoalbuminemia, ascites, failure to thrive, and diarrhea), more aggressive radiographic and surgical small bowel testing may be needed to determine whether the eosinophilic disease may involve areas beyond the mucosal layer, notably, the muscularis and serosal layers.

PATHOPHYSIOLOGY

EGE is less well understood than EoE. Many patients are recognized to have both an IgE and non-IgE-mediated inflammatory response with similar cytokines, such as interleukin-5, playing an important role. It is also recognized that specific genetic mutations may give rise to these unique eosinophilic conditions of the GI tract. In addition, the pathophysiology depends on the varying causes of eosinophilic GI disease shown in *Table 13.1*.

TREATMENT

With regard to effective therapies, there is a paucity of clinical experience and no randomized clinical trials to date to guide clinicians as to which therapies are most effective. Effective management also depends on identifying the correct etiology.

For patients with food antigen driven disease, strict dietary elimination by either food allergy test directed or empiric elimination remain the mainstay of therapy. The management is the same as described for EoE. EGE is distinct from EoE in that elemental diets are not uniformly successful for all patients.

As is true for nearly all GI inflammatory conditions, corticosteroids can be very effective in inducing and maintaining remission. However, the known risks of systemic

Table 13.1 Differential diagnosis of eosinophilic gastrointestinal disease

i. Food-mediated allergy

ii. Infectious:

Ancylostoma caninium (Hook worm)

Anisakis

Ascaris

Epstein–Barr virus

Eustoma rotundatum

Giardia lambila

Helicobacter pylori

Schistosomiasis trichus

Stercoalis

Strongyloides

Toxocara canis

Trichinella spiralis

iii. Noninfectious

  A. Disease states:

    Celiac disease

    Connective tissue diseases/vasculitis

    Systemic lupus erythematosus

    Scleroderma

    Churg–Strauss syndrome

    Polyarteritis nodosa

    Hypereosinophilic syndrome

    Inflammatory bowel disease (especially in younger children)

    Inflammatory fibroid polyp

    Malignancy

    Adrenal insufficiency

    Autoimmune disease

    Immune deficiency

  B. Medications*:

    Antibiotics

    Azathioprine

    Carbamazepine

    Enalapril

    Tacrolimus

*Many other medications have been described

steroids do not make them a desirable long-term option. Beclamethasone-containing capsules and budesonide have been used successfully as topical steroid formulations with less systemic toxicity. Success with immunomodulator therapy for maintenance of remission, used much in the same way as for inflammatory bowel disease remission, has been reported.

Cromolyn sodium and montelukast have been reported in the literature to be effective therapies, but the data are very limited. Th2 cytokine inhibitor (suplatast tosilate) and an antihistamine (ketotifen) have also been reported as treatments for EGE. Future therapies may include biologic medications such as human interleukin-5 antibodies.

At present, serial endoscopy with biopsy is the only modality for monitoring disease progression and response to therapy.

PROGNOSIS

The long-term outcomes for EGE remain poorly characterized and are dependent on the underlying etiology. The recognition that EoE is a chronic condition that requires long-term therapy is likely also true for EGE. In the appropriate clinical context, when food-mediated allergy has been excluded, it is especially important to consider inflammatory bowel disease, immune deficiencies, and hypereosinophilic syndrome.

CHAPTER 14

Gastric Infections

Mirza B. Beg, Archana Ramaswami

- • **Introduction**
- • *Helicobacter pylori* **gastritis**
- • **Bacterial gastritis**
- • **Viral gastritis**
- • **Fungal gastritis**
- • **Parasitic gastritis**
- • **Granulomatous gastritis**
- • **Conclusion**

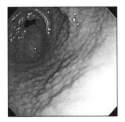
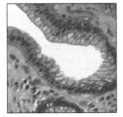
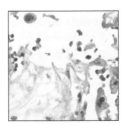
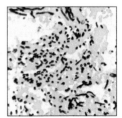

Introduction

The stomach is a muscular, hollow, dilated part of the digestion system which lies between the esophagus and duodenum. Although the acidic environment provides some protection against infections, a number of pathogenic micro-organisms can affect the stomach. These infections can extend to the esophagus proximally and duodenum and small intestine distally. Gastric infections can cause two common conditions – gastritis and gastroenteritis.

Gastritis describes gross and microscopic inflammation of the stomach mucosa due to a number of possible causes, with *Helicobacter pylori* infection being among the leading organism. Other pathogens include viruses, fungi, and parasites. This chapter will focus on infectious gastritis and its clinical implications.

Helicobacter pylori gastritis

DEFINITION AND PATHOPHYSIOLOGY
In 1983, Drs. Barry Marshall and Robin Warren successfully cultured the spiral organisms from human gastric antrum. Initially called *Campylobacter pyloridis*, it is now known as *H. pylori*.

H. pylori is a gram-negative bacterium. It produces urease, has a spiral like conformation, is microaerophilic and is motile because of the flagella. Flagella and urease are very important for colonization of the gastric mucosa. Urease neutralizes gastric acidity, converting the gastric urea to ammonium ions, and flagella help the bacterium pass from the acidic gastric lumen into the gastric mucus layer. Two of the most important genes of *H. pylori* are *VACA* and *CAGA*. The *VACA* gene encodes the Vac-A cytotoxin, a vacuolating toxin, and the *CAGA* gene codes for Cag-A protein, which seems to stimulate the production of neutrophil chemotactic factors by the gastric epithelium of the host.

H. pylori is the major cause of gastritis worldwide. Infection occurs more frequently in developing countries than in industrialized countries. An estimated 50% of the world population is infected with this ubiquitous organism but an exact prevalence is not known, mostly because accurate data are not available from developing countries. Caucasians are infected with *H. pylori* less frequently than persons of other racial groups. The percentage rate of infection is approximately 20% in Caucasians, 54% in African Americans, and 60% in Hispanic persons.

The most common route of infection is either oral-to-oral or fecal-to-oral. Parents and siblings seem to play a primary role in transmission. *H. pylori* infection may be acquired at any age. According to some epidemiologic studies, this infection is acquired most frequently during childhood. Children and females have a higher incidence of reinfection compared to adult males.

The natural history and histologic findings of *H. pylori* gastritis in children differ from the adult population. Spontaneous clearing and reacquisition of the gastric infection in preschoolers has been reported in the literature.

Acute gastritis associated with this organism is mild, transient and mostly asymptomatic and is rarely encountered clinically. Histologically it is characterized by degenerative changes of the epithelium, including infiltration by polymorphonuclear leukocytes.

Most commonly *H. pylori* infection causes chronic active gastritis which is characterized by a striking infiltrate of the gastric epithelium and the underlying lamina propria by neutrophils, T and B lymphocytes, macrophages, and mast cells. *H. pylori* may be detected in approximately 90% of individuals with peptic ulcer disease; however, less than 15% of infected individuals develop chronic active gastritis.

CLINICAL PRESENTATION

Clinical features of *H. pylori* infection may differ depending on geography and race. No specific clinical signs or symptoms have been attributed specifically to patients with *H. pylori* infection. Some patients may have dyspepsia, abdominal discomfort, or epigastric pain while others may only have halitosis. Chronic *H. pylori* infection can cause gastric and duodenal ulcers leading to hematemesis and anemia. Upper endoscopy may show nodularity of gastric mucosa (**14.1**).

The risk of gastric cancers, including non-Hodgkin lymphoma (e.g. mucosa-associated lymphoid tissue [MALT]) and adenocarcinoma is high in adults but it is nearly absent in children.

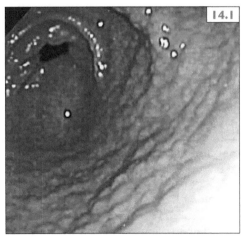

14.1 Endoscopic view of lymphoid nodular hyperplasia of the gastric antrum in a child with *Helicobacter pylori*.

DIAGNOSIS

Diagnostic work-up can be divided in to two broad categories:
- Noninvasive methods include *H. pylori* fecal antigen test, carbon-13 urea breath test, and *H. pylori* serology.
- Invasive tests include endoscopy for histologic assessment of antral biopsy, rapid urease tests, and culture of endoscopic biopsies.

Urea breath test

This diagnostic modality was shown to have the best sensitivity (100%) in testing older children. Isotopic urea (^{13}C) ingestion relies on abundant *H. pylori*-derived urease activity in the stomach as it releases carbon-13 (^{13}C) which is qualitatively detected in the expired air indicative of active infection. It is useful for initial diagnoses and follow-up of eradication therapy.

Serology test

Serology is a relatively inexpensive test with a limited application because of its poor specificity and sensitivity.

Stool antigen test

In accuracy, this test is almost equal to the urea breath test and is gaining widespread acceptance as a modality for initial diagnosis in all age groups.

Rapid urease test

This is a simple and convenient method done at the time of the upper endoscopy where antral and fundus biopsy tissue are embedded in a gel medium of urea and incubated for 24 hours. Testing relies on generating ammonia by enzymatic degradation of urea.

A color change due to alkaline pH is indicative of urease activity consistent with an active *H. pylori* infection. False negative results can occur in patients with a recent gastrointestinal bleed, antibiotic use, or proton pump inhibitor (PPI) therapy. False-positive results can be seen with *Helicobacter heilmannii* (formerly *Gastrospirillum hominis*) with a similar clinical presentation as *H. pylori*, but histologically larger organism linked to zoonotic transmission (**14.2–14.4**).

Histology

Biopsy specimens from endoscopy stained with Giemsa stain usually demonstrate a variable number of *H. pylori* organisms adhering to the gastric epithelium, both coating the gastric wall and lining the gastric glands. A large inflammatory infiltrate with lymphocytes, neutrophils, and a variable number of mast cells is present. Other stains, such as Genta, Warthin–Starry silver, immunohistochemical stain, and the classic hematoxylin and eosin (H&E) stain, can be used to identify the presence of an organism on gastric mucosa biopsies (**14.5–14.7**).

Culture

Bacterial culture from gastric tissue is difficult and is not used for routine diagnosis. It is recommended after failure of second-line therapy to check drug sensitivity.

TREATMENT

The goals of pharmacotherapy are complete eradication of the micro-organism, prevention of complications, and morbidity reduction. The US Food and Drug Administration has approved several antibiotics regimens, which are now accepted internationally. These regimens are known as 'triple therapies', are used worldwide and have reported cure

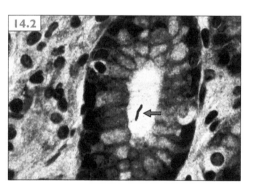

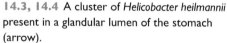

14.2 Gastrospirilium in the gastric crypt (arrow). (Courtesy of Dr. Rafal Kozielski, MD; Department of Pathology and Anatomic Sciences, Women & Children's Hospital of Buffalo.)

14.3, 14.4 A cluster of *Helicobacter heilmannii* present in a glandular lumen of the stomach (arrow).

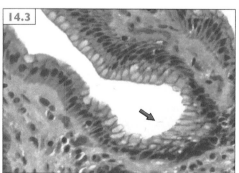

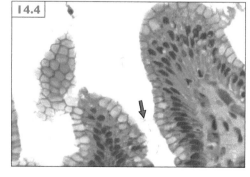

rates of 85–90%. A typical triple therapy is composed of high-dose PPI with two antibiotics for a duration of 2 weeks, followed by an extended period of acid suppression. The antibiotic choice may involve amoxicillin, clarithromycin, metronidazole, tetracycline, and levofloxacin. A number of factors, such as duration of treatment, choice of antibiotics, new drug combinations, and improved patient compliance, may help to improve the eradication rates.

Empiric treatment of *H. pylori* is not indicated for functional abdominal pain, asymptomatic children, nonulcer dyspepsia, children residing in chronic care facilities, and children at increased risk for acquisition of infection. Routine screening of asymptomatic children with a family history of gastric cancer or recurrent peptic ulcer disease is also not recommended.

Bacterial gastritis

Other bacterial pathogens causing gastritis include *Streptococcus*, *Staphylococcus*, *Lactobacillus*, *Bacteroides*, *Klebsiella* spp., and *Escherichia coli*. These organisms reside within the oral cavity and are thought to be swallowed and rarely have any clinical significance except under special circumstances, such as ischemia or immunosuppression, where they may produce increased morbidity. Gastric colonization with these bacteria can cause an intense acute inflammatory response with mucosal ulceration and abscess formation. These patients often present with nausea, vomiting, and upper abdominal pain and usually have neutrophilic leukocytosis in blood. The acute form of bacterial gastritis is exceedingly rare and has a high mortality.

14.5 *H. pylori* organisms can be seen adherent to the mucosal surface and crypt (arrows).

14.6 Chronic active gastritis of the antrum.

14.7 Warthin–Starry stain for *H. pylori* organisms. Black rod-shaped structures can be seen lining the gastric pits (arrows).

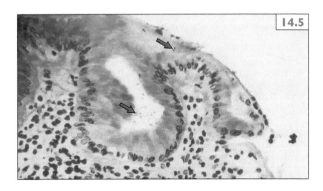

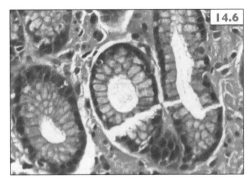

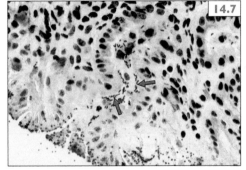

Viral gastritis

DEFINITION

Viruses commonly involved are cytomegalovirus (CMV) and herpes simplex virus (HSV).

CMV gastritis

The esophagus and the colon are the most frequent sites of CMV infection in the gastrointestinal (GI) tract; however, gastric as well as biliary, hepatic, and pancreatic CMV infections have been reported. Most patients present with nausea, vomiting, diarrhea, and occasionally significant epigastric pain. Gastric CMV infections are usually seen in the fundus with contiguous involvement of the esophagus and gastroesophageal junction. The distal stomach and antrum are less commonly involved, although there have been a few reported cases of CMV infection presenting as an antral mass. The mechanism of injury in CMV infection is believed to be due to infection of the endothelial cells, causing a small-vessel vasculitis that can lead to focal ischemia and necrosis (**14.8–14.10**).

While significant gastric ulcerations may occur, life-threatening complications, such as perforation caused by CMV, are more often seen in the thinner-walled small and large intestines.

CMV- induced Ménétrier disease can present with a variety of clinical features including epigastric pain, substantial weight loss, nausea, vomiting, and diarrhea in an otherwise immunocompetent patient. Occult GI bleeding may occur, but overt bleeding is unusual. Affected patients develop

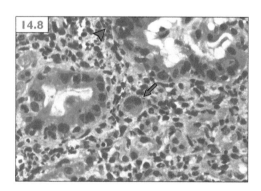

14.8 Cytomegalovirus gastritis in an immunocompromised patient postrenal transplant showing inflammatory cells in the lamina propria (arrowhead) and a cytomegalovirus-infected cell (arrow). The infected cell is enlarged, and contains both nuclear and cytoplasmic inclusions.

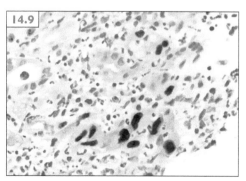

14.9 Positive immunostaining for cytomegalovirus antigens.

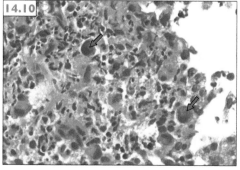

14.10 Large epithelial cells and eosinophilic intranuclear inclusion bodies (arrows) of a cytomegalovirus-infected gastric mucosa.

protein-losing gastropathy accompanied by hypoalbuminemia and edema. Diagnosis of this disease is established by the morphologic appearance of enlarged gastric folds seen on endoscopy or barium radiography. These gastric folds are usually enlarged symmetrically and confined to the body and fundus. A gastric biopsy is usually required for diagnosis, which shows foveolar hyperplasia and glandular atrophy, with replacement of chief and parietal cells with mucous glands.

Multiple medical treatments including antacids, anticholinergic drugs, prednisone, H2- blockers, and PPIs have been used for patients with this disease but none has proven to be consistently beneficial. A high-protein diet should be recommended to replace protein loss in patients with hypoalbuminemia. Surgery is indicated for patients with intractable pain, hypo-albuminemia with edema, hemorrhage, pyloric obstruction, and for those in whom malignancy cannot be excluded. In children it generally has a self-limited course.

HSV gastritis

GI involvement with HSV has been reported to occur in the esophagus and liver; however isolated gastric involvement is very rarely seen. Clinical features are indistinguishable from other etiologies of chronic gastric infection. Endoscopic evaluation may reveal discrete small raised plaque lesions with ulcerated tips. The best method of diagnosis is endoscopic appearance and examination of brush cytology specimen from gastric mucosa, which shows numerous single cells and clumps of cells revealing both 'ground glass' nuclei and well-formed eosinophilic intranuclear inclusion bodies surrounded by halos. These findings are characteristic of HSV infection (**14.11, 14.12**).

Other viruses that cause gastritis include rotaviruses, adenoviruses, caliciviruses, astroviruses, Norwalk virus, and noroviruses. Viral gastritis is usually a benign, self-limited illness unless it leads to severe dehydration from vomiting and diarrhea. Viral gastritis is highly contagious and is usually spread through contact with contaminated food, beverage, and close contact with infectious persons. Preventing severe dehydration caused by rapid loss of fluids from vomiting and diarrhea is the single most important aspect in managing viral gastritis.

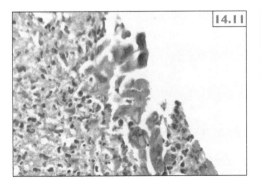 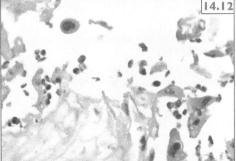

14.11, 14.12 Gastric biopsy with herpes gastritis.

Fungal gastritis

DEFINITION AND PATHOPHYSIOLOGY

Candida species (candidiasis), *Histoplasmosis capsulatum* (histoplasmosis), *Mucorales* species (mucormycosis), and *Paracoccidioides brasiliensis* (South American blastomycosis) are reported in the literature as pathogens causing gastric infections. Most fungal cases of gastritis tend to occur in patients who are immunocompromised as is seen in human immunodeficiency virus (HIV) infection, transplant patients, and uncontrolled diabetes mellitus. Signs and symptoms may include abdominal pain, frequently described as a dull, gnawing pain, bloating-sensation of fullness, belching, nausea and vomiting.

DIAGNOSIS

Upper GI endoscopy with biopsies is the gold standard for the diagnosis. Endoscopy may reveal focal invasion of a benign gastric ulcer or whitish plaques scattered on the mucosa in diffuse mucosal involvement form (rare). Histologically in colonization of pre-existing ulcers, hyphae of *Candida* species can be seen at the base of these gastric ulcers (**14.13–14.15**). Histoplasmosis may appear as mass lesions, ulceration, or thickened folds. Microscopically these organisms can be identified with silver staining (Gomori methenamine silver nitrate [GMS] stain). Diagnosis is confirmed by a positive culture, presence of typical organisms in granulomas on biopsy, or by high-complement fixation titers.

TREATMENT

Treatment options include antifungal medications and probiotic therapy.

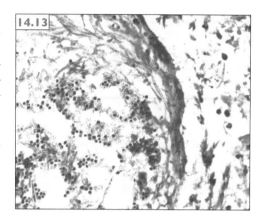

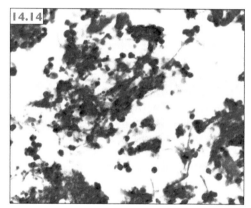

14.13, 14.14 Granulation tissue and numerous yeast consistent with *Candida albicans*.

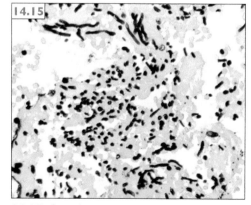

14.15 Granulation tissue, numerous yeast and pseudohyphal fungal forms on Gomori methenamine silver nitrate stain consistent with *Candida albicans*.

Parasitic gastritis

The stomach is not a preferred site for human parasite infection. *Strongyloides stercoralis*, schistosomiasis (*Schistosoma mansoni*, *S. japonicum*, *S. mekongi*, and *S. intercalatum*), and *Diphyllobothrium latum* may rarely infect the stomach. *Cryptosporidium* species can be observed in the lining of the gastric mucosa predominantly in immunocompromised individuals.

Anisakis spp. larvae transmitted by ingestion of contaminated raw fish may lead to gastric wall perforation. Eosinophilic infiltration with granulomatous resection surrounding the parasitic organisms can be seen in surgical resections.

Symptoms of parasitic gastritis include abdominal pain, bloating, indigestion, nausea, and vomiting, mimicking peptic ulcer symptoms. The most effective treatment involves administration of antiparasitic drugs.

Granulomatous gastritis

Granulomatous gastritis (GG) is a rare disease characterized by the presence of granulomas within the gastric mucosa or submucosa. Common causes of GG are Crohn disease, disseminated sarcoidosis, infections (tuberculosis, syphilis, fungal, parasitic), foreign bodies, underlying malignancy, chronic granulomatous disease, or vasculitis. *H. pylori* has been associated with GG in some case reports that resolve after treatment. Diagnosis is based on clinical information and histology. Treatment of GG should be carefully individualized with close follow-up.

Conclusion

Gastric infections are common causes of upper gastrointestinal symptoms and are often difficult to recognize clinically. Infectious gastritis is divided into acute and chronic forms. Symptoms are usually nonspecific. Endoscopy with biopsy and histologic examination can often identify a specific pathogen. *H. pylori* infection is the most common cause of chronic gastritis. Other forms of infectious gastritis include GG, chronic gastritis associated with parasitic infections and viral infections, such as CMV and HSV infection. Opportunistic gastric infections may be caused by numerous fungi, parasites, and viruses. Pharmacologic intervention has to be tailored to a specific organism causing gastritis.

ACKNOWLEDGMENTS
Many thanks and appreciations go to my colleagues Sanjay Mukhopadhyay, MD, Steve Landas, MD, and Manoochehr Karjoo, MD for providing pictures and pathology slides used in this chapter.

Gastroparesis

Ajay Kaul, Jose M. Garza

DEFINITION AND PHYSIOLOGY

Gastroparesis is a motility disorder of the stomach that is characterized by slowed emptying of gastric contents, in the absence of mechanical obstruction (**15.1**).

The stomach is a hollow muscular organ divided into the fundus, body, and antrum. Each functional segment plays a differing but complementary role in gastric emptying. The fundus serves as a reservoir for food due to its properties of accommodation and receptive and adaptive relaxation. It also demonstrates slow, phasic contractions which contrasts those of the antrum, responsible for mixing and trituration or grinding. As a result, the fundus facilitates gastric emptying of liquids while the antrum plays a greater role in gastric emptying of solids.

In addition to the intrinsic enteric nervous system (myenteric and submucosal plexuses), the stomach also receives innervation from the vagus nerve (parasympathetic) and the celiac ganglia (sympathetic). The vagus regulates fundic accommodation, antral contractions, and pyloric relaxation while the sympathetic input counters or inhibits these motor activities. The repertoire of neurotransmitters and signaling molecules in

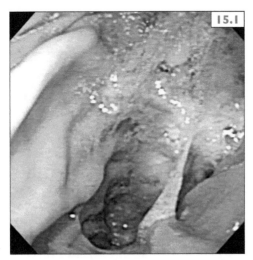

15.1 Endoscopic picture showing retained food in a patient with gastroparesis.

the stomach, both excitatory and inhibitory, are very similar to that found in the brain. The interstitial cells of Cajal (ICC), also known as 'pacemaker cells', constitute a unique group of cells (several subtypes) that are embedded within the wall of the stomach in close proximity to the enteric nerves. The ICC generate electrical slow waves that are eventually coupled to a smooth muscle contraction. Peristaltic contractions (3 cycles per minute) are initiated in the 'pacemaker region' in the proximal gastric body on the greater curvature and propagate distally to the antrum.

Nutrient delivery from the antrum to the duodenum is regulated closely at a rate of 1–4 kcal per minute. This is primarily the result of inhibitory feedback from the interaction of nutrients with the luminal receptors in the small intestine. This interaction is mediated by both neural and hormonal mechanisms. Several gut hormones secreted in response to ingested nutrients have the capacity to influence gut motor and sensory function. These include cholecystokinin (CCK), peptide YY, glucagon-like peptide-1 (GLP-1), and ghrelin.

CLINICAL PRESENTATION

Gastroparesis has phenotypic variability with age, gender, type of symptom onset, and severity of symptoms. The predominant symptoms include nausea, vomiting, bloating, early satiety, abdominal pain, and gastroesophageal reflux. Symptoms are typically worse after eating. It should be noted that both rapid ('dumping syndrome') and delayed gastric emptying (gastroparesis) can cause similar symptoms. About 50% of patients present acutely, mostly after an infectious prodrome. Younger children with gastroparesis tend to present more with vomiting, a feeding disorder, and poor weight gain. There does not appear to be a significant gender predilection in younger children but in adolescence and adults there is a clear female predominance. There is a higher prevalence of psychologic dysfunction, such as anxiety and depression in older children and adults, which is associated with symptom severity but not etiology or degree of gastric retention. Other comorbidities include migraine headaches, constipation, fibromyalgia, and chronic fatigue syndrome.

There is an overlap between gastroparesis and functional dyspepsia. There are some patients that have a clinical presentation and course that is indistinguishable from those with gastroparesis but have normal gastric emptying.

In milder cases of gastroparesis there may not be any evident findings on clinical examination. Those with more severe involvement may have epigastric or diffuse tenderness on palpation and succession splash on auscultation over the abdomen. There may also be dehydration and weight loss.

ETIOLOGY AND PATHOPHYSIOLOGY

The Gastroparesis Clinical Research Consortium (GpCRC) published their data in 2011 on the clinical features of more than 400 adult patients with gastroparesis enrolled in their registry (established in 2006). Of all patients with delayed gastric emptying, 61% had idiopathic gastroparesis and 32% had diabetic gastroparesis. The remainder included those that had undergone gastric surgery or had underlying Parkinson disease, collagen vascular disease, and intestinal pseudo-obstruction.

Postinfectious or postviral gastroparesis is regarded as a subgroup of idiopathic gastroparesis and a host of viral agents have been implicated including rotavirus, Norwalk virus, and Epstein–Barr virus. It is postulated that the infecting agent either directly affects the enteric nerves and ganglia causing a neuropathy or induces an immunologic and inflammatory response in the gastric wall.

Pathogenesis of diabetic gastroparesis is multifactorial and is the result of a neuro-myopathy. Increased oxidative stress, from low heme-oxygenase-1 levels and decreased insulin and insulin-like growth factor-1 signaling, lead to loss of interstitial cells of

Cajal. This in turn causes abnormal electrical slow waves, disordered peristalsis, and atrophy of smooth muscle.

Postsurgical gastroparesis is usually the result of vagus nerve trauma following upper gastrointestinal surgery (fundoplication, bariatric surgery) as well as after chest surgery (cardiac surgery, lung transplantation). Medications, such as tricyclic antidepressants and others with anticholinergic effects, can also cause gastroparesis. Slow gastric emptying can also be seen in children with mitochondrial disorders and hypothyroidism.

DIAGNOSIS

Blood tests should be tailored towards findings on history and physical examination and to rule out other potential comorbid conditions.

There are currently three modalities used for assessing gastric emptying: gastric emptying scintigraphy (GES), wireless motility capsule (WMC), and breath test. Scintigraphy is the most widely used test to diagnose gastroparesis. The American Neurogastroenterology and Motility Society and the Society of Nuclear Medicine have published their collective consensus standards for the performance of GES for adults. No such standardization exists for pediatrics yet. The recommended protocol is to consume two large egg whites with two slices of bread and jam with water after an overnight fast and discontinuation of medications that affect gastric motility for 48–72 hours prior to the test. Blood glucose in diabetic patients should be < 280 mg/dl (2.8 g/l) before starting the test. The meal is labeled with technetium-99m sulfur colloid and imaging is performed at 0, 1, 2, and 4 hours after meal ingestion. If there is >90% gastric retention of the meal at 1 hour, >60% retention at 2 hours and >10% retention at 4 hours the test is considered diagnostic for delayed gastric emptying. If gastric emptying is normal at 2 hours it is recommended that imaging be extended to 4 hours. In symptomatic patients, extending the study to 4 hours detects more abnormal

gastric emptying (**15.2**). A delayed gastric emptying test confirms gastric dysmotility but does not prove causality. Gastric emptying for solids is more representative of gastroparesis than liquid emptying. The latter is often used in postsurgical conditions as there can be discrepancy in liquid and solid gastric emptying after gastric surgery or vagal injury. Criteria for rapid emptying are

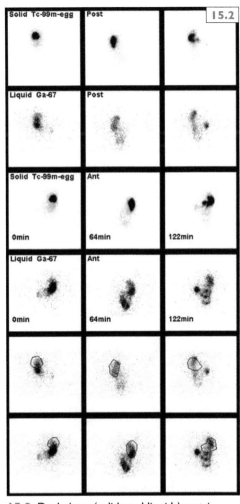

15.2 Dual phase (solids and liquids) gastric emptying scan showing severely delayed gastric emptying for both (2% emptying for solids at 2 hours and 1% emptying for liquids at 2 hours).

not standardized but <38% retention at 60 minutes is suggestive of accelerated gastric emptying.

The WMC has been approved by the United States Food and Drug Administration (FDA) for the evaluation of gastric emptying and colonic transit in adults. The WMC is ingested immediately following a standardized meal comprising a nutrient bar (255 calories, 2.2% fat) and 50 ml water. The subject is not permitted to eat or drink anything for the next 6 hours. Gastric emptying is defined as the duration of time from ingestion of capsule to an abrupt rise in pH as the capsule passes from the acidic stomach to the alkaline duodenum. The sensitivity and specificity of WMC in detecting delayed gastric emptying based on 4 hour scintigraphic data were 0.87 and 0.92, respectively. The cut-off point for delayed emptying for clinical use was determined to be 300 min in adults (**15.3**). The capsule is relatively large, similar in size to a video capsule, and not likely to be swallowed by younger children.

The gastric emptying breath test entails ingestion of a meal (egg) labeled with a stable radioactive isotope (^{13}C) after an overnight fast. This is usually the medium chain fatty acid 13c-octanoic acid or the blue-green algae (^{13}C-*Spirulina platensis*). The ^{13}C-containing substrate is absorbed after being emptied from the stomach, assimilates in the body's bicarbonate pool, and is excreted by the lungs as ^{13}CO$_2$. The content of this is measured in the breath at fixed time points (45, 150, 180 min) using mass spectrometry. Linear regression analysis is used for the interpretation as it has the highest concordance correlation coefficient with scintigraphic results. Other less expensive infra-red devices that can be used in the office are also commercially available and have been validated.

Ultrasonography and magnetic resonance imaging have also been used to measure gastric emptying in research settings. The technique using electrodes positioned on the abdominal skin to pick up gastric rhythmic slow wave activity (generated by the ICC) is called electrogastrography (EGG). The EGG parameters studied include dominant frequency/power, % of normal rhythm, % of bradygastria, % of tachygastria, instability coefficient, and power ratio. Clinical relevance and significance of EGG recording is controversial and gastric motility disorders are not usually diagnosed based only on an abnormal EGG.

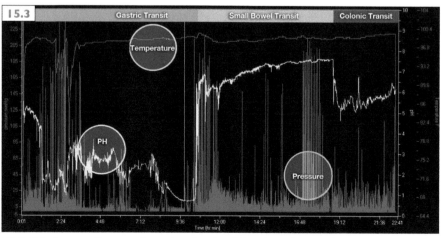

15.3 Wireless motility capsule tracing showing delayed gastric emptying.

TREATMENT

The clinical severity of symptoms of gastroparesis can be graded as grade 1 (mild), when symptoms are easily controlled and the patient is able to maintain weight on a regular diet; grade 2 (compensated), when symptoms are moderately severe and partially controlled on daily medications and the patient is able to maintain weight on a modified diet; and grade 3 (gastric failure), when symptoms are refractory and uncontrolled despite medications and dietary adjustments. Grade 3 gastroparesis is associated with frequent office or emergency room visits and/or inability to maintain hydration and nutrition orally.

Principles of management include: 1) identification and treatment of underlying disorder (diabetes mellitus) and/or discontinuation of incriminating medications; 2) addressing hydration and nutrition; and 3) alleviation of symptoms.

Diet

This intervention involves adjustment of meal content and frequency. Small and frequent meals primarily consisting of liquids should be encouraged, making sure the diet meets nutritional goals and weight is maintained. Gastric emptying of liquids is often preserved in gastroparesis. Fats and nondigestible fibers should be restricted as they retard emptying and high fiber containing fruits and vegetables may predispose to phytobezoar formation. Vitamin supplements should be added if the patient only tolerates blenderized meals and is not meeting daily requirements. The use of a dietician with knowledge of gastroparesis is essential.

Pharmacotherapy

Prokinetic agents that promote gastric emptying include metoclopramide, domperidone, and erythromycin. Metoclopramide is a substituted benzamide derivative and primarily a dopamine D2 receptor antagonist but also stimulates 5-HT4 receptors. It increases antral contractility, fundic tone, and antroduodenal peristalsis. It can cross the blood–brain barrier and cause extrapyramidal movement disorders. For this reason, metoclopramide is used with great caution. Parents should be made aware of this potential side-effect.

Domperidone is a benzimadole derivative and is a peripheral dopamine D2 receptor antagonist. Its mechanism of action is similar to metoclopramide but because it does not cross the blood–brain barrier, the central side-effects are minimal. Since the pituitary gland is not protected by the blood–brain barrier, both drugs can cause hyperprolactinemia which can result in breast enlargement, galactorrhea, and menstrual irregularities. Domperidone is widely available except in the United States where it is only approved on an investigational basis.

Erythromycin is a macrolide that acts on motilin receptors. In smaller doses it increases smooth muscle contractions in the stomach and proximal intestine thereby facilitating gastric emptying. It can also cause abdominal cramps and can prolong the QT interval. In neonates, its use has been associated with pyloric stenosis. Tachyphylaxis occurs over time making the drug less efficacious when used long term. Other 5-HT4 receptor agonists, such as cisapride and tegaserod (both previously FDA approved), have been withdrawn from the market, due to risk of death from cardiac arrhythmia and ischemic events. Newer prokinetic agents, with more efficacy and better safety profiles, are in various stages of clinical trials and their approval is much anticipated.

Antiemetic agents are widely used for symptomatic relief of nausea and vomiting, and these include phenothiazine derivatives (prochlorperazine), 5-HT3 receptor antagonists (ondansetron), dopamine receptor antagonists (metoclopramide, domperidone), H-1 receptor antagonists (diphenhydramine, promethazine), and benzodiazepines (lorazepam). These agents act peripherally and/or centrally on the chemoreceptor trigger zone of the area postrema (fourth ventricle).

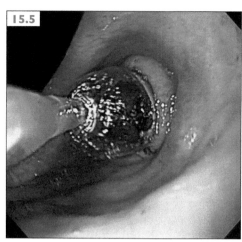

15.4 Endoscopic intrapyloric botulinum toxin injection.

15.5 Endoscopic balloon dilation of pylorus.

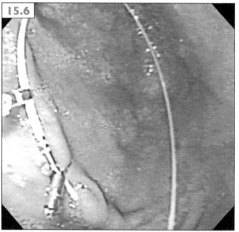

15.6 Endoscopic temporary gastric stimulator.

Prophylactic acid suppression with a proton pump inhibitor may be prescribed to prevent secondary acid damage to the esophageal mucosa from reflux or vomiting.

Surgery

Surgical intervention is reserved for those patients who have persistent symptoms not adequately controlled by dietary modifications and medications. These interventions include endoscopic therapy, such as botulinum toxin injection of the pylorus (**15.4**) and balloon dilation (**15.5**), surgical placement of a jejunostomy (or gastrojejunostomy) tube, pyloroplasty or pyloromyotomy, gastric electrical stimulation (temporary [**15.6**] or permanent) or, in the most severe cases, esophagojejunostomy (Roux-en-y). There is no consensus or guidelines for what patients or when such patients should receive which procedure.

Advances in stem cell-based therapies may offer more treatment options for gastric failure in the future.

PROGNOSIS

Most cases of postinfectious (idiopathic) gastroparesis in children resolve over time. When associated with mitochondriopathy, pseudo-obstruction, neurodevelopmental or psychiatric disorders, the symptoms may persist long term.

CHAPTER 16

Gastric Foreign Bodies

Thomas L. Sutton

DEFINITION

Foreign body ingestions commonly occur throughout the world. The majority of these ingestions involve children and include various items. Once past the esophagus, most objects will pass through the remaining gastrointestinal (GI) tract without difficulty. However, numerous complications have been reported with retained foreign bodies in the stomach. Therefore, understanding the indications for endoscopic removal of gastric foreign objects as well as the limitations of endoscopic modalities due to the smaller patient size is critical.

CLINICAL PRESENTATION

The clinical presentation can vary dramatically. Though medical care is most commonly sought after a witnessed ingestion, 40% of pediatric ingestions are not witnessed by the caregiver.

Presenting symptoms depend upon the type, location, size, and duration of the foreign body ingestion. Up to 50% of all confirmed pediatric foreign body ingestions are asymptomatic. However, a child can present with varying degrees of abdominal pain, nausea, vomiting, anorexia, abdominal distension, bleeding, or fever, possibly indicating GI obstruction, ulceration, perforation, or volvulus.

EPIDEMIOLOGY

The exact incidence of foreign body ingestion is not known. However, in the United States, the American Association for Poison Control Centers reported more than 116,000 ingestions in 2010. Of these, more than 70% occurred in the pediatric population. The most common ages were children under 6 years of age with a peak incidence between 6 months and 3 years. In these younger ages, 98% of these ingestions were accidental and there was an equal distribution between male and female. However, with the increasing age of a patient, frequency of intentional ingestions increased, particularly in children with developmental delay, psychiatric illness, alcohol use, or secondary gain. Furthermore, gender distribution in older patients with foreign body ingestion favors males.

The type of foreign body ingested varies with age and geography. In children from North America and Europe, coins represent up to 80% of foreign body ingestions. Other items commonly include toys, toy parts, sharp objects, batteries, magnets, fish or chicken bones, and other food items. In Asia and other areas where fish comprise a significant part of the diet, fish bones are the most commonly ingested foreign body followed by coins.

DIAGNOSIS

As with any medical concern, a detailed history and physical examination are critical in making a timely diagnosis and guiding therapeutic interventions. Key historical features include the following:

- Foreign body characteristics:
  - Type: coin, blunt, sharp, long, magnet, battery.
  - Size.
  - Contents/composition: plastic, wood, lead, or caustic chemicals.
  - Coingested materials.
  - Example of swallowed object (parents may be able to bring in a similar object to the one that was swallowed, for the medical team to examine).
- Timing of ingestion.
- Symptoms.
- Last meal eaten.
- Past medical history:
  - Previous foreign body ingestions.
  - Systemic illness.
  - GI surgeries or congenital anomalies.
  - Medications and drug allergies.
  - Mental health history.

The detailed physical examination should focus on indicators of complications.

Since most ingested foreign bodies are radiopaque, immediate biplanar radiographs of the neck, chest, and abdomen are recommended in order to determine the location, size, shape, and number of ingested foreign bodies as well as signs of perforation or other complications (**16.1**). Of note, fish and chicken bones, wood, plastic, glass, and thin metal objects may not be easily identified with radiography and endoscopic evaluation should be performed if there is a significant clinical suspicion of ingestion.

Expert recommendations discourage the use of contrast studies to identify foreign bodies because of the associated risk of aspiration as well as coating of the foreign body and GI mucosa which may preclude and delay endoscopic studies and retrieval.

Computed tomography with 3D reconstruction has been used to identify radiolucent foreign objects.

TREATMENT

Once the object reaches the stomach, management differs significantly from esophageal foreign bodies. The need for endoscopic removal of a gastric foreign body depends upon characteristics of the patient (age, size, and clinical condition) as well as the foreign body (type, size, location, and duration since ingestion and its ability to traverse the pylorus, duodenal sweep, and ileocecal valve).

For most asymptomatic patients, a conservative outpatient regimen of 'watchful waiting' is appropriate. However, some foreign bodies do require early endoscopic removal including sharp, large, or long objects; magnets, and disk batteries. These objects are discussed later in the chapter.

Endoscopy is typically performed with a flexible upper endoscope. Due to the increased airway compliance in younger patients and risk of obstruction, tracheal intubation is typically performed during the procedure. Retrieval devices include retrieval forceps, retrieval nets, polypectomy snares, polyp graspers, retrieval baskets, magnetic probes, banding caps, and sutures (*Table 16.1*, **16.2**). If the patient is large enough, the use of an overtube will help to protect the airway, facilitate multiple passages for removal of several objects or piecemeal removal of a bezoar, and protect the GI tract during removal of sharp or long objects. Currently, there are no pediatric-sized overtubes. Protecting the mucosa from further injury during the removal of a sharp item can also be performed with the use of a latex hood or friction fit adaptor.

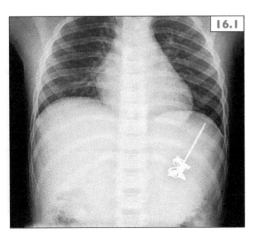

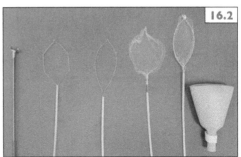

16.1 Radiographs can be used to locate ingested foreign bodies, such as this butterfly hair clip located in the stomach.

16.2 Several devices can be used to aid in successful retrieval of a foreign object including forceps, snares, baskets, and so on.

Table 16.1 Methods for extraction of foreign bodies

Type of foreign body	Retrieval devices
Coins	Forceps, baskets
Short, blunt objects	Forceps, snares, nets, baskets, suture
Sharps	Overtube, latex hood, friction fit adapter, banding cap
	Forceps, snares, nets, baskets
Batteries	Baskets, nets, polpectomy snares
Magnets	Forceps, nets, baskets, magnetic probes
Long objects	Overtube, latex hood, or friction fit adapter with dual operating channel endoscope
	Polypectomy snares, baskets, suture

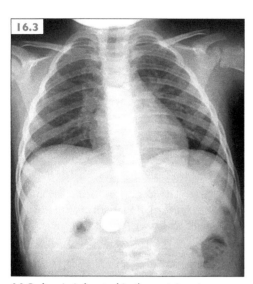

16.3 A coin is located in the gastric antrum.

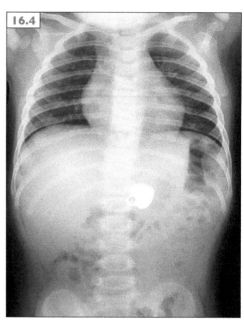

16.4 A heart-shaped locket is identified in the stomach.

Coins

Coins are the most frequently ingested foreign body in North America and Europe. Two-thirds of swallowed coins are already in the stomach upon initial medical evaluation (**16.3**). Although most coins pass without complication, gastric transit may be impaired in a very small child, especially if there is associated previous gastric surgery or the presence of an underlying disease. Once a gastric location is confirmed in an asymptomatic patient, parents can observe the child's stool to confirm passage of the coin. If coin passage is not observed, follow-up radiographs should be performed weekly to verify GI passage. Endoscopic removal of the coin would be warranted for the following reasons:

- Symptoms of obstruction or gastric injury (nausea, vomiting, distension, abdominal pain).

- Ingestion of a large diameter coin in relation to the child's size.
- Gastric retention of the coin for 3–4 weeks regardless of the lack of symptoms.

Short blunt objects

Short blunt objects may include marbles, rings, balls, toys, and other similar items (**16.4**). Similar to coins, the majority of these objects will pass without difficulty. Indications for endoscopic removal of a blunt object are similar to those for coin ingestion:

- Symptoms of obstruction or gastric injury.
- Ingestion of a large caliber object in relation to the child's size:
  - Child, object >1 × 3 cm.
  - Adult, object >2 × 5 cm.
- Gastric retention of the object for 3–4 weeks regardless of the lack of symptoms.

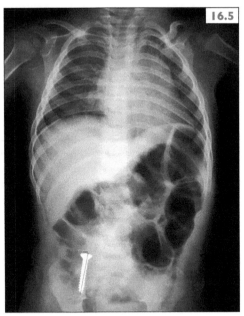

16.5 A screw is identified in the intestine in this radiograph.

If the object has passed beyond endoscopic reach, then observation for passage is recommended with weekly radiographs. If the object remains in the same intestinal location for >1 week, surgical referral would be indicated for possible removal.

Sharp objects

The ingestion of sharp objects poses a significant risk. Most commonly swallowed items include straight pins, needles, straightened paper clips, safety pins, toothpicks, fish bones, and chicken bones (**16.5**). The risk of GI complications following sharp foreign body ingestion has been reported to be as high as 35%. Because of this significantly higher risk, early endoscopic removal of all sharp objects within endoscopic reach is recommended. Caution must be taken if the ingestion involves a radiolucent object, such as a fish bone. Endoscopic evaluation should be performed in any patient with a suspected ingestion.

Preventing further injury during removal of the sharp foreign body is important. Care during removal can be accomplished by various techniques. In larger patients, the use of an overtube, latex hood, or friction fit adapter will prevent further injury. In smaller patients where passage of the above devices is not practical, orienting the object so that the sharp point is trailing during removal is critical.

Open safety pins may result in perforation during removal. Closure of the safety pin has been reported within the stomach. By using an endoscope with two operating channels or a single channel in combination with an orogastric tube, the open pin can be stabilized by grasping it with the forceps and then closing it with a small polypectomy snare. The pin can then be grasped by the circular spring end and removed. If this is not possible, then careful removal is advised with use of a hood or other device (**16.6, 16.7**).

If the sharp object has already passed the duodenal sweep, then daily follow-up radiography is recommended to confirm transit of the object. Surgical referral is required if the object remains in the same place for more than 3 days or the child develops any symptoms: such as abdominal pain, vomiting, fever, hematemesis, or melena.

Batteries

Battery ingestion has increased in direct correlation with their increased use in remote controls, toys, watches, hearing aids, cameras, and other electronic devices. Disk batteries are the most commonly swallowed batteries in pediatrics, with >60% of ingestions occurring prior to 5 years of age. Ingestion by a child typically occurs while a parent is replacing an old battery. Although batteries are similar in size to coins, their management is drastically different due to the intrinsic nature of the battery, its caustic contents, and its possible electrical discharge potentially resulting in necrosis and perforation, especially within the esophagus. Once the battery reaches the stomach, these risks, although still present, decrease substantially.

Upon presentation, immediate radiography needs to be performed to determine the location of the battery (**16.8**). If it is within the esophagus, emergent removal is indicated. Removal of a gastric cylindrical or disk battery is indicated for the following reasons:

- Symptoms of gastric injury.
- Large battery size or diameter in relation to the patient's size making passage through the pylorus, duodenal sweep, or ileocecal valve unlikely:
  - Battery >15 mm diameter in a child <6 years old.
  - Battery >15–20 mm diameter in adolescent or adult.
- A >15 mm diameter lithium or mercury containing battery.
- Coingestion of a magnet.
- Retention in the stomach for longer than 48 hours.

If an asymptomatic battery is not removed, follow-up radiographs should be obtained immediately if the child becomes symptomatic. Otherwise, one should be obtained every 3–4 days to document the battery's passage. Once past the duodenal sweep, 85% of disk batteries will pass within 72 hours.

Magnets

Like disk batteries, the incidence of magnet ingestions also is increasing in proportion to their popular use in toys, jewelry, and alternative medicines. Although the ingestion of one magnet is associated with minimal risk, the ingestion of two or more magnets, especially if ingested separately, can result in severe GI injury and death, arising from the mutual attraction of the magnets or other co-ingested metal objects, across intervening mucosal barriers resulting in ischemia of the compressed tissue. This process can lead to formation of a gastroenteric or enteroenteric fistula, obstruction, perforation, volvulus, or peritonitis.

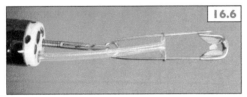
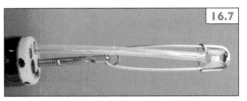

16.6, 16.7 In order to close a gastric safety pin, it is grasped using forceps (**16.6**). A snare can then be used to encircle the open pin. As the snare is tightened, the safety pin closes (**16.7**).

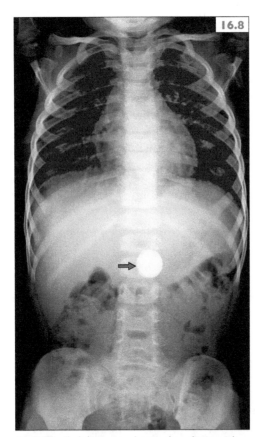

16.8 The 'halo' sign can be used to distinguish a gastric disc battery from a coin. The arrow demonstrates the double circle around the circumference consistent with a battery.

Upon presentation, immediate radiography needs to be performed to determine the location and number of magnets ingested (**16.9, 16.10**). Current expert recommendations advocate early endoscopic removal of all magnets located in the stomach and proximal small bowel.

If the magnet is beyond endoscopic reach, then careful monitoring to ensure passage is warranted. Surgical consultation may be required if there is a lack of progression through the GI tract or the child becomes symptomatic.

Long objects

The ingestion of long foreign bodies does not commonly occur in the young pediatric age range. However, the incidence increases in the adolescent and adult where ingestion is typically intentional. Accidental ingestions have been reported to involve dental instruments during procedures or toothbrushes used to induce vomiting (**16.11**). Long objects are associated with a significantly increased risk of complications usually involving impaction at the pylorus, duodenal sweep, or ileocecal valve.

Removal of all ingested long objects is indicated. However, the length of the foreign body requiring removal varies according to the age and size of the patient:

- In an infant, an object longer than 2–3 cm is unlikely to traverse the GI tract successfully and must be removed.
- In a child under 2 years of age, an object longer than 3 cm should be removed.
- In adolescents, since 50% of objects longer than 5 cm can become trapped at the ileocecal valve, foreign bodies longer than 5 cm must removed.
- In adults, an object longer than 6 cm must be removed.
- If the object is >2 cm in thickness, the maximum length of retained gastric bodies in adults requiring endoscopic removal decreases to 5 cm.

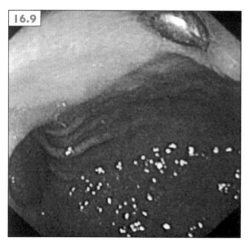

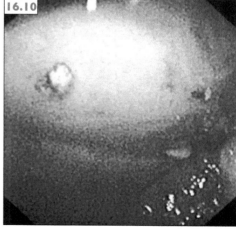

16.9, 16.10 After ingesting two, small, spherical magnets, this patient experienced immediate onset of abdominal pain. Endoscopic evaluation revealed that the two magnets adhered together across the intervening mucosal barriers (16.9) resulting in a small ulcer identified after removal of the gastric magnets (16.10).

Endoscopic removal of a long object is best accomplished by orienting it along its long axis. The best technique to achieve this depends on the shape of the object. Techniques that have been used include grasping the object and moving it into an overtube in larger patients, double snaring the object through a double channel endoscope, or using the 'suture' technique for those objects with a hole. If retrieval is unsuccessful, referral to surgery may be indicated.

Lead

Though lead intoxication is more commonly associated with the ingestion of lead-based paint, several reports have linked lead intoxication with the ingestion of lead-based objects: toys, key chain emblems, clothing accessories, fish sinkers, weights, curtain weights, lead shot, air rifle pellets, and so on. Early endoscopic removal of any lead-containing object is recommended. If the object is beyond endoscopic reach, consideration of serial radiographs and serologic lead levels should be considered. Treatment with bowel irrigation of isotonic electrolyte solution or chelation therapy has been reported.

Bezoars

A bezoar is a concretion or mass of foreign material located within the GI tract, in this case within the stomach. There are various types of bezoars: lactobezoars are made of milk and are usually seen in infants; phytobezoars are made of vegetable matter; trichobezoars are made of hair (**16.12**). Pharmacobezoars consist of medications, e.g. sucralfate, extended release nifedipine, and sodium alginate. Other bezoars include shellac, fungus, cement, tissue paper, to name a few. Symptoms usually have a gradual onset depending on the shape and size of the bezoar and include bloating, dyspepsia, nausea, vomiting, early satiety, anorexia, weight loss, and halitosis. Potential complications include GI perforation, intussusceptions, pancreatitis,

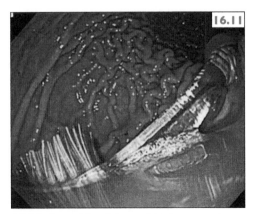

16.11 A toothbrush located in the stomach visualized during endoscopic retrieval.

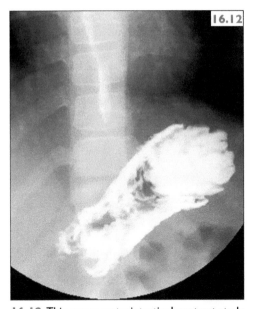

16.12 This upper gastrointestinal contrast study demonstrates a large gastric trichobezoar.

malnutrition, esophagitis, protein-losing enteropathy, and steatorrhea.

The treatment depends on the type of bezoar. Lactobezoars will typically resolve without significant treatment. Endoscopic removal is recommended for phytobezoars which can be removed slowly with forceps or baskets. Dissolution of the phytobezoar with cellulase or cola has been used to aid in endoscopic removal. Cautery with a polypectomy snare may help break the bezoar into smaller pieces. Trichobezoars are typically surgically removed.

PROGNOSIS

Foreign body ingestion occurs frequently in the pediatric population. If the foreign body reaches the stomach, the vast majority (89%) will pass through the GI tract without difficulty and conservative outpatient management can be followed. Although endoscopic removal is only required in 10–20% of ingested foreign bodies, urgent endoscopy is recommend in all symptomatic patients. Severe complications requiring surgery occur in less than 1% of patients and mortality is extremely rare (less than 1 in 1000). Early endoscopy is recommended in all ingestions retained in the stomach involving sharp objects, lead, long or large objects, magnets, or batteries in the stomach longer than 48 hours.

Once the object is in the stomach, >80% of such objects will pass through the remaining GI tract within 4 days. Factors which may increase the likelihood of gastric retention include the age and size of the patient in relation to the ingested object, as well as a past history of gastric surgery, underlying illness, GI malformation, or medications. Sharp objects have the highest risk for complications with rates reported as high as 35%. Complications include complete bowel obstruction, stricture, abscess, perforation, migration to extraintestinal site, peritonitis, ischemia, and volvulus.

Duodenal Ulcer

Samuel Bitton, Melanie Greifer

DEFINITION

Peptic ulcer disease of the duodenum, as in the stomach, is ultimately the result of an insult to the surface epithelium's mucosal defense. A duodenal ulcer is characterized by a break in the duodenal mucosa that has depth (**17.1**). Duodenitis, or inflammation of the duodenal mucosa, may accompany or precede an ulcer. Duodenitis is more often associated with erosions, which can appear endoscopically as smaller superficial lesions of the mucosa.

CLINICAL PRESENTATION

The presentation of duodenal ulcers is not unlike that of gastric ulcers, and children may have abdominal pain as the chief complaint. Children, unlike adults, may not express specific complaints and therefore a complete history is necessary. Pediatric abdominal pain, when the child is capable of expressing their pain, may be localized to the epigastric abdominal area. However, periumbilical pain, along with other symptoms also can be associated with an ulcer.

Associated symptoms of a duodenal ulcer may include postprandial pain, regurgitation, bloating, belching, nausea, and vomiting. Some may experience pain relief while eating. Pain that awakens a child at night can be elicited as well. No clinical features can differentiate gastric from duodenal ulcers reliably. Less often, a child may present with upper gastrointestinal (GI) bleeding, occult blood in the stool, and weight loss. Many times, there is a family history of peptic ulcer

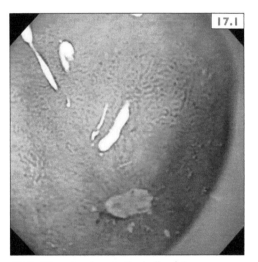

17.1 Discrete ulcer in the bulb of the duodenum in a pediatric hemophiliac patient who presented with hematemesis.

disease and even *Helicobacter pylori* infection in other family members.

Since the aforementioned symptoms are nonspecific, it is important to consider other possible medical conditions such as parasitic infections, pancreatitis, inflammatory bowel disease, biliary/hepatic disease, lactose intolerance celiac disease, and functional abdominal disorders like irritable bowel syndrome.

ETIOLOGY AND EPIDEMIOLOGY

Duodenal ulcers can be considered as primary or secondary conditions. Primary duodenal ulcers are idiopathic events with no identifiable cause, whereas secondary ulcers can be a result of infection (most commonly identified as *H. pylori*) (**17.2**), medication (such as nonsteroidal anti-inflammatory drugs [NSAIDs], corticosteroids, and bisphosphonates), chronic diseases (e.g. Crohn disease) (**17.3**), overproduction of gastric acid, older age, tobacco smoking, and alcohol consumption. In general, these etiologies are known to cause duodenal ulcers by increasing gastric acid production or weakening the intestinal epithelium's mucosal barrier.

Zollinger–Ellison syndrome is a more specific example of a condition that is associated with duodenal ulcers due to extreme acid production. In this condition, uncontrolled release of gastrin by a neuroendocrine tumor stimulates the production of excessive amounts of gastric acid causing multiple ulcerations in the stomach, duodenum, and jejunum. It can be part of the multiple endocrine neoplasia (MEN) 1 syndrome, a genetic syndrome in which gastrin-secreting tumors are associated with pituitary tumors (e.g. prolactinoma) and hyperparathyroidism. In most cases, there are no associated metastases; however, in 25% of people with gastrinomas, it may display an aggressive growth pattern that involves metastases to the liver most commonly.

Chronic use of NSAIDs (such as aspirin, ibuprofen, and naproxen) is thought to act directly on the mucosa as a chemical irritant and diminishes the production of protective prostaglandins that help maintain the mucosal barrier. High-dose corticosteroids are thought to inhibit prostaglandin production as well as impair healing. Cigarette smoking contributes to peptic ulcer disease by impairing mucosal blood flow and the ability of the mucosa to heal.

Another condition that is associated with duodenal ulcers is the situation when hypercalcemia induces gastrin production, as in chronic renal failure and hyperparathyroidism. Recently, a center in Turkey studied a small group of children with chronic renal failure on peritoneal dialysis with endoscopic peptic disease and found that they had significantly elevated gastrin levels when compared to age-matched patients with endoscopic peptic disease, without renal disease.

In adults, alcoholic cirrhosis and chronic obstructive pulmonary disease are known to be frequently associated with duodenal ulcers.

Peptic ulcers are four times more commonly found in the duodenal bulb than in the stomach. They are usually found on the anterior wall of the duodenum within a few centimeters of the pyloric valve. The typical peptic ulcer is a round to oval, sharply punched-out defect with a white base. The mucosal margin is usually at the same level as the surrounding mucosa. Malignant lesions tend to be characterized by 'heaped-up' margins. Malignant transformation of peptic ulcers is rarely found in adults and children, and such findings likely represents early carcinomas which were mistaken to be peptic ulcerations. An exception can be seen in patients who have received organ transplants, who are susceptible to post-transplant lymphoproliferative disorder (PTLD), and can present with volcanic or 'heaped up' ulcers.

Historically, gastric and duodenal ulcerations occur infrequently in children. Although the incidence of duodenal ulceration reaches 200,000–400,000 cases per year in adults, it has historically been reported as only 5.4 new cases per year in large pediatric medical centers. Most of these data were collected prior to *H. pylori* predominance as the most important cause of gastroduodenal ulceration. However, as countries have become more developed and eradication therapies for *H. pylori* have become more successful, the proportion of non-*H. pylori* duodenal ulcers is thought to be increasing.

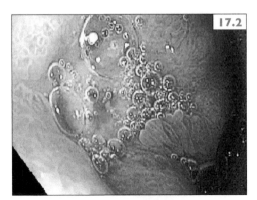

17.2 Duodenal bulb ulcer in a pediatric patient who presented with hematemesis, associated with antral biopsies that showed *H. pylori* infection.

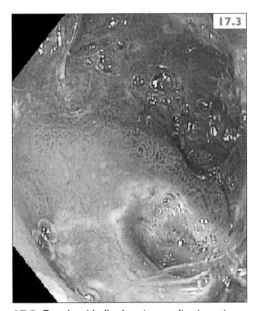

17.3 Duodenal bulb ulcer in a pediatric patient with Crohn disease.

DIFFERENTIAL DIAGNOSIS

Duodenal ulceration can be the initial presentation of inflammatory bowel disease, tuberculosis, or opportunistic infections, such as cytomegalovirus. Duodenal ulcers in the distal duodenum are highly suspicious for a nonpeptic etiology, and a further work-up should ensue.

DIAGNOSIS

In most cases, the physical examination is normal. Epigastric tenderness can sometimes be elicited. A complete examination in a patient with peptic symptoms should include a fundoscopic examination for those children complaining mainly of vomiting in order to assess for increased intracranial pressure.

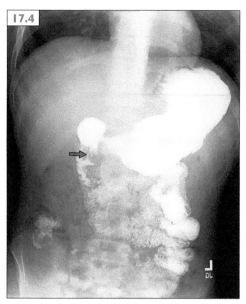

17.4 **A large duodenal bulb ulcer in a 16-year-old male with severe abdominal pain seen on barium upper gastrointestinal series (arrow).**

An oropharyngeal examination may find pertinent aphthous ulcers, that may prompt an investigation for an inflammatory process. Hepatic and splenic size should be assessed, since an increase in size usually indicates a different medical condition, like a malignant process. A rectal examination to assess for perianal disease and stool examination for occult blood should always be performed.

- Radiographic studies, such as barium contrast upper GI examinations (**17.4**), have not been shown to detect the presence of duodenal ulcers reliably, especially in children.
- Upper endoscopy is a more sensitive test. In addition, endoscopy can distinguish actively bleeding ulcers from healed ulcers and can diagnose *H. pylori* on antral biopsies.

Among noninvasive tests for *H. pylori*, serologic assays are not used in children due to a wide variation in sensitivity and specificity of the assays. Monoclonal antibody assays used to detect *H. pylori* stool antigens have been shown to have a higher sensitivity (96.6–98%) and specificity (94.7–100%) before treatment, and can be used after treatment to verify eradication. This can be especially useful in children who present with a perforated duodenal ulcer and who are not ideal candidates for an endoscopy.

Special testing
Zollinger–Ellison syndrome manifests classically as the triad of fulminating peptic ulcer disease, gastric acid hypersecretion, and nonbeta islet cell tumors of the pancreas. However, current studies have found that up to 50% of gastrinomas are located in the duodenum, usually in the proximal duodenum. The majority of gastrinomas are found within the defined area named the 'gastrinoma triangle', formed by the junction of the cystic and common bile ducts, the junction of the second and third part of duodenum, and the junction of the neck and body of the pancreas. The presence of the gastrinoma tumor produces extraordinary amounts of gastrin that leads to stimulation of gastric acid production, up to five times more than normal, and eventually multiple peptic ulcers, that can lead to life-threatening complications. The syndrome should be highly suspected when multiple duodenal ulcers are found, especially when associated with diarrhea. This diagnosis should be verified by an elevated fasting serum gastrin level. However, false-positive elevations in gastrin levels can be seen in individuals with chronic use of proton pump inhibitor (PPI) medications, which are known to cause hypergastrinemia that falls in the range of those with Zollinger–Ellison syndrome. Therefore, fasting gastrin level should be performed after stopping the PPI for at least 1 week. Other conditions that can cause physiologic hypergastrinemia include atrophic gastritis, *H. pylori* infection, pernicious anemia, chronic renal failure, and following gastric acid reducing surgery.

Celiac disease is an immune-mediated systemic disorder elicited by gluten antigens which is principally characterized by small bowel enteropathy. Rarely, multiple nonpeptic ulcers of the proximal duodenum can be associated with celiac disease. These ulcers are readily treated by initiating a gluten-free diet and, depending on the severity, a short course of corticosteroids.

Other disease processes that have been reported in the pediatric literature known to be associated with duodenal ulcers include rotavirus infection, eosinophilic enteritis (**17.5**), Hermansky–Pudlak syndrome, and sarcoidosis.

TREATMENT

In general, an effort should be made to discontinue the offending or ulcerogenic agents. When possible, NSAIDs and corticosteroids should be discontinued. Adolescents should be made aware that in addition to the well known detrimental effects of cigarette smoking and chronic alcohol abuse, their use impairs ulcer healing and increases relapse of symptoms.

Duodenal ulcers heal well with acid suppression; however, they will reoccur if therapy is discontinued or if the *H. pylori* organisms are not eradicated. PPIs, by and large, have replaced histamine-2 receptor-blockers as first-line treatment of peptic ulcer disease. Most ulcers heal after a 4 week course of PPI therapy, which can be documented by repeat upper endoscopy if necessary. Sucralfate, a cytoprotective agent, adheres to injured mucosa in the duodenum to allow further regeneration of the ulcerated tissue. However, sucralfate requires an acidic environment to be active and is contraindicated in children who have renal failure. Anticholinergic agents, which do decrease gastric acid secretion, have fallen from favor due to their unfavorable side-effect profile, such as dry mouth, constipation, blurred vision, and urinary retention.

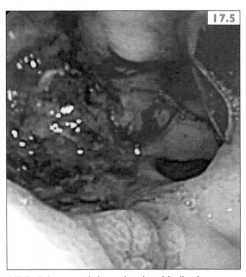

17.5 A large and deep duodenal bulb ulcer seen on endoscopy that corresponds to the findings on the barium study in Figure 17.4.

H. pylori eradication is indicated in children with *H. pylori*-positive peptic ulcer disease. Eradication of *H. pylori* greatly reduces the relapse rate of ulcer formation and ulcer-related bleeding. First-line eradication regimens include the following: triple therapy with a PPI, amoxicillin and clarithromyin or an imidazole; or bismuth salts with amoxicillin and an imidazole (e.g. metronidazole); or sequential therapy. Tetracycline can be used in patients above 8 years of age, who are penicillin allergic or in areas of clarithromycin resistance. However, its use is complicated by four times daily dosing. Treatment usually is prescribed for 10–14 days, and the PPI is continued to complete a 4–6 week course. A reliable noninvasive test for eradication, such as detection of stool *H. pylori* antigen, is recommended at least 4–8 weeks following completion of therapy. The stool *H. pylori* antigen test should be obtained at least 4 weeks after discontinuing antibiotics and 2 weeks after discontinuing PPI therapy,

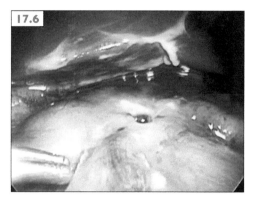

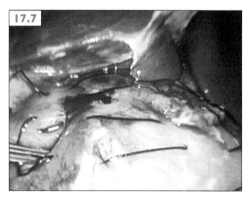

17.6–17.8 Diagnostic and therapeutic laparoscopy of a 16-year-old male who presented with severe epigastric pain of sudden onset that woke him from sleep. Abdominal computed tomography scan indicated abdominal free air and concern for a duodenal ulcer. Patient was found postoperatively to be positive for *H. pylori* infection, diagnosed by stool *H. pylori* antigen testing. **17.6**: Perforation of the anterior surface of the duodenum; **17.7**: sutures placed in preparation for a Graham patch (an omental patch); **17.8**: tongue of omentum is secured over the duodenal perforation, to complete the Graham patch.

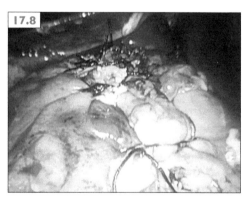

greatly diminished owing to the effective treatment available to eradicate *H. pylori* and the availability and reliable healing rates associated with PPI use.

PROGNOSIS

In most cases the cause of duodenal ulcers remains elusive and idiopathic duodenal ulcers, compared to *H. pylori*-positive ulcers, have been found to recur despite PPI therapy. However, the prognosis of duodenal ulceration is excellent when the cause is identified and targeted therapy is available. When *H. pylori* infection is eradicated, the ulcers are unlikely to return unless resistant organisms are present or reinfection from asymptomatic infected family members occurs. Ulcer bleeding and perforation are the most severe complications. Gastric outlet obstruction from chronic duodenal ulceration due to peptic and nonpeptic causes can rarely lead to pyloric stenosis.

since false-negative results may occur due to decreased bacterial load without true eradication.

Surgery is indicated for duodenal ulcer perforation (**17.6–17.8**), which is considered an emergency. Otherwise, the role of surgical intervention in elective situations has

CHAPTER 18

Pediatric Functional Gastrointestinal Disorders

Katja Kovacic, B U.K. Li

DEFINITION

Functional gastrointestinal disorders (FGIDs) are common among children and adolescents. FGIDs comprise a constellation of gastrointestinal symptoms such as abdominal pain, bloating, nausea, regurgitation, vomiting, constipation, and diarrhea (*Table 18.1*). Historically, the term 'functional' refers to a spectrum of disorders not explained by structural or biochemical abnormalities. Recurring abdominal pain is one of the most frequent complaints to both general pediatricians and pediatric gastroenterologists. Pain-predominant FGIDs include functional abdominal pain (FAP), irritable bowel syndrome (IBS),

---

Table 18.1 Childhood functional gastrointestinal disorders (FGIDs) by Rome III criteria

Abdominal pain-related FGIDs	Vomiting and aerophagia	Constipation and incontinence
Irritable bowel syndrome	Adolescent rumination syndrome	Functional constipation
Functional dyspepsia	Cyclic vomiting syndrome	Nonretentive fecal incontinence
Abdominal migraine	Aerophagia	
Childhood functional abdominal pain		

functional dyspepsia, and abdominal migraine (*Table 18.2*). These disorders present with a combination of recurrent symptoms including abdominal pain that has no identifiable cause. This chapter will focus on the pain-predominant FGIDs, in particular IBS, as these are most commonly encountered in clinical pediatric practice.

Over the last two decades, the understanding of FGIDs has rapidly evolved from a view of it being a psychosocial diagnosis to mounting evidence of abnormalities in multiple systems. Aberrations in motor, sensory, autonomic, immunologic, endocrine, genetic, and psychosocial function are now acknowledged to play a role in a resulting disordered brain–gut communication. The Rome criteria, now in its third edition, were established as a symptom-based classification tool to diagnose FGIDs. Although the Rome criteria group FGIDs into distinct disorders, a fair degree of overlap exists. Some studies have found limited utility and reliability of the Rome criteria as used in the clinical setting. There is also evidence of low concordance between the criteria and inter-physician reliability, suggesting the need for further refinement and education on the Rome criteria.

EPIDEMIOLOGY

Recurrent abdominal pain is often the central complaint in pain-predominant FGIDs. According to Apley's classical study of 1,000 schoolchildren, approximately 10% of children suffer from recurrent abdominal pain. Prevalence studies on recurrent abdominal pain vary greatly, with prevalence rates ranging from 0.3% to 19%. Methodological limitations, such as selection

---

Table 18.2 Abdominal pain-predominant functional gastrointestinal disorders (FGIDs) by Rome III criteria

Pain-predominant FGIDs	Irritable bowel syndrome	Functional dyspepsia*	Abdominal migraine	Functional abdominal pain**
Symptoms at least once/week for minimum of 2 months	+	+		+
Two or more associated symptoms***			+	
No evidence of organic process	+	+	+	+
Pain or discomfort in upper abdomen		+		
Altered bowel movements****	+			
Interferes with activities			+	
Discrete pain episodes			+	+/–

*Need to exclude irritable bowel syndrome.

**Need to exclude other FGIDs.

***1) anorexia; 2) nausea; 3) vomiting; 4) headache; 5) photophobia; 6) pallor.

****Abdominal pain + *two or more* of the following: 1) improvement with defecation; 2) associated with change in stool frequency; 3) associated with change in stool form.

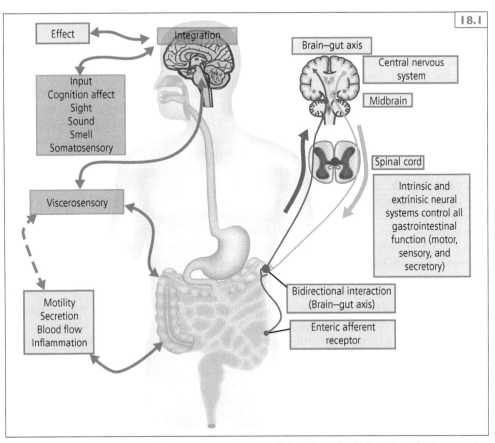

18.1 Biopsychosocial model of functional gastrointestinal disorders: the bidirectional brain–gut axis.

bias and different diagnostic criteria, may explain some of this wide variation. A prospective study by Saps *et al.* in 2009 found a weekly prevalence of abdominal pain in 38% of school-aged children. About one-quarter of these children reported persistent abdominal pain lasting more than 2 months. Symptoms typically peak between 4 and 6 years and early adolescence, with a female preponderance during the adolescent years. The estimated prevalence of IBS, the most prevalent of the pain-predominant FGIDs, ranges from 6% to 14% in children and from 22% to 36% in adolescents.

PATHOPHYSIOLOGY

The pathogenesis of FGIDs is multifactorial and is the result of complex interplay between genetic, environmental, physiologic and psychosocial factors. This forms the basis for the biopsychosocial model which is essential to understanding and treating FGIDs. This model proposes that psychosocial factors interact with the gut to form the brain–gut axis: a bidirectional communication between the brain and the enteric nervous system (ENS) (**18.1**). In this model, emotions, thoughts and perceptions widely influence gastrointestinal (GI) sensation, motility, immunity, mucosal inflammation and permeability. Conversely, GI factors can affect conscious perception and behavior. A dysregulated brain–gut axis is thought to underlie most functional GI disorders. Numerous studies have tried to assess whether psychosocial distress is a cause or consequence of the dysregulated brain–gut axis. However, it appears that psychosocial morbidity is just as prevalent before as after the medical presentation.

During health, the brain receives afferent signals from the GI tract that activate autonomic responses. In patients with FGIDs, the afferent information is consciously perceived and associated with autonomic nervous system output and emotional changes. An abnormal interplay between the ENS and the central nervous system (CNS) may lead to heightened responses to noxious stimuli or even to normal physiologic stimuli, such as gastric distention from a meal. This heightened perception, termed visceral hypersensitivity, appears augmented by psychologic stress and is likely to be a major contributor to the manifestations of functional GI disorders.

Inflammatory insults to the GI tract in childhood such as cow's milk allergy, Henoch–Schönlein purpura, or acute GI infections, may alter pain perception and have been proposed to play a role in the development of FGIDs later in life. Rodent studies show that acute infections of the colon and surgical procedures result in the development of persistent, long-term visceral hypersensitivity following the insult. This pathophysiology mirrors the scenario in which postinfectious IBS ensues from ongoing low-grade inflammation that induces visceral hypersensitivity. According to recent findings, gut microbiota are thought to influence not only the ENS but also the CNS and the brain–gut axis through neural, neuroendocrine, immunologic, and humoral mechanisms.

Pain-predominant FGIDs and the Rome Criteria

Abdominal pain-predominant FGIDs are divided into four separate categories based on Rome III criteria: FAP, IBS, functional dyspepsia, and abdominal migraine (*Table 18.2*). IBS is one of the most commonly diagnosed FGIDs in clinical practice. In the Rome III criteria, childhood IBS is defined as abdominal discomfort or pain occurring at least once per week for a minimum of 2 months. The abdominal pain must have two or more of the following features 25% of the time: relief with defecation; onset associated with a change in frequency of stool; and/or onset associated with a change in the form of stool. In addition, there should be no evidence of structural or biochemical abnormalities to explain the symptoms. Childhood functional dyspepsia differs from IBS in that the pain is centered in the upper abdomen and symptoms are not associated with changes in stooling pattern. The Rome criteria for functional dyspepsia are thus fairly nonspecific, likely accounting for the high frequency of overlap with IBS.

On the contrary, the classification of abdominal migraine includes a more specific clinical symptom pattern. Abdominal migraines are characterized by intense, discrete episodes of periumbilical pain, lasting at least 1 hour and with associated features (two or more) of anorexia, nausea, vomiting, headache, photophobia, or pallor. The pain is severe enough to interfere with the child's activities and characterized by intervening periods of normal health. Childhood FAP represents those patients who do not meet the criteria for any other pain-predominant FGID. It is defined as continuous or episodic abdominal pain, not explained by an organic process or another FGID, and occurring at least once per week for a minimum of 2 months.

Although these criteria share many clinical features and may not distinguish FGIDs from organic etiologies of pain, a thorough history focusing on pain frequency, location, severity, timing, and associated bowel disturbances is key to elicit the correct diagnosis.

DIAGNOSIS

The evaluation of recurrent abdominal pain and diagnosis of potential FGIDs frequently present a diagnostic dilemma to the clinician. The Rome criteria require exclusion of organic disease and, in the past, extensive investigations including esophagogastroduodenoscopy (EGD) have often been performed. The North American Society for Pediatric Gastroenterology, Hepatology, and Nutrition recommendations conclude that EGD has low yield in the absence of alarm symptoms and a systematic review similarly has reported a low yield of EGD in children with abdominal pain. Specific reported alarm symptoms and signs from a large single center cohort, predicting organic disease in patients with chronic abdominal pain include anemia, hematochezia, and weight loss. Vomiting and night-time awakening from pain were not found to be predictors of organic disease.

In the current approach, the absence of alarm symptoms allows the clinician to make a symptom-based diagnosis and avoid an extensive, costly, and invasive exclusionary diagnostic work-up. When the index of suspicion for an organic illness is low, the Rome criteria will help determine a positive diagnosis of a functional disorder. In addition, exploring psychosocial influences should always be considered in the evaluation of patients with FGIDs.

EXPLANATORY MODEL

Explaining the diagnosis of a functional disorder to the patient and family is often difficult. This may be due to misconceptions of both the physician and the family, that a functional disorder is primarily a psychologic problem. It is thus important to emphasize to families that symptoms are not imagined but due to altered physiologic cross-talk between the brain and the gut. The brain–gut axis can

be explained in simple terms. Some examples include discussing 'the big brain' (i.e. CNS) communicating with 'the little brain' (i.e. ENS) and sending wrong messages; 'the sensitivity dial' being turned up like the volume on a radio (visceral hyperalgesia); or a pain signal that was turned on by an infection and the body 'forgot how to turn it off'.

Clinicians should also emphasize the positive value of a diagnosis established on symptom-based criteria and the need to avoid extensive diagnostic testing, which may even be counterproductive for treating FGIDs. Simultaneously, the physician must help validate the symptoms and recognize the distress and possible adverse impact of a FGID on quality of life.

TREATMENT

There are many strategies for the treatment of FGIDs, including pharmacologic, dietary, cognitive-behavioral, and complementary approaches (*Table 18.3*). Because data on specific treatments for pediatric FGIDs are sparse, empiric therapy is typically employed. Management should be tailored to each individual patient's specific symptoms and focused on promoting overall functioning and rehabilitation. Psychotherapeutic techniques, such as relaxation, hypnotherapy, biofeedback, and cognitive-behavioral therapy, can help develop coping skills and improve the child's ability to self-manage symptoms.

Various food substances appear to be implicated in exacerbating symptoms of FGIDs and dietary manipulations are often effective. Gluten-free diets or low carbohydrate intake may improve symptoms in IBS. Reduced intake of poorly absorbed short-chain carbohydrates and monosaccharides, the so-called FODMAP diet (Fermentable Oligo-, Di-, Monosaccharides and Polyols), may be beneficial in IBS. Rapid bacterial fermentation of these substances that results in colonic luminal distention is the proposed underlying mechanism. Supplemental fiber can either

Table 18.3 Treatment options for irritable bowel syndrome (IBS) and functional abdominal pain

Treatment	Type	Dose	Comment
Fiber supplementation	Psyllium (ispaghula husk)	5–30 g	Adult data from six RCT; NNT=11
Probiotic	*Lactobacillus rhamnosus GG*	3×10^9 CFU × 4–8 weeks	Conflicting studies but two RCTs showing moderate treatment success versus placebo
FODMAP	Low fructose/fructans diet		Limited pediatric data; RCT in adults with IBS and fructose malabsorption showing symptom improvement.
Antispasmodic	Peppermint oil	1–2 enteric-coated capsules 3×d	Reduced pain but no effect on other IBS symptoms; 40% placebo response rate
Tricyclic antidepressants	Amitriptyline	10–30 mg qhs × 4–8 weeks	Multi-center RCT in pain-predominant FGIDs: 63% response rate but comparable placebo effect; RCT in pediatric IBS: improved overall quality of life and pain
SSRI	Citalopram	10–40 mg daily × 12 weeks	Open-label, flexible dose trial in recurrent abdominal pain; improvement in pain and co-morbid anxiety/depression but methodological limitations
Alternative treatments	Cognitive behavioral therapy	Various	Five randomized trials showing statistically significant improvement in pain; small studies and methodological limitations

CFU: colony forming units; FGID: functional gastrointestinal disorder; FODMAP: fermentable oligo-, di-, monosaccharides and polyols; NNT: number needed to treat; RCT: randomized controlled trial; SSRI: selective serotonin reuptake inhibitor.

play a positive or negative role in treating IBS. Probiotics may have a role in the treatment of children with FGIDs, possibly through restoring altered gut flora and down regulating mucosal inflammation. Although results from pediatric studies are conflicting, *Lactobacillus rhamnosus* GG (LGG) use in children improved abdominal pain in 72% of subjects with IBS and FAP, compared to 53% in the placebo group. A meta-analysis concluded that LGG moderately increases treatment success, particularly in IBS. A study of LGG in children with FAP, functional dyspepsia, and IBS found that the probiotic significantly reduced abdominal pain in the IBS patients. Antispasmodic agents, such as peppermint oil and hyoscyamine, have also been shown to be helpful for IBS and FAP, presumably through reduction of GI smooth muscle spasms. These are all treatment options with few side-effects that should serve as first-line options.

When first-line treatments fail or symptoms are severe and adversely affect the quality of life (e.g. school attendance and extracurricular participation), antidepressants may be tried empirically. Both tricyclic antidepressants (TCAs) and selective serotonin reuptake inhibitors (SSRIs) have been found to be beneficial in treating adults with FGIDs, with no significant differences observed between them. Proposed mechanisms of action for these medications include reduced afferent pain signaling and perception, anticholinergic effects on the GI tract, and improvement in mood and anxiety. Amitriptyline is a commonly used TCA for the treatment of various FGIDs such as IBS, FAP, abdominal migraine, and cyclic vomiting syndrome. A few studies in children demonstrate improved quality of life in adolescents with IBS and reduced anxiety scores in children with pain-predominant FGIDs, but marginal reduction in pain symptoms. However, these studies are limited by a substantial placebo effect, short duration of treatment, and a single low, fixed dose of antidepressant. Future studies are needed to further clarify the efficacy of amitriptyline in childhood FGIDs. Similarly, literature on the use of SSRIs in pediatric FGIDs is sparse. One study that evaluated citalopram showed benefit in 84% of patients on a global improvement scale. However, further studies are needed to confirm this effect.

PROGNOSIS

Despite the benign nature of functional GI disorders, long-standing symptoms can adversely and profoundly affect quality of life and school performance. Multiple studies confirm that FGIDs impair health-related quality of life to the same extent as organic GI disease. A long-term outcome study in children with FAP with mean follow-up of 9 years, showed that most children with the more intense GI symptoms at baseline met criteria for a FGID at follow-up. One major prognostic factor for the persistence of abdominal pain into adulthood includes having a parent with GI complaints. Pediatric FGID patients are found to have higher levels of anxiety and depression, lower self-worth perception, and more negative life events leading to poorer long-term outcomes. To prevent these long-term consequences, it is vital that pediatricians recognize FGIDs at an early stage, understand the biopsychosocial model, and use multimodal and individualized treatment approaches.

JEJUNUM AND ILEUM

CHAPTER 19

Malabsorption

Simon S. Rabinowitz

DEFINITION AND EPIDEMIOLOGY

The major function of the digestive system is the absorption of virtually all energy and nutrients from the diet. Any condition that interferes with this process is referred to as 'malabsorption'. Fat and carbohydrate are both absorbed through the small bowel but each has unique pathways with multiple required steps.

Carbohydrate malabsorption is most often encountered in intestinal diseases. However, lipid absorption requires extensive digestion by pancreatic enzymes and the presence of bile salts. The bipolar bile salts are required to form mixed micelles which allows these water insoluble nutrients to be absorbed. Thus, besides small bowel pathology, fat malabsorption is commonly encountered in pancreatic or biliary pathology.

The clinical sequelae of malabsorption, the failure to utilize ingested nutrients, can be identical to malnutrition which is the failure to ingest required nutrients. Aside from widespread small bowel disease as in the short bowel syndrome, protein malabsorption rarely is a clinical concern. However, certain children with intestinal diseases that result in malabsorption also may have protein-losing enteropathy. In this condition, protein that has already been synthesized by the body is inappropriately lost. This condition can yield chronic protein depletion defined as kwashiorkor.

Since malabsorption is a heterogeneous term, the incidence is dependent on which nutrient one is examining. In addition, in the developing world where the burden of intestinal infections is high, the proportion of people with malabsorption is also much greater.

Enteric infections result in intestinal dysfunction (diarrheal illnesses) yielding malabsorption. The lack of nutrients further compromises intestinal function, thus further escalating the initial insult. While there are no accurate epidemiologic data on malabsorption, there is some related information.

A common cause of both carbohydrate and fat malabsorption, celiac disease, can be screened for with serum tests such as the tissue transglutaminase and anti-endomysial immunoglobulin (Ig)A antibody titers. Utilizing this approach on large numbers of stored bloods has revealed that the prevalence of celiac disease is reportedly slightly more than 1 in a 100 people in the United States, Europe, and large parts of Asia.

Since celiac disease only contributes to a fraction of all patients with malabsorption, the prevalence for malabsorption is much higher than this number. Estimates in the United States for the incidence of malabsorption are about 5%. In the developing world, the percentage is much higher and is a major contributor to mortality.

The most common form of malabsorption is from the milk sugar, lactose. About 90% of adults throughout the world are believed to have lactose malabsorption. While few infants and toddlers have this problem, children approach adult values of lactose malabsorption during the early school years.

CLINICAL PRESENTATION

In children, the most apparent presentation for malabsorption is failure to thrive and if malabsorption continues long enough, short stature. Malabsorbed carbohydrates enter the colon, where they are fermented by bacterial flora to yield a watery, acidic, osmotic diarrhea. This can cause a *Candida* spp. diaper (nappy/napkin) rash, bloating, distension, and excessive gas.

Malabsorption of fat is often accompanied by deficiencies in fat soluble vitamin(s) with a prevalence in part related to their relative hydrophobic state, including vitamins E, D, K, and least likely A.

Vitamin E deficiency leads to loss of deep tendon reflexes, due to posterior column defects. Vitamin D is required to prevent rickets (bowing of legs, flaying of knees and wrists) in younger children, and osteopenia (frequent or atypical fractures) in adolescents. Figure **19.1** shows the characteristic radiographic findings of rickets with flaying of the distal ends of the long bones. Inadequate amounts of vitamin D interferes with the normal deposition of calcium and phosphate into growing bone, leading to creation of the structurally abnormal and weaker bone. Our understanding of vitamin D activity is expanding and deficiencies have been identified with many diseased states.

Vitamin K deficiency causes excessive bleeding with documentation of coagulopathy. As vitamin K is synthesized by enteric flora rather than ingested in our diet, other conditions can alter the bacterial source of this vitamin.

Vitamin A depletion results in exophthalmia, dry conjunctiva and skin, and impaired night vision. In the developing world it is associated with impaired immune function and increased morbidity due to infectious agents.

ETIOLOGY AND PATHOPHYSIOLOGY
Small intestinal disease (carbohydrate and fat malabsorption)

In these conditions the villi are usually shortened which compromises the absorptive surface. Besides having less surface area to absorb nutrients, there is a reduction or absence of villi tips that contain the disaccharidases (lactase, sucrase, isomaltase, and maltase) that are required to digest the disaccharides into the monosaccharides (glucose, galactose, and fructose) that are then absorbed. Figure **19.2** show the morphologic appearance of the compromised small intestine mucosa as seen on endoscopy. The folds are reticulated rather than smooth and there is subtle notching noted. Figure **19.3** shows the histopathologic appearance with a blunting of the normally much longer,

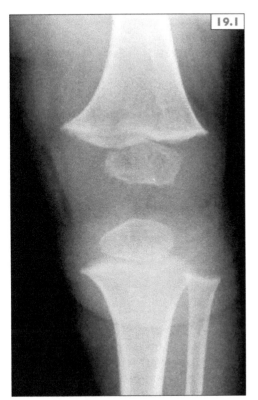

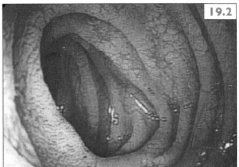

19.1 Rickets. Bone changes with flaying of the distal ends of the long bones in a child with vitamin D deficiency.

19.2 Duodenal scalloping seen with intestinal mucosa inflammation and malabsorption.

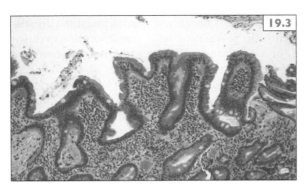

19.3 Blunted villi in the duodenum with decreased surface absorptive area.

slender villi which results in less surface area for absorption.

If the insult is moderate, there could be a drop out of lactase, found exclusively on the ends of the villi, leading to exclusive lactose malabsorption. If the insult is more severe, there could be a transient decrease in the level of sucrase–isomaltase also, which leads to malabsorption of additional dietary sources of carbohydrate. There are also genetic diseases that can affect these enzymes. It is extremely rare to be born with alactasia or primary loss of the lactase gene. A primary or congenital form of the sucrase–isomaltase gene deficiency is seen much more frequently, but still not often.

Inflammatory

Celiac disease, also known as gluten enteropathy, is an immunologic disorder triggered by wheat, rye, or barley exposure in individuals with the genetic profile to have this condition which includes human leukocyte antigen (HLA) DQ2 and HLA-DQ8.

Postviral enteropathy is a prolonged immune response following clearance of the infectious organism. Human immunodeficiency virus (HIV) infection frequently results in malabsorption, but in addition to this mechanism, there may be repeated infectious insults and additional undefined problems that interfere with villi regeneration.

Cow milk and/or soy protein allergy can lead to immune-mediated damage that will reappear with reintroduction of these antigens.

Chronic enteric infections (especially in the face of immune dysfunction which compromises the intestine's ability to clear the pathogen) result in prolonged villous damage. This includes parasitic infections (*Giardia lamblia*, *Isospora belli*, *Strongyloides stercoralis*) and bacterial agents in special circumstances, such as tropical sprue and bacterial overgrowth related to compromise

in intestine anatomy, peristalsis, or gastric acid production.

Crohn disease involving the small bowel frequently leads to inadequate energy absorption and growth compromise. In addition, children with Crohn disease will have decreased calorie intake which further contributes to growth failure and short stature.

Noninflammatory conditions yielding compromised absorption

- Infiltrative disorders that compromise the absorptive capacity including lymphoma, Whipple disease, abetalipoproteinemia, *Mycobacterium avian intracellulare*.
- Severe iron or zinc deficiency (acrodermatitis herpetica seen with celiac disease) presumably compromises the usual rapid turnover of villi seen in the normal small bowel.
- Radiation enteritis and blind loop syndromes also can be accompanied by bacterial overgrowth that worsens the extent of absorption dysfunction.
- Edema of the small bowel as can be seen in right-sided congestive heart failure.
- Short bowel syndrome from congenital anomalies or surgical resection decreases the total length of bowel available for absorption.

Small intestinal disease yielding fat malabsorption exclusively (compromised enterohepatic circulation)

Crohn disease or necrotizing enterocolitis (NEC) of the terminal ileum can severely impair the absorption of bile acids resulting in depletion of the bile acid pool. If the liver cannot increase synthesis to exceed the excessive losses through the intestine, there is inability to form micelles and consequently fat malabsorption.

Primary or secondary lymphangiectasia interferes with the delivery of the bile salts into the proximal small bowel where they are required for nonpolar fat absorption.

Extraintestinal causes of malabsorption (pancreatic exocrine insufficiency)

Cystic fibrosis, an autosomal recessive disease caused by mutations to the gene for the chloride transporter, is by far the most common etiology for this condition. Pulmonary problems are an even more serious aspect of this disease along with hepatobiliary disease, sweat abnormalities, nasal polyps, and limited reproductive ability.

Other rarer forms include Shwachman–Diamond syndrome, Johanson–Blizzard syndrome, Pearson syndrome, and isolated pancreatic enzyme deficiencies.

DIAGNOSIS

Carbohydrate malabsorption can be most directly documented by finding an excessive amount of sugar in the stool, measured by reducing substances in the stool. Other methods commonly employed are an increased generation of hydrogen or methane gas measured on breath testing, or finding an acidic pH of the stool which results from bacterial fermentation in the colon of unabsorbed sugar.

Once carbohydrate malabsorption is documented then the approach below is employed to determine the etiology of this condition.

Congenital or acquired neonatal conditions such as NEC, bowel resection, and enzymatic or mucosal dysfunction, can lead to nutrient malabsorption. A history of previous or current infections with gastrointestinal, sinopulmonary, dermatologic, or systemic organisms should be sought. Family history is critical when considering causes such as Crohn disease, celiac disease or cystic fibrosis. Physical examination findings of hepatomegaly, clubbing, and pulmonary, musculoskeletal or dermatologic diseases can provide important clues in evaluating the pathophysiology of malabsorption.

Potential noninvasive testing includes serology for celiac disease, serologic evaluation for immune function, food allergy testing (IgE or skin prick testing); sweat testing; and possibly mutational analyses for cystic fibrosis. Fecal testing for pH, reducing substances, guaiac, fat, and leukocytes is inexpensive and often elucidating. Additional stool investigations would identify the presence of infectious agents, and measurement of fecal elastase is used as a marker for pancreatic exocrine sufficiency. If there is evidence for compromised protein status a fecal specimen for alpha-1-antitrypsin as a marker for protein-losing enteropathy would be indicated.

Radiographic studies can further support diagnosis of Crohn disease, NEC stricture, and anatomic abnormalities that can lead to small bowel overgrowth.

Endoscopy and biopsy of the duodenum is required to diagnose celiac disease, Crohn disease of the small bowel, Whipple disease, abetalipoproteinemia, certain enteric infections, and lymphoma of the small bowel.

TREATMENT

The treatment for malabsorption is disease specific, and typically involves some degree of nutritional support. Most children with malabsorption will require supplemental and/or simpler forms of nutrients to prevent deficiencies. It is important to analyze which nutrients may be affected. Malabsorption or deficiencies of carbohydrate, protein or fat will vary in clinical presentation and biochemical profile. Treatment of fat malabsorption related to bile acid deficiency, may require medium chain triglycerides which can be absorbed directly through the intestine without relying on micelle formation.

Malabsorption related to pancreatic exocrine insufficiency can be corrected by providing the child with pancreatic replacement enzymes which are taken with meals. This permits adequate digestion of the ingested food so that complete absorption can occur.

Small bowel diseases that lead to malabsorption are the most challenging and require adequate treatment of the underlying condition to yield adequate absorptive surface area to avoid deficiencies.

Celiac disease (gluten), cow milk protein allergy, and soy protein allergy require removal of the triggering antigens to allow the bowel to heal fully.

Enteric infections may require prolonged treatment regimens especially when immune dysfunction is contributing to the chronicity. In addition, chronic highly active antiretroviral therapy for HIV, antituberculosis medications for enteric tuberculosis, and intravenous immunoglobulin (IVIG) replacement for some B cell immune deficiencies may allow for reconstitution of the villi.

Therapy for specific illnesses such as Crohn disease or intestinal lymphoma will be required when these conditions contribute to intestinal malabsorption. In certain cases, where malabsorption cannot be corrected, amino acid-based diets with glucose polymers are used to permit adequate nutrient absorption.

Finally, the child with extensive small bowel disease such as severe short bowel syndrome and motility disorders may have to receive parenteral nutrition when all efforts to provide adequate enteral nutrition are unsuccessful. A subset of these children can ultimately develop enough intestinal function through intensive intestinal rehabilitation programs. The remainder of such patients are candidates for small intestine transplantation.

PROGNOSIS

Identifying the exact nutrient(s) that is/are not being adequately absorbed suggests that a strategy to overcome the deficiency can be developed to attenuate adverse effects. The degree of malabsorption can become severe enough that special diets and special programs are required. The more serious the underlying problem, the worse the long-term prognosis is.

Intestinal rehabilitation programs are now reporting that a high proportion of children who enter such programs are able to be discharged on long-term enteral therapy, although some will still require supplemental parenteral nutrition.

For children who require intestinal transplant, survival rates have been reported as high as 97% at 1 year and 74% at 3 years post-transplantation. However, only a small proportion of those patients who are on the waiting list will ultimately be able to live long enough to find a suitable donor.

CHAPTER 20

Celiac Disease

Justin Hollon, Alessio Fasano

DEFINITION

Celiac disease is a T-cell-mediated chronic inflammatory enteropathy with an autoimmune component. This potentially systemic disease is triggered by the ingestion of gluten in genetically susceptible individuals. Unique as an immune-mediated disorder, the primary environmental trigger is not only known, but lifelong removal of this dietary trigger leads to remission of the disease.

CLINICAL PRESENTATION

The highly variable manifestations of celiac disease lead to a broad spectrum of clinical presentations. The classic (malabsorptive) form of celiac disease seen in infants and young children, with chronic diarrhea, muscle wasting, and weight loss, is seen less commonly than those presenting with extraintestinal symptoms or less overt signs of intestinal pathology.

Presenting gastrointestinal (GI) symptoms include abdominal discomfort, bloating, weight loss, anorexia, nausea, vomiting, diarrhea, and constipation. A lack of apparent GI symptoms does not equate to a lack of malabsorptive disease, and presumably asymptomatic patients may present with the consequences of malabsorption such as short stature, delayed puberty, osteoporosis, or isolated nutritional deficiencies. In fact, iron deficiency anemia, resistant to oral iron supplementation, is the most common extraintestinal manifestation. Other non-GI or 'atypical' signs include dermatitis herpetiformis, permanent-tooth enamel hypoplasia, hepatitis, epilepsy, peripheral neuropathy, and arthritis.

Associated diseases

There is an increased association with autoimmune and immune-mediated diseases in general, with a strong association in those with type 1 diabetes, thyroiditis, or selective immunoglobulin (Ig) A deficiency. In addition to screening asymptomatic children with these conditions, the 2005 North American Society for Pediatric Gastroenterology, Hepatology and Nutrition (NASPGHAN) celiac disease clinical guideline recommends screening asymptomatic children with Down syndrome, Turner syndrome, and Williams syndrome due to a higher prevalence of celiac disease in these children.

ETIOLOGY AND EPIDEMIOLOGY

Celiac disease is common in the United States, with a reported seroprevalence in both adults and children of roughly 1 in 100. While this rate is similarly ~1% in the European adult population, European studies have demonstrated an even higher prevalence in children, and the seroprevalence in symptomatic children in the United States is as high as 1:25. Although this disorder is less common in individuals of non-European descent, the prevalence among symptomatic minorities in the United States still remains high. Likewise, the disease is increasingly recognized in the Middle East, India, north Africa, south Asia and Mexico. As with most autoimmune diseases, females are diagnosed two to three times more frequently than males.

Celiac disease is triggered by the ingestion of gluten-containing grains (including wheat, rye, and barley) in genetically susceptible persons. The fact that someone may not develop celiac disease until late adulthood despite being on a lifelong gluten-containing diet, argues for the involvement of environmental cofactors.

Dietary trigger

Wheat, and the taxonomically related rye and barley, serve as the environmental trigger in celiac disease patients. Wheat gluten is a protein composite that remains after starch is washed from wheat flour dough. In baking, gluten is responsible for dough elasticity, viscosity (thickness), and increased moisture absorption; however, it is also used as a stabilizing agent in nonbaking products, such as ice cream and ketchup, and as an excipient in many medications. Gluten is a protein composite of gliadins (monomers) and glutenins (polymers), with the gliadin protein being the primary immunogenic and toxic fraction. Barley and rye both possess prolamin fractions equivalent to wheat gliadins (hordeins and secalines, respectively) and demonstrate the same toxic properties in celiac patients.

Genetic factors

Genetics play a significant role in disease susceptibility. The concordance rate for celiac disease among monozygotic twins is 75%, with a roughly 10% concordance among dizygotic twins. Likewise, the prevalence of celiac disease among first-degree relatives is as high as 10% in the United States. Genetic linkage studies have shown that susceptibility to celiac disease is strongly associated with human leukocyte antigen (HLA) DQ genes, specifically the DQ2 variant HLA-DQA1*05/DQB1*02 and the DQ 8 variant HLA-DQA1*03/DQB1*0302. Approximately 95% or more of celiac patients have the DQ2 allele, with

the remainder of celiac patients being almost exclusively DQ8 positive. As 30% of the general/control North American population carries the DQ2 allele, the presence of either the DQ2 or DQ8 gene is essential but not predictive; clearly other non-HLA genes must be involved.

Environmental cofactors

Additional environmental factors that may contribute to the development of celiac disease include infant feeding practices and intestinal infections. During a pediatric epidemic of celiac disease in Sweden, a case–control study demonstrated that the risk of celiac disease was reduced in children, particularly infants, still being breast-fed when gluten was introduced, and that the introduction of large amounts of gluten at infancy increased the risk of celiac disease. Timing of the introduction of gluten in infants may also be important. A United States prospective observational study of at-risk infants demonstrated a decreased risk of celiac disease in children exposed to gluten between 4 and 6 months of life. Whether changing dietary habits reduces the overall risk of disease or simply postpones disease onset is unclear, but it has been hypothesized that the switch from gluten tolerance to that of an immune response depends heavily on the developing intestinal microbiota of infants. Recent research regarding the intestinal colonization of infants has demonstrated a strikingly immature gut microbiota within the first 2 year of life in DQ2/DQ8 infants compared to the genetically unsusceptible, with a relative absence of fecal Bacteroidetes. Intestinal infections may also contribute to triggering onset of disease, presumably through a rise in small bowel permeability.

DIAGNOSIS

Celiac disease autoantibodies are used to identify individuals who should undergo biopsy-confirmation, strengthen the diagnosis of those with histological findings suggestive of celiac disease, and monitor dietary compliance after diagnosis. The most highly predictive IgA autoantibodies tests are the antiendomysial (EMA) and the antitissue transglutaminase (tTG) assays. Because tTG is the main autoantigen recognized by anti-EMA antibodies, either test may be performed, based on availability and lab experience/expertise. In symptomatic individuals, the positive predictive value of these tests approaches 1.00. Although generally inferior to EMA or tTG testing, measurement of antigliadin antibodies (AGAs) should also be performed in children less than 18 months old, as an increased proportion of children this age lack tTG or EMA antibodies. As the frequency of selective IgA deficiency in celiac disease is roughly 2%, and routine serologic assays for celiac disease use IgA antibodies, total serum IgA should be measured at initial celiac screening; if low, patients should undergo IgG testing of either EMA or tTG.

Current North American guidelines require duodenal biopsies, while on a gluten-containing diet, to make the diagnosis of celiac disease. The European Society for Pediatric Gastroenterology, Hepatology, and Nutrition (ESPGHAN), on the other hand, has recently revised their guidelines to allow omission of duodenal biopsies in the symptomatic pediatric patient with a tTG IgA greater than 10 times the upper limit of normal, provided they are EMA and HLA positive. Those not meeting these conditions must still demonstrate the histologic features indicative of celiac disease in order for diagnosis. As the characteristic histologic lesions may be patchy, a minimum of four biopsies should be obtained from the second or more distal duodenum and additional biopsies should be obtained from the duodenal bulb, as isolated disease of the bulb has been well demonstrated and bypassing the bulb may lead to a missed diagnosis in up to 10% of patients.

Endoscopic markers of villous atrophy (**20.1, 20.2**) include a mosaic pattern of the duodenal mucosa, nodular mucosa, scalloping of the duodenal folds, loss of these circular folds, and atrophic mucosa with visible vessels. While these findings are fairly specific for villous atrophy, the sensitivity of these markers is roughly only 50%. Therefore, endoscopic visualization of villous atrophy should not be relied upon for identification of celiac disease. This highlights the utility of pre-endoscopic screening and the necessity of duodenal biopsies, regardless of the presence of these endoscopic markers.

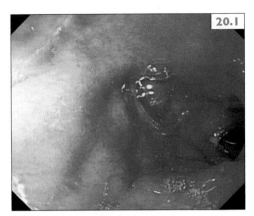

20.1 Loss of circular folds on endoscopic evaluation in celiac disease.

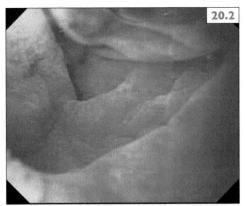

20.2 Immersion technique demonstrating loss of villi and scalloping of the duodenal folds in celiac disease.

The Marsh–Oberhuber classification is used to characterize the various histologic degrees of injury, with villous atrophy, or Marsh type 3, being a characteristic feature of celiac disease (**20.3**). Diagnosis of less straightforward cases, such as those showing infiltrative changes with crypt hyperplasia but no villous atrophy (Marsh 2), may be strengthened by other supporting criteria such as serologic and HLA testing. Symptom resolution on a gluten-free diet and reversion of positive serologic tests both support the diagnosis and suggests dietary compliance. Initial absence of serologic markers or failure to improve on the gluten-free diet warrants consideration of other causes of villous atrophy to include eosinophilic disease, infectious enteritis, and small bowel bacterial overgrowth.

PATHOPHYSIOLOGY

The immunogenic gliadin peptides in gluten are resistant to intraluminal digestion. Via a combination of impaired mucosal integrity attributable to increased zonulin release (the paracellular route) and interferon-gamma-regulated transcytosis (the transcellular route), the enhanced gut permeability of celiac patients allows these undigested peptides to cross the intestinal epithelium. Once in the lamina propria, the gliadin peptides undergo deamidation by tTG, significantly increasing the affinity of these gliadin fragments for HLA-DQ2/DQ8 molecules and leading to enhanced antigen presentation and CD4+ T cell response. These CD4+ T cells drive a TH1 predominant cytokine response, resulting in intraepithelial lymphocytosis, crypt hyperplasia, and villous atrophy. Additionally, tTG is the target celiac autoantigen of the autoimmune response. Although valuable in the screening and diagnosis of celiac disease, the role of these celiac-specific anti-tTG antibodies in disease pathogenesis is not well established. These autoantibodies may contribute to mucosal damage by inhibition of extracellular membrane-bound tTG functions and subsequent cytoskeleton changes and actin redistribution.

TREATMENT

Treatment of children diagnosed with celiac disease removes the increased cancer risk of enteropathy-related T-cell lymphoma associated with celiac disease in adulthood. Moreover treatment is protective against the consequences of enteropathy to include osteoporosis and growth failure. Although not proven, treatment may also decrease the likelihood of acquiring other autoimmune disorders associated with celiac disease, such as Type 1 diabetes and thyroid disease. The sole current treatment for celiac disease is a lifelong strict gluten-free diet, excluding wheat, rye, and barley. Oats are non disease-inducing in the vast majority of celiac patients, although there is risk for wheat contamination during processing. While the Food Allergen Labeling Consumer Protection Act of 2004 mandates packaged food labels to identify wheat, the United States Food and Drug Administration (FDA) currently has not implemented a rule for 'gluten-free' labeling. At this time, the FDA is working on a proposal based on a 'gluten-free' threshold of less than 20 parts per million (ppm) of gluten, based on a combination of evidence-based research, assay sensitivity, and the experience with current commercial 'gluten-free' products. If adopted, this law will bring the United States in line with Canada and the European Union, where the 20 ppm threshold is the standard for 'gluten-free' labeling.

Regardless of labeling, involvement of an experienced dietician is crucial for both initial dietary counseling and future compliance assessment. Serial measurement of tTG antibody levels, used in combination with nutritional assessment, initially at 6 months and then annually, is a reliable method for monitoring dietary compliance. Lastly, strict gluten avoidance requires attention to medication and pharmacy assistance, as some excipients used as binding agents may contain gluten.

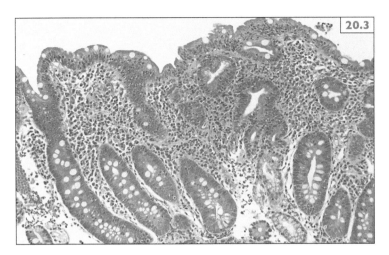

20.3 Marsh 3 with villous atrophy, increased intraepithelial lymphocytes, and hyperplastic crypts in celiac disease.

Small Bowel Infections

Niraj Patel

DEFINITION

Infections of the small intestine, including the duodenum, jejunum, and ileum, generally result from the ingestion of contaminated food or water. The majority of infections are caused by *Escherichia coli*, rotavirus, *Giardia lamblia*, and *Cryptosporidium parvum*. Other microbes have been associated with small bowel infections including *Vibrio cholerae*, *Salmonella* spp., *Shigella* spp., and *Entamoeba histolytica*.

EPIDEMIOLOGY

Annual incidence for infections of the small intestine varies according to the pathogen. Giardiasis has an annual incidence of 2 million people worldwide. The annual incidence for enterotoxigenic *E. coli* (ETEC) is estimated at 200 million people. Enteropathogenic *E. coli* (EPEC) accounts for around 5–10% of pediatric diarrheal illnesses in the developing world. *Giardia lamblia*, which causes giardiasis, occurs worldwide and is the most commonly identified intestinal parasite in the United States. The prevalence is highest in children aged 1–9 years, with a prevalence of 0.1–23.5 cases per 100,000 population in the United States. Cryptosporidiosis occurs worldwide, but is more prevalent in underdeveloped countries with infection rates as high as 32%. Rotavirus is the most common cause of diarrhea among infants and children worldwide, with more than 125 million cases of infantile diarrhea occurring each year. The development of the rotavirus vaccine has greatly reduced the incidence of rotavirus disease worldwide.

CLINICAL PRESENTATION

ETEC and EPEC present with watery diarrhea that is usually self-limited. The incubation period is 6–48 hours. Persistent diarrhea with ETEC and EPEC is uncommon. Infection with *Giardia* spp. is often asymptomatic; however, a broad spectrum of clinical symptoms can occur including diarrhea, malaise, abdominal distension, weight loss, abdominal cramps, and flatulence. Less common symptoms include vomiting, fever, and constipation. The incubation period averages 3–25 days, with a median of 7–10 days.

Cryptosporidiosis is manifested as profuse watery diarrhea, although the infection can be asymptomatic. Crampy abdominal pain, vomiting, and diarrhea can occur, but fever is uncommon. The diarrhea can contain mucous, but rarely contains white or red blood cells. Biliary tract disease, characterized by fever, right upper quadrant pain, nausea, vomiting, and diarrhea, can occur in immunocompromised patients. The incubation period is 2–14 days.

Rotavirus gastroenteritis results initially with vomiting followed by watery diarrhea. Low-grade fever may be present. Dehydration is common with severe illness. The incubation period is approximately 2 days.

ETIOLOGY AND PATHOPHYSIOLOGY

ETEC are the most common cause of gastroenteritis in travelers in developing countries. ETEC are ubiquitous in developing countries and usually follow consumption of contaminated food or water. Infants can become ill after introduction of food. ETEC utilize fimbrial colonization factor antigens to adhere to the small bowel mucosa (**21.1**). ETEC subsequently produce enterotoxins which increase secretion of fluid and electrolytes from the mucosa of the small bowel. The vehicle that transmits EPEC is unknown, but a high incidence occurs in infants less than 6 months of age and not exclusively fed breast milk in developing countries.

EPEC colonize the intestine by a bundle forming pilus, then induce an attaching and effacing lesion which disrupts the apical skeleton, and finally induce secretion of fluid from intestinal cells.

In giardiasis, *Giardia* spp. cysts are ingested and produce trophozoites, which colonize the small intestine. Subsequent damage to the intestinal epithelial cells and their brush borders occurs, leading to diarrhea. As few as 10–100 cysts are sufficient for infection, and person-to-person transmission has been reported in childcare centers.

Spread of oocysts of *Cryptosporidium* spp. occurs by person-to-person transmission or from contaminated food or water. Zoonotic transmission has also been reported. Following ingestion of infectious oocysts, sporozoites are released and invade the intestinal epithelial cells. Inside the cells, the parasite multiplies and gets released as infectious oocysts.

Rotavirus is transmitted by the fecal–oral route, and the highly concentrated virus can be found at 10 trillion infectious particles per gram of stool. Malabsorption and diarrhea, occurring after ingestion of infectious rotavirus particles, result from a variety of mechanisms including direct destruction of the intestinal enterocytes and toxins that increase chloride secretion and disrupt reabsorption of water.

DIFFERENTIAL DIAGNOSIS

- *Campylobacter* spp.
- *Clostridium perfringens*.
- *Cryptosporidium parvum*.
- *Cyclospora cayetanensis*.
- *Giardia lamblia*.
- *Isospora belli*.
- *Plesiomonas shigelloides*.
- *Salmonella* spp.
- *Shigella* spp.
- *Vibrio cholerae*.
- *Vibrio parahemolyticus*.
- *Yersinia enterocolitica*.

DIAGNOSIS

Isolation of *E. coli* from the stool requires distinguishing it from other nonpathogenic bacteria by a variety of biochemical methods as well as nucleic and non-nucleic acid detection methods for identification of phenotype. Diagnosis of giardiasis is established by detection of trophozoites or cysts in stool specimens, duodenal fluid, or tissue from small bowel (**21.2**). Cryptosporidiosis can be detected by enzyme immuonoassays or immunofluorescent assays. Definite diagnosis of crytposporidial infection is made by identifying oocysts in feces or body fluids, or along the epithelial surface of biopsy tissue (**21.3**). Diagnosis of rotavirus gastroenteritis is most commonly made by detection of the virus by enzyme immunoassay. Other detection methods include identifying viral particles by electron microscopy (**21.4**) and polymerase chain reaction.

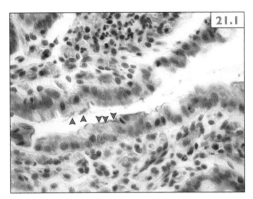

21.1 Enterotoxigenic *Escherichia coli* adhering to the brush border of the small intestinal mucosa (arrowheads).

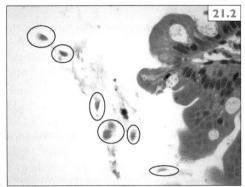

21.2 *Giardia* spp. trophozoites in the lumen of the small intestine (circled).

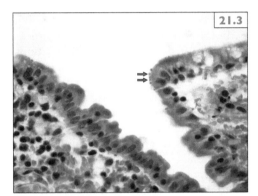

21.3 Cryptosporidiosis, showing small round bodies on the surface of the epithelium (arrows).

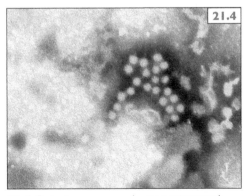

21.4 Rotavirus seen on electron micrograph.

TREATMENT

Fluid and electrolyte management is the most important step in management of patients with infection with ETEC or EPEC. Antimicrobial therapy for ETEC and EPEC in adults includes an oral flouroquinolone. In children, alternative therapy includes trimethoprim/sulfamethoxazole for ETEC or EPEC, or cefixime for ETEC. Duration of oral therapy is generally 5 days. Antimicrobial therapy should be withheld if enterohemorrhagic *E. coli* (EHEC) cannot be ruled out given that data suggest an increased risk for hemolytic uremic syndrome with usage of antimicrobials. Also, antimicrobial therapy has not been shown to alter the course of diarrhea due to EHEC.

Antimotility agents may be beneficial in patients with ETEC, but are generally contraindicated in patients with diarrhea due to EHEC. Treatment for giardiasis includes correction of dehydration and electrolyte abnormalities. The drugs of choice include metronidazole, tinidazole, or nitazoxanide for 5–7 days. Furazolidone and quinacrine are alternatives, while albendazole and mebendazole are also effective.

Most infections with *Cryptosporidium* spp. are self-limited and require no therapy except hydration. In immunocompromised individuals however, nitazoxanide is approved for the treatment of cryptosporidiosis. Clarithromycin, azithromycin, roxithro–mycin, and paromomycin have been reported to be successful against *Cryptosporidium* spp. Antidiarrheal agents, such as kaolin plus pectin, loperamide, diphenoxylate, bismuth subsalicylate, or opiates, have improved symptoms.

The mainstay of therapy for rotavirus gastroenteritis is maintenance of hydration. In 2004, the World Health Organization recommended use of a low-osmolarity oral rehydration solution and zinc supplementation for dehydration caused by acute diarrhea.

PROGNOSIS

With aggressive fluid and electrolyte management, prognosis remains excellent for diarrheal infections with ETEC and EPEC, and disease is usually self-limited. The cure rate for infections with *Giardia* is high, with relapses occurring most commonly in immunocompromised individuals who may require prolonged treatment. Most infections with *Cryptosporidium* spp. are self-limited in immunocompetent individuals. When rotavirus gastroenteritis is managed effectively with rehydration, prognosis is excellent.

Short Bowel Syndrome

Rajasekhar Bodicharla, Amber Daigre, Alan Delamatar, Debora Duro

DEFINITION AND EPIDEMIOLOGY

Short bowel syndrome (SBS) is a clinical definition used to describe those complications caused by the loss of at least 50% of the small intestine either congenitally or acquired. These complications include diarrhea, malabsorption, and malnutrition. If severe, SBS can cause intestinal failure which occurs when nutrition/fluid must be supplied using parenteral nutrition (PN). Those patients with SBS and long-term PN dependency are at risk of other complications including intestinal failure-associated liver disease (IFALD) and catheter-related infections.

Overall reported incidence of SBS is 1200/100,000 live births. Survival rates in pediatric SBS ranges from 73% to 89%, based on various factors such as the degree of shortened bowel. Furthermore, the availability of a multidisciplinary program specializing in SBS can improve survival rates and help wean SBS patients from PN.

CLINICAL PRESENTATION

Clinical manifestations of SBS in children are as follows:
- Diarrhea and steatorrhea.
- Weight loss.
- Anemia related to iron and/or vitamin B12 malabsorption.
- Bleeding diathesis related to vitamin K malabsorption.
- Osteoporosis/osteomalacia related to vitamin D and calcium malabsorption.
- Hyponatremia, hypokalemia.
- Hypovolemia.
- Macronutrient or micronutrient deficiency states.

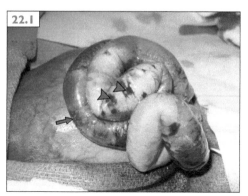

22.1 Severe necrotizing enterocolitis (NEC-totalis). This 3-week-old, former 28 week gestational age neonate developed significant abdominal distension, feeding intolerance, and severe acidosis. At laparotomy, significant pneumatosis (arrow), bowel infarcts (arrowheads), and necrosis was discovered. The entire bowel was affected from the ligament of Treitz to the mid-transverse colon; unfortunately, this child did not survive. (Courtesy of Shawn Larson, MD; Department of Surgery, University of Florida.)

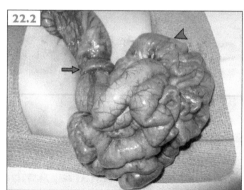

22.2 Malrotation with mid-gut volvulus. This 4-month-old infant presented to the emergency department with bilious emesis and poor peripheral perfusion. At laparotomy, a mid-gut volvulus was discovered (arrow) with ischemic bowel (arrowhead). The volvulus was reduced with adequate perfusion of the bowel. Malrotation with mid-gut volvulus is a significant etiology for short bowel syndrome. (Courtesy of Shawn Larson, MD; Department of Surgery, University of Florida.)

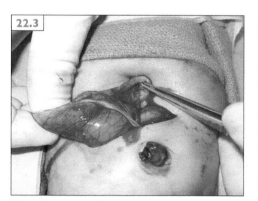

22.3 Newborn infant with jejunal atresia. This term infant was noted to have distended stomach and proximal intestinal loop. At laparotomy, a Type IIIa jejunal atresia was noted with a significant mesenteric defect and short bowel. (Courtesy of Shawn Larson, MD; Department of Surgery, University of Florida.)

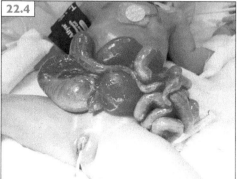

22.4 Newborn infant with gastroschisis (pre-silo reduction). This former 35 weeks gestational age infant was born with a 4 cm abdominal wall defect with stomach, large and small intestine, bladder, and ovary eviscerated. Note the mild inflammatory peal present on the intestinal loops. This child underwent silo placement, subsequent reduction and closure with delayed bowel function (prolonged enteral feeding intolerance and poor absorption).

ETIOLOGY

The most common cause for SBS in children is necrotizing enterocolitis (**22.1**), although midgut volvulus (**22.2**), intestinal atresia (**22.3**), and gastroschisis (**22.4**) are also seen. In adults, causes include Crohn disease, malignancy, radiation, and vascular insufficiency. Risk factors include a progressive underlying diagnosis such as Crohn disease or cystic fibrosis. Other important factors include the length, type, and function of the available bowel as well as the presence of the colon and ileocecal valve which may protect against bacterial overgrowth.

Complications of SBS are related to the degree of shortened bowel as well as the need for PN and adaptation of the remaining bowel. Acute complications include dehydration and electrolyte disturbances such as hyponatremia. Catheter-related problems include central venous thrombosis and sepsis which can be rapid onset and fatal. More chronic complications include IFALD. IFALD is seen in 40–60% of children receiving PN and can be seen as early as 2–4 weeks after starting PN. Although liver biopsy is considered the gold standard for diagnosing IFALD, laboratory testing is more frequently used including hepatic transaminases, total and conjugated bilirubin, albumin, prothrombin time, and gamma-glutamyl transferase.

A serum direct bilirubin concentration >2 g/dl (34 μmol/l) is associated with 20% survival compared to 80% survival rates in infants without cholestasis, suggesting a higher mortality rate in infants unable to be weaned off PN. The pathophysiology of IFALD is multifactorial and possibly related to immature liver function associated with prematurity or inflammatory mediators associated with catheter-related sepsis. Recent ongoing studies on parenteral fats enriched with omega-3 fatty acids, such as omegaven and SMOF lipids (soybean oil, medium chain triglycerides, olive oil, and fish oil), have shown potential benefit in regards to IFALD. Management strategies for IFALD include early enteral feeding, reducing the frequency/duration of PN infusion, strict aseptic techniques while handling central lines, and usage of ethanol, antibiotic, or antimicrobial locks which has been shown to decrease the rate of line infections and the need for catheter changes in these patients. Oral ursodeoxycholic acid improves bile flow and may lessen bile stasis. In children with end-stage liver disease, liver transplantation may be required. Other chronic complications include bacterial overgrowth, D-lactic acidosis, enteric hyperoxaluria, anastomotic ulcers, and nutritional deficiencies. Children with SBS exhibit a high prevalence of micronutrient deficiencies during the PN weaning process.

DIAGNOSIS

SBS is a clinical diagnosis dependent on the history and nature of intestinal loss coupled with symptoms suggestive of malabsorption. Diarrhea is the most common symptom although cramping, bloating, and weight loss frequently occur as well.

TREATMENT

Role of a multidisciplinary team in intestinal rehabilitation

There are many potential facets to the management of SBS, and it is important to recognize that each case is unique. Furthermore, the multiple and varied issues and complications related to SBS can make treatment very challenging. Therefore, a multidisciplinary approach to the care of SBS patients is preferred. The multidisciplinary team (MDT) focuses on intestinal rehabilitation and reversing, when possible, intestinal failure.

This approach to management includes monitoring for complications such as electrolyte disturbances or minimizing risk of IFALD. The inclusion of several disciplines, such as gastroenterology, surgery, nutrition, nursing, pharmacy, social work, and psychology, help treat the entire child rather than a specific aspect of their disease. Nutritional deficits can be prevented more easily, surgical and medical aspects discussed more openly, and with more resources and available data on hand to make the best decision for the child.

Psychologic considerations

Beyond the medical considerations that are imperative to the treatment of children with SBS, child psychology involvement can be very important. Prolonged hospitalizations during early life are associated with delays in motor, speech, and cognitive development. Given the extended length of hospital stays associated with intestinal failure, it is important that developmental milestone achievement be addressed in the clinical setting and that the appropriate referrals are made when delays are noted. Speech milestones may also be delayed as a function of decreased oral stimulation associated with intestinal failure, since many patients receive either PN or enteral nutrition (EN) rather than using the oral route. Prematurity, prolonged hospitalization, and enteral feeding also increase the risk of oral and food aversion. Behavioral interventions provided by the psychologist can address these aversions within the clinic setting and can provide parents with strategies for use within the home, such as lip stimulation, inclusion in mealtimes, and exposure to varied food textures to increase tolerance and expand dietary repertoire. In addition, identifying and helping to minimize the parental stress that is common to families of chronically ill children further improves long-term management of children with SBS.

Enteral feeding

The initial period following intestinal resection is focused on stabilization and maintenance of a good nutritional status through administration of PN and gradual introduction of EN. This initial period may be complicated by large volume fluid and electrolyte losses, needing careful fluid and electrolyte management. Gastric hypersecretion following intestinal resection may be associated with pancreatic enzyme deactivation, altered nutrient and drug absorption, and increased intestinal fluid loss. Proton pump inhibitors have been shown to be effective in reducing fluid losses and improving absorption and acid suppression in SBS. Once the infant's fluid and electrolytes are stable, enteral feeds should be introduced slowly to enhance intestinal adaptation. Initially, continuous feeds via a gastrostomy tube are preferred over bolus feeds. Several enteral formulas are available commercially and can be selected based on individual patient characteristics. Breast milk or protein hydrolysate formula may be used initially as they are hypoallergenic, but some infants may need elemental formulas composed of simple amino acid monomers.

In general, hypoallergenic formulas are well tolerated and absorbed better compared to regular formulas in SBS patients. Older children generally may not need elemental formulas as protein allergy is uncommon at this age. Fiber supplementation may be helpful in preventing high fluid losses in SBS patients with a remaining colon, as fiber can decrease stool volume and can be useful in infants with perianal skin breakdown. Medium-chain triglycerides can be supplemented because of better absorption compared to long-chain triglycerides due to bile acid or pancreatic insufficiency. Lactose restriction is usually not necessary in children with SBS; however, it should be restricted in the presence of intolerance. Higher oxalate-containing foods (beets, cocoa, spinach, and rhubarb) may need to be restricted to prevent kidney stone formation. Vitamin and trace element replacement may be considered based on the blood levels of these nutrients. PN should be gradually tapered as the enteral intake increases. Indications for continued PN include poor weight gain and fluid and electrolyte imbalances which cannot be replaced orally.

Factors affecting resumption of oral diet

- Length of remaining intestine: immediate postsurgical bowel length is a poor indicator of whether the child will need PN by itself. Proximal small intestine is mostly responsible for absorption of proteins, carbohydrates, and fats.
- Presence of colon and intact ileocecal valve: loss of colon along with extensive small bowel resection is associated with long-term PN requirement as the colon plays an important role in water and electrolyte absorption. The ileocecal valve serves as a barrier to colonic bacteria and delays small bowel transit which improves nutrient absorption. Loss of the ileocecal valve is associated with rapid intestinal transit and bacterial translocation in the small bowel with subsequent bacterial overgrowth.
- Intestinal adaptation: the ileum can adapt to proximal small bowel resection, and resection of ileum can be problematic since the jejunum has limited adaptability. The ileum is associated with vitamin B12 and bile acid absorption, and resection can lead to vitamin B12 and bile acid malabsorption. Bile acid malabsorption, consequently, can cause fat soluble vitamin deficiency and cholerheic enteropathy. Gastric emptying is also delayed by the presence of unabsorbed lipids in an intact ileum, and ileal resection causes the loss of this compensatory mechanism which can contribute to diarrhea in SBS. Intestinal adaptation involves lengthening of intestinal villi rather than upregulation of specific transporters. Small bowel dilation and lengthening of intestinal villi increases the absorptive surface area. Enteral feeds facilitate intestinal adaptation by stimulating both biliary and pancreatic secretions as well as enterocyte-derived mediators such a glucagon-like peptide. Intestinal adaptation will not occur if there is total reliance on PN. Intestinal adaptation is less likely if <15 cm small bowel is remaining, the ileocecal valve is removed, or the colon is removed and primary anastomosis cannot be performed.

Indirect assessment of intestinal adaptation may be obtained by measuring citrulline, an enterocyte-produced amino acid. Citrulline has been studied as a marker for enterocyte mass and as a predictor for PN dependence. Decreased levels of this biomarker indicate bowel loss/dysfunction while increasing levels may reflect intestinal adaptation and ability to discontinue PN.

Surgery

Various surgical interventions are needed to establish full EN in infants with SBS. These procedures include placement of a gastrostomy tube or gastroduodenal/gastrojejunal tube in patients with motility disorders involving the stomach or duodenum. These enteral tubes ensure access to the gastrointestinal (GI) tract as most of these infants have poor oropharyngeal reflexes and abnormal swallowing. Many infants with SBS have proximal small intestinal ostomies, and intestinal continuity should be established as soon as medically/surgically feasible. Continuity of bowel ensures maximal contact and absorption of nutrients, fluid, and electrolytes.

Intestinal lengthening procedures have been used to lengthen the dilated small bowel to increase the length of intestine and the absorptive surface. The Bianchi procedure involves longitudinal intestinal lengthening where the lumen is recreated by formation of two narrow channels which are approximated in series to potentially double the length of intestine. The serial transverse enteroplasty (STEP) procedure involves applying a surgical stapler at right angles to the bowel in successive, alternating sides so as to create a zig-zag formation of a longer and narrower channel (**22.5**). The STEP procedure also increases intestinal length and absorptive area while decreasing the risk of small bowel bacterial overgrowth and D-lactic acidosis (**22.6, 22.7**).

Intestinal transplantation

Intestinal transplantation has been primarily used only as a life-saving therapy for intestinal failure patients who fail PN therapy and for those patients with life-threatening abdominal pathology. Failure of PN therapy is characterized as significant liver injury with elevated transaminases and cholestasis, multiple line infections, thrombosis of two of the central veins, and/or frequent episodes of dehydration. Absolute contraindications to small bowel transplantation include profound neurologic disability, life-threatening and other irreversible diseases that are unrelated to the GI system, and nonresectable malignancies. There are three different kinds of intestinal transplantation: intestine alone, liver plus intestine, and multivisceral that contains stomach, duodenum, pancreas, intestine, and liver. Transplantation still carries significant morbidity and mortality, including the need for life-long immune suppression and associated complications due to infection and rejection.

Tissue engineering

Functional tissue engineering of the GI tract is a complex process aiming to aid the regeneration of structural layers of smooth muscle, intrinsic enteric neuronal plexuses, specialized mucosa, and epithelial cells as well as interstitial cells.

The final tissue-engineered construct is intended to mimic the native GI tract anatomically and physiologically. This modality has been increasingly explored as it would potentially prevent the complications associated with transplant as well as the need for immune suppression. Over the last decade, significant advances have been made to mitigate adverse host reactions. These include a quest for identifying autologous cell sources such as embryonic and adult stem cells, bone marrow-derived cells, neural crest-derived cells, and muscle derived-stem cells.

ACKNOWLEDGMENT

The authors would like gratefully to acknowledge the contributions of Thomas G. Diamantidis, Pharm.D, Rod Okamoto, RPh., and Andrea Hershorin, ARNP in the preparation of this material.

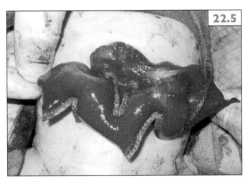

22.5 Newborn infant with jejunal atresia. A tapering enteroplasty was performed followed by anastomosis. A serial transverse enteroplasty was then performed in an attempt to lengthen the remaining intestine.

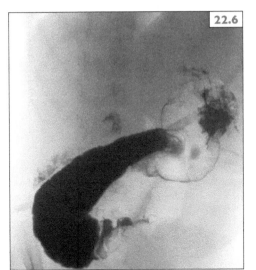

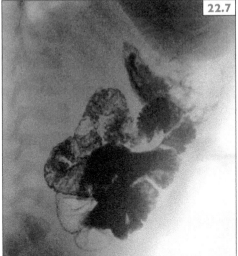

22.6, 22.7 Serial transverse enteroplasty (STEP). **22.6**: Pre-STEP radiograph showing shortened, dilated small intestine relative to post-STEP radiograph (**22.7**) demonstrating lengthened, narrower bowel.

Protein-Losing Enteropathy

Khalid Khan, Zohreh Movahedi

DEFINITION

Protein-losing enteropathy (PLE), defined as the abnormal loss of protein from the gastrointestinal (GI) tract, occurs in many diseases through pathologic processes that involve the enteric, vascular, and lymphatic systems. In healthy adults, about 1–2% of plasma albumin is lost daily from the enteric system; in individuals with symptomatic PLE, however, that rate increases to 40–60%.

CLINICAL PRESENTATION

The cardinal features of PLE are edema and hypoalbuminemia, lymphopenia, and loss of T cells and immunoglobulins. Lymphopenia may appear years after the onset of protein loss and in variable ways. Asymmetric peripheral edema may signify a lymph disorder that precedes PLE.

Children with intestinal lymphangiectasia typically have diarrhea; other symptoms include fatigue, fever, weight loss, and abdominal pain. Growth retardation is common in chronic cases of PLE. In general, manifestations are variable and depend on the underlying disease processes (malabsorption, inflammation, infection, or malignancy).

ETIOLOGY
Primary intestinal lymphangiectasia
Intestinal lymphangiectasia, an uncommon condition, is characterized by diffuse or localized ectasia of the enteric lymphatics (**23.1–23.3**), often in association with

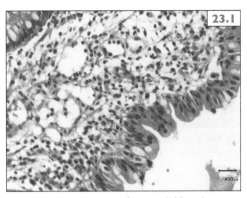

23.1 Duodenal mucosa from a child with protein-losing enteropathy showing dilated lacteals. Eosinophilia is also present.

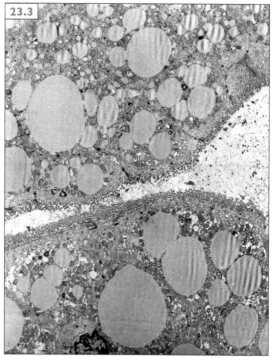

23.2 Duodenal mucosa from a child with protein-losing enteropathy showing ectatic lymphatics (arrow).

23.3 Electron microscopy of enterocytes, from **23.1** and **23.2** showing fat globules.

lymphatic abnormalities elsewhere that may present at any age.

Secondary lymphangiectasia

Lymphatic obstruction occurs in a wide range of disorders. In children, certain syndromes are associated with intestinal lymphangiectasia, most notably Turner, Noonan, and Klippel–Trénaunay–Weber syndromes. Intestinal lymphangiectasia has also been reported in families.

Lymphatic obstruction can be seen in patients with infiltrative processes (such as lymphoma, tuberculosis, and sarcoidosis). Elevated lymph pressure can occur from mechanical obstruction (as in malrotation) or can have more remote origins (due to structural heart defects, constrictive pericarditis, cardiomyopathy, following cardiac surgery, or transplant). The Fontan procedure is a well-known precursor of PLE, which sometimes appears years after the procedure itself.

Mucosal disease and enterocyte dysfunction

Erosion, ulceration, and inflammation of the intestinal mucosa causing PLE may be the result of infectious or noninfectious disorders. Infectious causes include bacterial overgrowth, malaria, viruses, and parasites. In children, measles and rotavirus are known causes, and PLE may be part of a postviral syndrome. Hirschsprung disease and necrotizing enterocolitis – causes of PLE that may, in part, be related to the microbiological environment – are specific to children; in contrast, peptic and immune-related inflammation may develop at any age.

PLE is very occasionally a feature associated with cow's milk protein allergy. Other enteropathic processes that can cause PLE include celiac disease and eosinophilic disease. Severe malnutrition, systemic vasculitidies (including Henoch–Schönlein purpura), congenital disorders of glycosylation, and

phenobarbital toxicity may be seen in the pediatric population while hypertrophic gastropathy (Ménétrier disease) and the Zollinger–Ellison syndrome are both causes of PLE although extremely rare causes in children.

PATHOPHYSIOLOGY

Primary lymphangiectasia is characterized by ectatic lymphatics located in the mucosa, submucosa, or subserosa. Lymphatic occlusion or agenesis results in an increase in pressure and rupture, with loss of proteinaceous lymph from the lacteals in mucosal microvilli. In patients with cardiac disorders, chronically elevated systemic venous pressure and increased thoracic duct pressure may be implicated in the development of PLE.

In patients with lymphatic disorders, mucosal pathologic changes include alteration in the enterocyte basal membrane glycosaminoglycans. In patients with PLE, loss of proteoglycans from the intestinal epithelium may be the result of increased lymphatic pressure or inflammation. Furthermore, in patients with congenital glycosylation defects (characterized by loss of heparan sulfate proteoglycans) PLE may be secondary to increased intestinal permeability.

Primary mucosal disorders involve the release of proinflammatory cytokines, resulting in disruption of mucosal cells and in increased intestinal permeability to proteins. Matrix metalloproteinases degrade components of the extracellular matrix in ulcer formation. The degradation of epithelial proteoglycans may be implicated in protein leakage, epithelial permeability, hyperemia, and disruption of the mucosal integrity.

DIAGNOSIS

A child with edema and hypoalbuminemia, who is otherwise well-nourished and who does not have renal or liver disease, should undergo evaluation for PLE. Cardiac disease may not

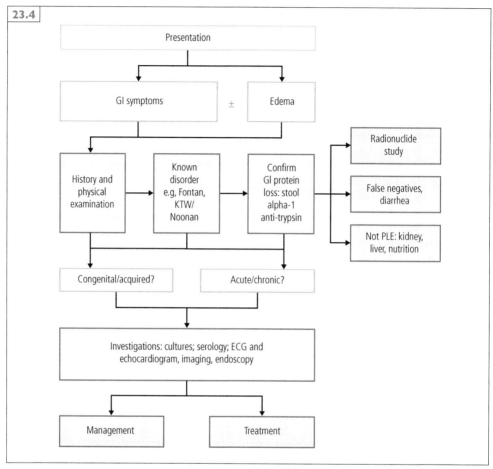

23.4 Proposed algorithm for the management of protein-losing enteropathy (PLE) in children. ECG: electrocardiogram; GI: gastrointestinal; KTW: Klippel–Trénaunay–Weber syndrome.

be evident from the history and physical examination; in unclear cases, it should be actively investigated (**23.4**).

Detection of intestinal protein loss

Stool concentration of the protease inhibitor alpha-1 antitrypsin (A1AT) is a marker of intestinal protein loss. It has a molecular weight similar to albumin and is not secreted, absorbed, or present in the diet. Resistant to digestion, it is detectable for up to 3 days in fecal samples. Fecal A1AT clearance (normal value, <24 ml/24 h) is a highly sensitive tool in diagnosing PLE in adults. However, it is *not* reliable in patients with gastric protein loss or GI blood loss, and A1AT undergoes degradation when the pH is <3. Intravenous administration of radiolabeled (chromium 51) albumin followed by a timed stool analysis is a standard method to assess enteric protein loss.

Localization of disease

Scintigraphy with technetium 99m-labeled albumin can be used to localize the intestinal site of protein loss. Lymphangiectasia in the small intestine may be identified with an enteral contrast study or computed tomography (CT). Magnetic resonance imaging (MRI) has been shown to be of value in the examination of the intestine (**23.5**), mesentery, thoracic duct, and mesenteric lymphatics as well as the peripheral limb. In diagnosing underlying disorders associated with PLE, both CT and MRI are indicated.

Endoscopy or enteroscopy with biopsy will reveal hypertrophic gastric folds of Ménétrier disease, inflammation, erosion, enteropathy, and certain infections. After a high-fat meal, endoscopy may show edema and the typical 'starry-sky' appearance of the mucosa with prominent villi (**23.6, 23.7**). Histologically, ectatic, dilated lacteals can be visualized in the mucosa (**23.1**). An enteric capsule study may be similarly useful to demonstrate PLE findings.

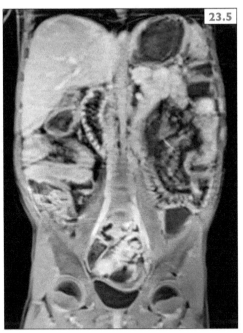

23.5 MRI showing abnormal enhancement of the small bowel (beaded appearance) on post-contrast T1 images of a 9-year-old patient with a diagnosis of protein-losing enteropathy and lymphangiectasia.

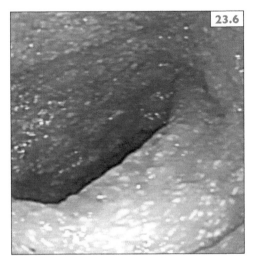

23.6 Endoscopic appearance of the small bowel in a child with protein-losing enteropathy showing a 'starry-sky' reflection pattern.

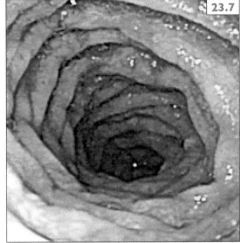

23.7 Endoscopic appearance of the small bowel in a child with protein-losing enteropathy showing an edematous small bowel and lymph engorged villi.

TREATMENT

A high-protein, low-fat diet supplemented with medium-chain triglycerides (MCTs) is the most suitable nutritional regimen for patients with PLE. MCTs are absorbed directly into the portal circulation, bypassing the enteric lymphatic system; as a consequence, lymphatic flow and pressure are reduced. Diuretics and supportive care (with stockings, limb elevation, and protection of the skin) may help avoid complications from peripheral edema. Intake of fat-soluble vitamins should be monitored and supplemented.

Management of the underlying disorder is a prerequisite for the treatment of PLE. In patients who develop PLE after heart surgery, administration of corticosteroids, heparin, and surgical intervention (baffle fenestration of a transplanted heart) have been successful. The mechanisms of such actions are thought to include stabilizing the capillary endothelium and reducing protein leakage into the extravascular space and gut lumen. In some patients, surgery for local intestinal disease may be the only option.

Crohn Disease

Michael Docktor

DEFINITION AND EPIDEMIOLOGY

Crohn disease (CD) is a chronic inflammatory bowel disease (IBD) which can cause transmural inflammation in a discontinuous distribution throughout the gastrointestinal (GI) tract from the oral cavity to the anus. The entity was first described in 1932 by Dr. Burrell Crohn and colleagues as a 'regional ileitis' characterized by subacute inflammation causing ulceration, a 'disproportionate connective tissue reaction', stenosis, and formation of multiple fistulas of the terminal ileum.

Similar to ulcerative colitis (UC), a form of IBD characterized by inflammation isolated to the mucosa of the colon, nearly 25% of patients with CD are diagnosed before the age of 16 years. Median age of diagnosis of CD was 12.9 years in a study of 379 children across the United Kingdom and Ireland. This same study noted an annual incidence of 3 per 100,000 children with a 62% male predominance.

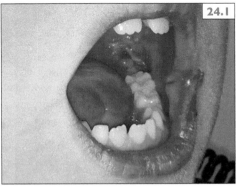

24.1 Common oral manifestations of Crohn disease include angular cheilitis and posterior mucosal tags. Other findings include painless labial swelling, recurrent aphthous lesions, mucogingivitis and cobblestoning of the buccal mucosa (not shown).

CLINICAL PRESENTATION

CD has an often insidious presentation, with average time to diagnosis of roughly 5 months from onset of symptoms in children. This delay is due to the vague and systemic symptoms that may mimic many other illnesses. Children with CD are most likely to present with abdominal pain (86%), while other classical symptoms include weight loss (80%), diarrhea (78%), blood in the stool (49%), perianal lesions (49%), fevers (38%), mouth ulcers (28%), and arthralgias (17%).

Particular attention should be paid to children with chronic or recurrent oral ulcerations/ inflammation and perianal disease such as large anal tags, recurrent abscesses, or fistulae (24.1, 24.2). The differential diagnosis with these particular findings is limited and may herald the diagnosis of CD years prior to the development of intestinal symptoms.

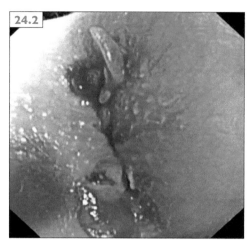

24.2 Perianal manifestations seen in Crohn disease. Note the large perianal skin tag at the 12 o'clock position with multiple small perianal fissures and fistulae present at the 7 o'clock position.

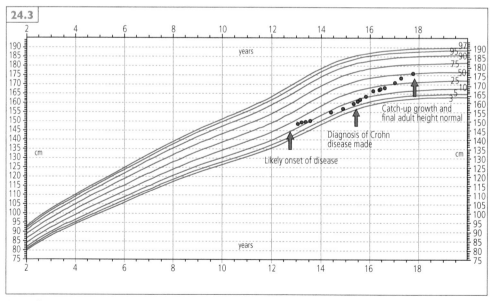

24.3 Growth chart of classical presentation of Crohn disease in a young male. Given insidious onset, a plateau of linear growth and crossing of percentiles is noted long before diagnosis is made. Note recovery of height velocity and achievement of near-expected adult height.

Table 24.1

Site	Extraintestinal manifestation
Musculoskeletal system	Arthritis: colitic type, ankylosing spondylitis, isolated joint involvement
	Hypertrophic osteoarthropathy: clubbing, periostitis
	Miscellaneous manifestations: osteoporosis, aseptic necrosis, polymyositis
Dermatologic and oral systems	Reactive lesions: erythema nodosum, pyoderma gangrenosum, aphthous ulcers, necrotizing vasculitis
	Specific lesions: fissures, fistulas, oral Crohn disease, drug rashes
	Nutritional deficiencies: acrodermatitis enteropathica, purpura, glossitis, hair loss, brittle nails
	Associated diseases: vitiligo, psoriasis, amyloidosis
Hepatopancreatobiliary system	Primary sclerosing cholangitis, bile duct carcinoma
	Associated inflammation: autoimmune chronic active hepatitis, pericholangitis, portal fibrosis, cirrhosis, granulomatous disease
	Metabolic manifestations: fatty liver, gallstones associated with ileal Crohn disease
Ocular system	Uveitis/iritis, episcleritis, scleromalacia, corneal ulcers, retinal vascular disease
Metabolic system	Growth retardation in children and adolescents, delayed sexual maturation
Renal system	Calcium oxalate stones

From: Levine JS, Burakoff R. Extraintestinal manifestations of inflammatory bowel disease. *Gastroenterology and Hepatology* 2011;**7**(4):235–241.

Given the systemic inflammatory nature of CD, nearly every system of the body may be affected by extraintestinal manifestations (*Table 24.1*). Furthermore, the toll of this disease has a profound impact on the growth and nutrition of developing children. This finding can be seen in the marked growth and pubertal arrest seen in CD (**24.3**). Circulating inflammatory cytokines in concert with inadequate caloric intake, increased loss from diarrhea, and malabsorption lead to dramatic losses in weight and bone density, and consequently linear growth. These issues are only compounded by corticosteroids, a frequently used induction therapy medication, which may further impair growth and bone mineralization.

ETIOLOGY

The precise cause of CD is unknown; however, it is thought to be a multifactorial process due to an aberrant interaction of the mucosal immune system with a complex array of food, microbial, and environmental antigens in genetically susceptible individuals.

Genetics

The study of the genetics of CD in particular has yielded much evidence to support its role in the pathogenesis of the disease. Nearly one-third of patients diagnosed with CD under 20 years of age have a positive family history of CD. Twin studies demonstrate an incredibly high concordance rate among monozygotic twins, as high as 58% when compared to 0–4.5% in dizygotic twins. Clustering within families has been widely recognized and led to many of the discoveries of specific susceptibility loci. Within ethnic groups, Jewish Americans have among the highest risk of developing IBD, with a two to nine times greater prevalence than that of their Caucasian, non-Jewish counterparts.

Identification of the first, specific susceptibility locus, NOD2/CARD15 has led to phenomenal discoveries in the etiopathogenesis of CD. This gene plays a role in the recognition of cellular components of bacteria and is found in one-third of Caucasians with CD. Those with two copies of the risk allele have a 20–40-fold increased risk of developing CD. Interestingly, a genotype/phenotype relationship is becoming increasingly evident with a striking association noted with ileal disease, earlier onset, and even stricturing behavior in multiple-allele carriers.

Immune system

Since the discovery of NOD2/CARD15, over 100 other susceptibly loci have been discovered, nearly one-third of which overlap with UC. These genes control cellular and immune regulation of autophagy, microbial recognition, and mucosal barrier function. At its core, CD appears to be a dysregulated immune response to the hundreds of millions of microbes, food, and environmental antigens interacting with the mucosal immune system and propagation of an aberrant inflammatory response.

Environment

Among the multitude of environmental factors contributing to the development of IBD, the role of diet may have the greatest impact. Studies have shown a marked increase in the incidence of CD in the setting of a westernization of the diet. This aspect is thought to be related to the increased intake of proinflammatory omega-6 polyunsaturated fatty acids (PUFAs), versus the anti-inflammatory omega-3 PUFAs found most commonly in fish. This finding is further supported by the robust clinical and histologic response to exclusive enteral therapy and its ability to induce remission in CD. The relationship with microbes and the diet also is becoming increasingly clear; however, whether the diet is modulating the microbes and thereby the immune system or *vice versa* remains an area of intense research.

DIFFERENTIAL DIAGNOSIS

Given the multitude of presenting symptoms in CD, the differential diagnosis is extensive and includes: infections such as *Mycobacterium tuberculosis*, *Yersinia enterocolitica*, and *Clostridium difficile*; inflammatory conditions such as UC; and vasculitis as seen in Henoch–Schönlein purpura and Behçet disease. Other etiologies including lymphoma, hidradenitis suppurativa and chronic granulomatous disease should be considered.

DIAGNOSIS

CD may have very subtle findings early in its course. As such, one must remain vigilant particularly in the setting of abdominal pain, a nearly universal complaint. Clues to a more insidious cause of abdominal pain may include concomitant growth failure, rectal bleeding, pubertal delay, weight loss, fatigue, anemia, or a family history of IBD. When CD is suspected, a thorough physical examination including careful inspection of the oral cavity and perianal area, should be performed. Physical examination should be followed by screening laboratory studies including a complete blood count, erythrocyte sedimentation rate, C-reactive protein, electrolytes, albumin, transaminases, and fecal occult blood. Normal laboratory values should not preclude one from further investigation if the suspicion remains high. Due to their relatively low sensitivity, IBD serologies such as anti-*Saccharomyces cerevisiae* antibodies (ASCA), along with perinuclear antineutrophil cytoplasmic antibodies

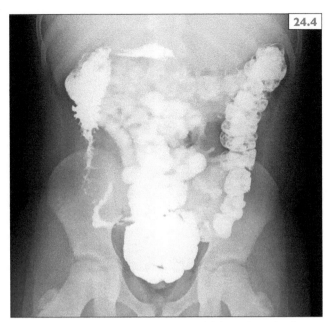

24.4 Upper gastrointestinal small bowel follow-through of patient with severe ileocecal Crohn disease. Note the string of contrast on the right representing stricturing of the terminal ileum and cecum. (Courtesy of Athos Bousvaros, MD, MPH; Boston Children's Hospital/Harvard Medical School.)

(ANCA) are generally discouraged as a screening tool.

A broad differential diagnosis should be considered given the often variable presentation and potentially normal laboratory findings. Prompt referral to a pediatric gastroenterologist should follow once the diagnosis of IBD is suspected. Contrast imaging, such as abdominal magnetic resonance imaging or an upper GI with small bowel follow-through barium study, may help define the presence of small bowel disease and help to differentiate CD from UC (**24.4**). Ultimately, endoscopic evaluation is necessary to define the extent and location of inflammation and to obtain biopsies to help diagnose and define IBD phenotype. Follow-up investigations should include assessment of extraintestinal manifestations including growth and pubertal status, nutritional and micronutrient deficiencies, and disease complications including stricturing and penetrating sequelae.

Classically, CD causes transmural, skip lesions throughout the GI tract commonly involving the terminal ileum. In a study of nearly 300 children with CD, 43% presented with ileocolonic and upper tract CD. Typical macroscopic features include a spectrum of ulcerations from superficial aphthous lesions which may progress, to deep penetrating linear ulcerations (**24.5–24.11**). Histologically, CD shows a basal plasmacytosis, transmural inflammation, and in roughly 20–40% of cases, a pathognomonic epithelioid granuloma (**24.12**).

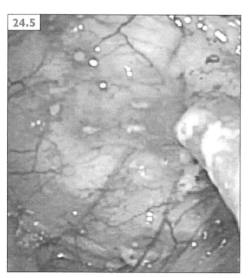

24.5 Several small, scattered aphthae of the cecum.

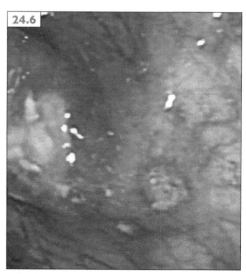

24.6 Larger solitary aphthous lesion.

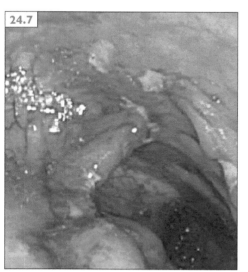

24.7 Several deeper, stellate ulcerations of the cecum.

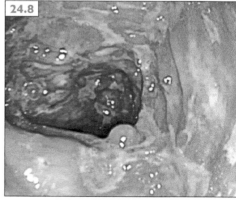

24.8 Classical Crohn ileitis with deep ulcerations, mucopurulent exudate, erythema, and edema.

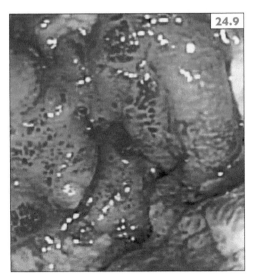

24.9 Petechiae and ulcerations with mucus seen in the terminal ileum of Crohn disease.

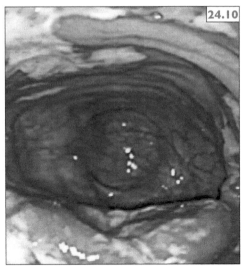

24.10 Inflamed and stenotic ileocecal valve at the 6 o'clock position, with deep linear ulcerations of the cecum. Note skip lesions and surrounding normal appearing mucosa.

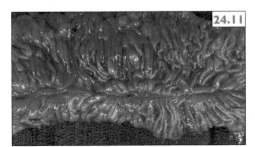

24.11 Deep linear ulceration across resected portion of small bowel with a bleeding vessel in the center.

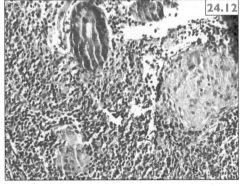

24.12 A typical noncaseating granuloma of Crohn disease. (Courtesy of Jeffery Goldsmith, MD; Children's Hospital Boston/Deaconess Medical Center.)

TREATMENT

CD is a heterogeneous inflammatory disorder, which may affect any area of the body in addition to the GI tract. Understanding the disease phenotype and with increasing importance, genotype, may allow the clinician to select the most appropriate therapy. Age of onset, location, behavior, and effects on growth are all key disease parameters outlined in the Paris classification of pediatric CD (*Table 24.2*). While clinical response and laboratory normalization is a desired end point, the more current concept of 'mucosal healing' has become a more sought after goal and has been shown to change the natural history of the disease with reduced rates of hospitalization and need for surgical resection.

Given the chronic and relapsing nature of CD, the maxim of therapy is to induce a robust and lasting remission. This aspect is paramount for children in particular, in order to maximize opportunity for growth, pubertal development, social development, and quality of life. To achieve this, one may require a combination of nutritional, surgical, and medical therapies. Much debate has centered around two concepts in medical treatment in CD, the 'step-up' *versus* 'top-down' approach. Ultimately, finding the most appropriate therapy for a patient and their family is a difficult decision that must take into account many factors. Among these are a child's specific disease phenotype, the presence of extraintestinal manifestations, and a child's growth, nutritional, and pubertal status. The risk of toxicity and side-effects of chosen therapies must be weighed and balanced with their known or theorized benefit. Therapeutic options comprise both induction and maintenance medications and include nutritional therapy, corticosteroids, 5-aminosalicylates, immunosuppressants and biologics, each with their own mechanism of action, risks, and benefits.

PROGNOSIS

Longitudinal studies on the natural history of CD demonstrate that the disease is a progressively destructive illness, which has more severe effects on children over a lifetime. By 20 years following diagnosis, as many as 80% of patients with CD will require intestinal surgery. The early induction of remission and prevention of disease progression to stricturing and penetrating events may ultimately lead to less morbidity and indeed mortality throughout a lifetime with CD. The ability to prognosticate disease behavior and tailor predictive therapy based on this is the hope of many of the investigations ongoing from genome-wide association studies to the microbiome and analysis of the host environment–immune interaction.

Table 24.2 Paris classification of Crohn disease

Age
- A1a: 0–<10 y
- A1b: 10–<17 y
- A2: 17–40 y
- A3: >40 y

Location
- L1: distal 1/3 ileum ± limited cecal disease
- L2: colonic
- L3: ileocolonic
- L4a: upper disease proximal to Ligament of Treitz
- L4b: upper disease distal to ligament of Treitz and proximal to distal 1/3 ileum

Behavior
- B1: nonstricturing nonpenetrating
- B2: stricturing
- B3: penetrating
- B2B3: both penetrating and stricturing disease, either at the same or different times
- p: perianal disease modifier

Growth
- G0: No evidence of growth delay
- G1: Growth delay

(From: Levine *et al.* Pediatric modification of the Montreal classification for inflammatory bowel disease: the Paris classification. *Inflammatory Bowel Diseases* 2011;**17**(6):1314–1321.)

Bacterial Overgrowth

Susan S. Baker

DEFINITION AND EPIDEMIOLOGY

Small intestine bacterial overgrowth (SIBO) is defined as a condition in which abnormally large numbers of bacteria are resident in the small intestine. SIBO is fairly rare, although its true prevalence and relationship to specific diseases and symptoms, such as irritable bowel syndrome, is in dispute. The proximal small intestine usually contains a small number of culturable bacteria that rarely exceeds 10^3 colony units (CFU)/ml in the jejunum. In about 33% of healthy individuals no bacteria can be cultured. It is important to note, however, that not all bacteria in the gastrointestinal (GI) tract can be cultured and that the application of molecular techniques to the study of small bowel ecology may change current understanding of SIBO. SIBO most commonly develops after surgery that creates a pouch or partial obstruction (**25.1**), when the small bowel has abnormal motility, or when the small bowel length is so short so that bacteria can increase substantially in number and even compete for nutrients.

CLINICAL PRESENTATION

The most common symptoms are diarrhea, abdominal pain/cramping, weight loss, bloating, nausea, vomiting, and constipation. Other symptoms, such as hypoalbuminemia, epigastric discomfort, edema, incontinence, vitamin deficiency,

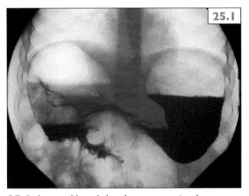

25.1 Large dilated duodenum proximal to a surgically caused stenotic area in the second portion of the duodenum.

abdominal distention, steatorrhea, flatulence, and protein-losing enteropathy, occur less frequently. Conditions that predispose to bacterial overgrowth include the use of acid reducing medications, diabetes, surgery, obstruction, chronic renal failure, resection of the ileocecal valve, chronic pancreatitis, and intestinal dysmotility.

SIBO can occur in the presence of other conditions, or other conditions may predispose to the development of SIBO. For example, Crohn disease with associated bowel dysmotility, fistulae, or perhaps surgical resection may predispose a child to SIBO. The symptoms of abdominal pain, bloating, and diarrhea are characteristic of irritable bowel syndrome as well as SIBO.

DIFFERENTIAL DIAGNOSIS

- Malabsorption.
- Short bowel.
- Functional GI disease (such as functional constipation or irritable bowel syndrome).

DIAGNOSIS

There are several tools to diagnose SIBO. Each, however, is fraught with inaccuracies and so care must be taken when SIBO is considered.

Culture

Culture of aspirated small bowel fluid from the jejunum is considered the 'gold standard' for diagnosis of SIBO. Several techniques are available to sample the GI tract for SIBO and include brushings and biopsies of the mucosa and aspiration of luminal fluid, each of which are then cultured. SIBO is generally defined as $\geq 10^5$ CFU/ml (colony forming units per milliliter); however, a recent systematic review of the literature concluded that there is no level of bacteria that can be considered diagnostic of SIBO. Care must be taken when using the aspiration technique that the fluid is obtained from the jejunum and not the second portion of the duodenum as the bacterial content is different. Studies using one technique cannot be compared to studies using a different technique. In addition, aspiration of luminal contents is invasive, time consuming, and risks contamination by oral and esophageal bacterial contents. Finally, many GI bacteria have not been or cannot be cultured.

Breath tests

Several possible breath tests are available to assess for SIBO including ^{14}C labeled bile acids and ^{13}C and/or ^{14}C D-xylose and hydrogen and/or methane breath quantitation. Hydrogen and methane breath tests are most commonly used and are based on the premise that nonabsorbed carbohydrate is fermented by bacteria in the gut lumen, generally anaerobic bacteria in the colon. When the carbohydrate reaches the colon and bacteria that are normally present produce hydrogen and/or methane gas, these gases are measured in the breath. A simple sugar, such as glucose, or a nonabsorbable carbohydrate, such as lactulose, is most commonly used. Several days prior to the breath test a low fiber diet must be followed to avoid a high baseline hydrogen/methane. After a 12 hour fast a baseline breath hydrogen/methane is obtained and then the sugar is administered. The breath analysis is then repeated every 15 minutes for several hours. An early rise in breath hydrogen/methane is used to indicate SIBO (**25.2**). However, several factors make this simplistic interpretation difficult at times to apply to clinical situations. If rapid transit is present, the carbohydrate can reach the colon in a very short time and the early rise in hydrogen/methane would not signal SIBO. Malabsorption, a high fiber diet, or oral flora can confuse interpretation of the breath test. Smoking and acid suppression, as well as performing the test in a nonfasted state affect hydrogen/methane levels in the breath. If the resident colonic bacteria do not produce hydrogen or methane, these gases will not be measured in the breath, whether SIBO is present or not. There is controversy over which carbohydrate reflects more accurately the presence of bacteria in the small bowel.

Diagnosis of SIBO based on breath testing is controversial. Some recognize a high baseline noting it represents ongoing fermentation by bacteria present proximally, others ascribe a high baseline to a nonfasting state, or continued consumption of a high fiber diet until the time of fasting. Some accept an increase within 90 minutes of ingestion of the carbohydrate of greater than 20 ppm above basal or an increase of greater than 20 ppm above basal hydrogen/methane within 180 minutes of ingestion of the carbohydrate. Most clinicians accept the following double peak description as a positive breath test: an early elevation in breath hydrogen/methane that signals bacteria in the small bowel and a later, second peak that marks metabolism of the carbohydrate by cecal bacteria.

Other tests

Imaging studies, urinary D-lactate levels, serum markers, such as bile acids, folic acid, and cobalamin, and a trial of antibiotics have been purported to identify SIBO. However, none of these strategies have been validated.

PATHOPHYSIOLOGY

SIBO occurs when normal defensive functions, such as gastric acid, pancreatic and biliary secretions, the presence of mucus, and intestinal motility, are disrupted and stasis ensues. Absence of the ileocecal valve in the distal small bowel, which acts as a mechanical barrier against the colonization of the small bowel with colonic bacteria, promotes SIBO.

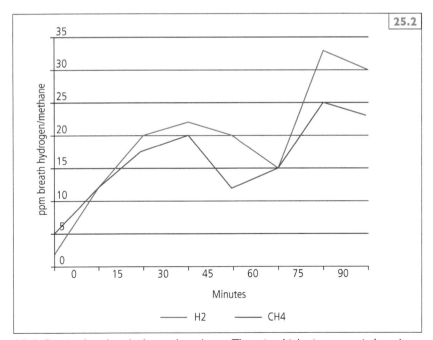

25.2 Positive lactulose hydrogen breath test. There is a biphasic pattern in breath hydrogen and methane levels with an early increase of at least 12 ppm, followed by a second much larger increase after 1 hour. In some instances the two peaks may merge as an early plateau.

TREATMENT

Because SIBO is a secondary phenomenon, treatment is focused on correcting the primary problem which may be an anatomic or physiologic abnormality or medication-induced physiological disruption such as acid suppression or dysmotility. If the primary GI abnormality cannot be corrected, then the risk of recurrent bouts of SIBO is high. Treatment is generally with an antibiotic, preferably a poorly absorbed one, such as neomycin or rifaximin. Metronidazole, trimethoprim–sulfamethoxazole and even liquid gentamicin can be used. However, without cultures, it is difficult to know if the chosen antibiotic is effective. For some patients who have a noncorrectable primary GI problem, such as short small bowel or dysmotility, repeated courses of antibiotics, usually the first week of every month, have been used. In this situation, the choice of antibiotic is often rotated to prevent the development of resistance.

Probiotics may be beneficial. However, no solid evidence exists to support their use unequivocally. Both the primary GI disease itself and SIBO may be associated with malabsorption. Mucosal damage has been associated with SIBO as has bacterial metabolism of nutrients. Careful attention to nutritional status of vitamins, protein, and energy is necessary in the treatment of SIBO to replete deficiencies and maintain the normal nutritional status.

PROGNOSIS

Eradication of the abnormal bacteria in the small bowel with antibiotics to which they are susceptible results in resolution of the problem and hence a good prognosis. However, SIBO most often occurs in the setting of a primary GI abnormality, and unless this abnormality can be corrected, it is likely that repeated bouts of SIBO will occur.

CONCLUSION

SIBO as a clinical entity is not clearly defined with multiple diagnostic modalities that are less than satisfactory. Despite limitations of diagnostic approaches, empiric treatment is often initiated. Because of these factors, the concept of SIBO as a distinct entity that requires treatment is challenged by some clinicians. In the next several years the study of the intestinal microbiome is likely to impact our understanding of this topic and potentially set a different foundation for therapeutic intervention.

Neoplasms of the Abdomen and Gastrointestinal Tract

Douglas C. Barnhart

TUMORS OF THE GASTROINTESTINAL TRACT

- **Gastrointestinal stromal tumors**
- **Carcinoid**
- **Colorectal carcinoma**
- **Gastric adenocarcinoma**
- **Lymphoma**

ABDOMINAL TUMORS NOT FROM THE GASTROINTESTINAL TRACT

- **Pancreatoblastoma**
- **Hepatoblastoma**
- **Wilms tumor**
- **Neuroblastoma**
- **Rhabdomyosarcoma**
- **Conclusion**

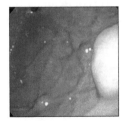
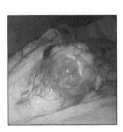
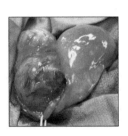
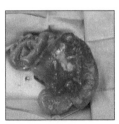

DEFINITION AND EPIDEMIOLOGY

Fortunately malignant neoplasms of the abdomen are uncommon in children. The most common pediatric intra-abdominal malignancies are neuroblastoma and Wilms tumor, each with an incidence of 7–8:1,000,000 per year. The incidence of hepatoblastoma is slightly less than 1 per million children per year. Tumors of the gastrointestinal (GI) tract are even less common. Despite the relative infrequency of these tumors, they are clinically important because they are often curable through combined modality therapy despite their grim natural history. Moreover, a broad understanding of these malignancies is important as they may present with nonspecific GI symptoms and may be mistaken for more common entities and should be specifically considered. These tumors are often initially diagnosed during evaluation of GI complaints.

CLINICAL PRESENTATION

Individual aspects of the presentation of individual malignancies will be discussed in the sections that follow but there are common aspects to many of these malignancies worth discussing. Intra-abdominal tumors often present as a painless abdominal mass detected by a caregiver during routine childcare. Similarly, parents may initially note abdominal distension in an otherwise healthy child. Therefore, based on symptoms, these tumors may initially be misinterpreted simply as constipation. Physical examination will often allow palpation of a distinct mass or a less distinct abdominal fullness. Either of these should prompt diagnostic evaluation with imaging studies.

DIAGNOSIS

If a palpable mass is not noted on physical examination, the first clear indication of an abdominal mass may be findings on a plain radiograph. These images may show a mass effect with displacement of the small bowel and colon. While these radiographs may provide initial recognition of an abdominal mass, they are not needed in children in whom the abdominal mass is palpable. It is also important to recognize that non-neoplastic diseases may also present as a palpable abdominal mass. These palpable lesions include massive hydronephrosis, polycystic kidney disease, omental cysts, ovarian cysts, and lymphatic malformations. Given the lifelong risk of malignancy associated with radiation exposure in children, computed tomography (CT) scans should be used judiciously. Abdominal ultrasound is the preferred initial study in a child presenting with a palpable abdominal mass. Most benign diagnoses can be made with the use of ultrasound alone and may never require a CT scan.

Cross-sectional imaging with either CT scan or magnetic resonance imaging (MRI) is an essential component of the evaluation of abdominal masses which have solid components. For the purposes of initial evaluation, CT scan with intravenous contrast with or without enteral contrast, and MRI with intravenous contrast are comparable. The advantages of CT scan are its wide availability and rapidity of the scan which can typically be done without sedation even in young children. The major disadvantage is exposure to ionizing radiation although modern scanning protocols seek to minimize this exposure. Alternatively, MRI provides cross-sectional imaging without radiation exposure but requires longer scan times. As a result of these longer scan times, sedation or general anesthesia is required for most children. Both CT and MRI allow characterization of the tumor's extent, characteristics, and relationship to visceral blood vessels. Given the adequacy of both techniques in terms of defining the tumor and the competing risks and benefits of each, the selection of one versus the other is often based upon local practice. Regardless of the local practice, however, abdominal tumors should rarely be biopsied, medically treated, or surgically resected without first obtaining cross-sectional imaging.

TUMORS OF THE GASTROINTESTINAL TRACT

Gastrointestinal stromal tumors

DEFINITION AND EPIDEMIOLOGY

Gastrointestinal stromal tumors (GIST) arise from the mesenchyme and may occur anywhere along the GI tract but are most common in the stomach. These tumors are rare in children with an estimated incidence of 0.08 per million. Given the rarity of these tumors, most clinical practice is based upon limited case series and extrapolation from experience with adult patients. It is critical to recognize, however, that pediatric GISTs are biologically distinct from those that occur in adults. Adult GIST tumors characteristically have a mutation in the tyrosine kinase receptor (c-KIT) or in the platelet-derived growth factor receptor (PDGFR) which are targets of therapy with imatinib, a tyrosine kinase inhibitor. Only 10 % of pediatric GISTs carry one of these mutations. Pediatric GIST may be associated with Carney's triad: GIST, paragangliomas (extra-adrenal pheochromocytoma), and pulmonary chondromas.

CLINICAL PRESENTATION

The median age of presentation is the early teens, and with female predominance, accounting for 70% of reported cases. Size of tumor at presentation is widely variable as are presenting symptoms. Over 80% of reported pediatric cases occurred in the stomach with upper GI bleeding being the most common presentation. Tumors are often multifocal and frequently have lymph node metastases at the time of diagnosis.

DIAGNOSIS

Given the frequency of GI bleeding at presentation, upper endoscopy may suggest a stromal tumor when an ulcerated mass is identified (**26.1, 26.2**). However, endoscopic biopsies are typically not deep enough

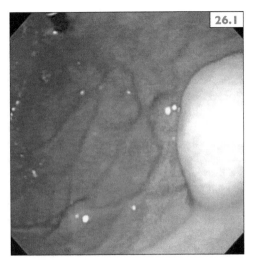

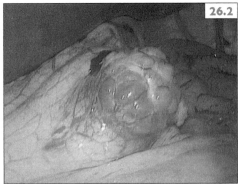

26.1, 26.2 Endoscopic view of gastric gastrointestinal stromal tumors (GIST).
26.1: Endoscopic view of gastric GIST;
26.2: laparoscopic view of same gastric GIST.

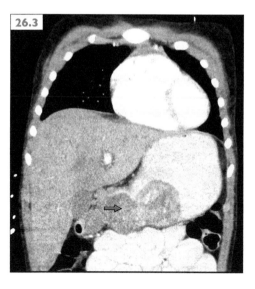

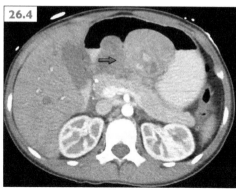

26.3, 26.4 Multifocal large gastric gastrointestinal stromal tumor (GIST). Coronal (**26.3**) and axial (**26.4**) images from a CT scan demonstrate large multifocal GISTs protruding into the gastric lumen (arrow).

to yield diagnostic tissue. While endoscopic ultrasound may provide additional delineation of the mass, a CT scan will provide adequate information to identify metastatic disease and plan operative intervention (**26.3, 26.4**).

TREATMENT

Surgical resection is the cornerstone of treatment (**26.5–26.7**). Given the relatively indolent course of this tumor, overly aggressive resections are not merited. The goal of resection is complete extirpation with a clear margin, which can often be achieved with wedge resections rather than a formal gastrectomy. Recurrences are common (70%) and typically occur as small nodules which can be resected. The surgeon must recognize that the risk of recurrence is unlikely to be affected by a more radical resection as long as negative margins are achieved, while realizing that more radical resections may significantly impact the child's postoperative quality of life and have nutritional consequences. The second most common site of GIST is the small intestine which can be treated with a segmental small bowel resection with

primary anastamosis. Obviously sites such as the gastroesophageal junction and esophagus require more extensive surgery to achieve negative surgical margins and functional reconstructions. All resected specimens should be analyzed for c-KIT and PDGFR mutations.

PROGNOSIS

Most children with GISTs survive long term but have courses typified by local recurrences and metastases. Patients who have undergone apparent complete resection are observed with surveillance imaging. Chemotherapy or radiation therapy is not typically used. Tyrosine kinase inhibitors may be considered for KIT/PDGFR mutation-positive patients, or for those with unresectable progressive disease. It is important to note, however, that unlike adult patients, most children will have wild-type KIT and therefore will be less likely to respond to tyrosine kinase inhibitors. Due to the fact that the tumors are slow growing and not physiologically active, symptomatic recurrent disease is typically managed with surgical resection.

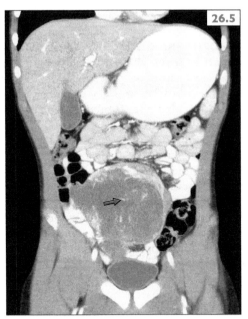

26.5 Coronal CT image of a gastrointestinal stromal tumor involving the jejunum (arrow).

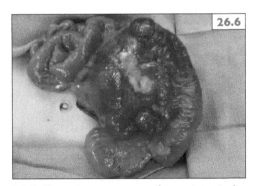

26.6 Operative appearance of gastrointestinal stromal tumor involving the jejuneum with extension into the small bowel mesentery.

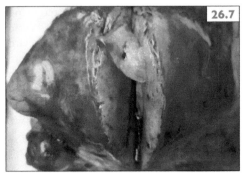

26.7 Cut surface of resected small intestine gastrointestinal stromal tumor.

Carcinoid

DEFINITION AND PATHOPHYSIOLOGY

GI carcinoid tumors arise from the neuroendocrine cells which are a part of the amine precursor uptake and decarboxylation system. Although carcinoid also may occur in the lungs, mediastinum, liver, bronchus, pancreas, and other organs, these tumors most commonly occur in the GI tract in children. GI carcinoid tumors are typically classified by whether they arise from the foregut, midgut or hindgut. The most common site is the appendix in which the tumor is typically located at the tip. While appendiceal carcinoid is typically identified as an incidental finding at appendectomy, most other sites are usually associated with disseminated disease at presentation.

CLINICAL PRESENTATION

Carcinoid syndrome is the most troublesome complication of carcinoid tumor. This syndrome of flushing, diarrhea, abdominal pain, tachycardia, hypertension, and altered mental status is caused by the active amines secreted by the tumor. The syndrome is associated with foregut tumors (due to decreased opportunity for first-pass clearance by the liver), larger tumors, and disseminated disease. This is particularly noted with liver metastases. Carcinoid syndrome is not known to occur with isolated appendiceal carcinoid tumors.

TREATMENT

Most appendiceal carcinoids are small (<2 cm) at the time of diagnosis and are adequately treated with resection of the appendix and mesoappendix. In these cases metastatic disease is rare, and no other treatment or diagnostic evaluation is required. An increased risk of recurrence is associated with tumor diameter >2 cm, cecal involvement, lymphatic invasion, lymph node involvement, extension into the mesentery, positive resection margins, cellular pleomorphism, and high mitotic index. Patients with these features should undergo right hemicolectomy with mesenteric lymphadenectomy.

In other locations in the GI tract, the goal is complete resection of the carcinoid with details of the operation varying by location. The overall slow growth rate of carcinoids supports resection of limited metastases.

Octreotide is used for symptomatic relief of carcinoid syndrome.

Colorectal carcinoma

Despite being the third most common cancer in adults, colorectal carcinoma is very rare in children, and therefore it is difficult to characterize risk factors. This pediatric cancer is likely different than adult colorectal cancer because premalignant adenomas are rarely seen in children with sporadic colorectal cancer. Presenting complaints are nonspecific and include vague abdominal pain, changes in bowel habits, weight loss, and anemia. Children typically present with advanced stage disease and other unfavorable risk factors. Treatment is based on the adult experience and includes resection with a 5 cm margin of bowel and lymphadenectomy. Chemotherapy and follow-up surveillance is similar to that of adults.

Gastric adenocarcinoma

Adenocarcinoma of the stomach is sufficiently rare so that all pediatric experience is limited to isolated case reports and a single small case series from a referral center. Pediatric specific risk factors, prognostic indicators, and recommended treatments cannot be defined with the limited number of cases. Resection via partial or total gastrectomy (dependent upon tumor size and location) with lympadenectomy is the cornerstone of treatment. The use of chemotherapy is individualized and without pediatric evidence to guide specific regimens.

Lymphoma

DEFINITION AND EPIDEMIOLOGY

Burkitt lymphoma and Burkitt-like lymphoma account for 40% of lymphomas in children. In developed western countries, Burkitt lymphoma most frequently presents with abdominal disease. These lymphomas are a B-cell lineage variety of non-Hodgkin lymphoma which have a characteristic c-MYC rearrangement with a translocation of chromosome 8 and 14. Burkitt–like lymphoma is an aggressive, rapidly growing non-Hodgkin lymphoma that shares features with diffuse large B-cell lymphoma and Burkitt lymphoma. It is treated like a Burkitt lymphoma. These tumors are the most rapidly growing neoplasms in children. The doubling time is 1 day, and as a result of this rapid growth, there is also a high rate of tumor cell death. Consequently metabolic derangements, such hyperuricemia and hyperphosphatemia, may occur before or during treatment and can cause secondary renal failure.

CLINICAL PRESENTATION

These lymphomas most often present with abdominal symptoms (**26.8–26.10**). Typically the presenting complaint is a palpable abdominal mass. As the lymphoma may involve the wall of the bowel as well as the mesenteric lymph nodes, children may also present with GI symptoms. Bowel obstruction may occur due to intussusception with the lymphoma serving as a lead point, or kinking or occlusion of the lumen by the tumor. If the tumor erodes through the mucosa, GI bleeding may occur. Due to the rapid cell turnover with these lymphomas,

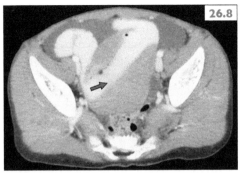

26.8 Axial image from CT scan showing Burkitt lymphoma involving the terminal ileum with partial bowel obstruction (arrow).

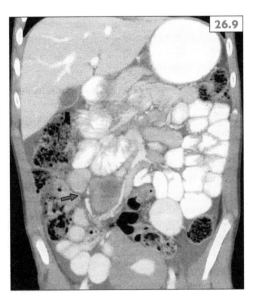

26.9 Coronal image from CT scan showing Burkitt lymphoma encircling the ileum and mesenteric lymphadenopathy (arrow).

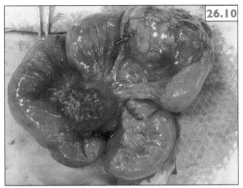

26.10 Burkitt lymphoma presenting with near obstructing lesion of the ileum, with involvement of the bowel wall and mesenteric lymph nodes (arrow).

GI perforation may occur. In such cases a portion of the bowel wall is replaced by tumor and subsequent tumor necrosis results in perforation. This necrosis and perforation may also occur as a consequence of the rapid cell death that occurs with treatment.

TREATMENT

Chemotherapy is the primary treatment of non-Hodgkin lymphoma, with surgery and radiotherapy having limited roles. With current regimens, outcomes for patients with Burkitt or Burkitt-like lymphoma are excellent with 5-year event-free survival approaching 100% in those with resected tumors and 86% in those with disseminated (stage 4) disease. Current treatment protocols include induction, consolidation, reintensification, and maintenance phases.

While chemotherapy is the cornerstone for cure of these lymphomas, surgical procedures often play a role in treatment of these children. Frequently diagnosis is made by biopsy of the abdominal mass. Additionally, operative treatment of complications, such as intussusception, may be necessary. In general, resection of these lymphomas should not be attempted. Typically there is extensive involvement of the mesentery, and complete resection has the potential for significant morbidity. Additionally, given the rapid rate of growth of these tumors it is critical to avoid procedures (such as bowel anastamosis) that would delay the initiation of chemotherapy if an incomplete resection is performed. Given the marked responsiveness of these tumors to chemotherapy, the extent of disease is more important than the completeness of resection in determining overall survival. However, in the infrequent cases in which complete resection can be done in straightforward fashion, resection may decrease the risk of complications (e.g. perforation due to necrosis) and improve event-free survival.

ABDOMINAL TUMORS NOT FROM THE GASTROINTESTINAL TRACT

Pancreatoblastoma

DEFINITION AND EPIDEMIOLOGY

Pancreatoblastoma is a rare malignancy which arises from the exocrine pancreas (**26.11, 26.12**). These usually occur in children under 8 years of age. Children with Beckwith–Weidemann syndrome and familial adenomatous polyposis syndrome are at increased risk.

CLINICAL PRESENTATION

The clinical presentation of children with these tumors is nonspecific. These tend to be slow growing and usually are quite large at presentation. Presenting symptoms may include a palpable abdominal mass, upper abdominal pain, and failure to thrive. Despite the fact that the head of the pancreas is the most common location, jaundice is less common than in adult pancreatic tumors. Some pancreatoblastomas are endocrinologically active and can cause Cushing syndrome or the syndrome of inappropriate antidiuretic hormone (SIADH). Alpha-fetoprotein (AFP) may be elevated as well.

DIAGNOSIS

Diagnostic imaging is essential in characterizing the extent of the mass and metastatic disease. These tumors may occur anywhere in the pancreas but seem to be more common in the head of the pancreas and are typically large at the time of presentation. Definitive diagnosis is obtained through biopsy as the appearance on CT scan may not be distinctive from other large retroperitoneal tumors of childhood (e.g. neuroblastoma, germ cell tumors, and rhabdomyosarcoma). Due to the proximity to the liver and an elevated AFP measurement, the presentation and appearance on imaging may overlap with hepatoblastoma until an operative exploration or biopsy is performed.

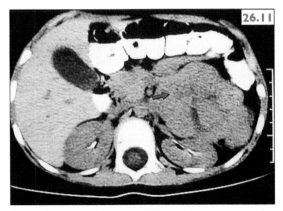

26.11 Pancreatoblastoma. CT scan shows mass in the tail of the pancreas of 3-year-old boy (arrow).

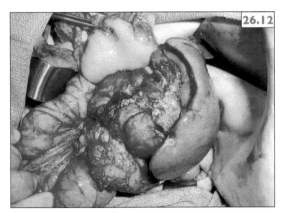

26.12 Intraoperative appearance of pancreatoblastoma after mobilization of the spleen and distal pancreas. Note that the stomach is retracted superiorly with the clamp, and the descending colon has been rotated medially.

TREATMENT AND PROGNOSIS

Complete surgical resection is the cornerstone of treatment, if feasible. Based on the location of the tumor this may be done with a distal pancreatectomy or a pancreaticoduodenectomy (Whipple procedure). Preresection chemotherapy is indicated if there is invasion of adjacent organs, encasement of blood vessels, or metastatic disease at presentation. A variety of regimens have been used, with cisplatin and doxorubicin being most common. Radiotherapy is not commonly used.

There is a high rate of recurrence even after complete resection but long-term survival is usually possible.

Hepatoblastoma

DEFINITION

Hepatoblastoma is the most common hepatic malignancy in preschool children (**26.13, 26.14**), but as children become older, hepatocellular carcinoma becomes predominant. Most children are diagnosed when they are discovered to have an apparently asymptomatic mass during routine care or on 'well-child' examination. Alternatively a minority of children present with nonspecific symptoms such as anorexia, weight loss, abdominal pain, fever, or fatigue. Hepatoblastoma may present with rupture and bleeding although this presentation is surprisingly uncommon despite the size of these tumors.

CLINICAL PRESENTATION AND ETIOLOGY

There are numerous nonmalignant causes of hepatic masses in children including vascular malformations, benign neoplasms (e.g. mesenchymal hamartomas, hepatic adenomas), cystic lesions, abscesses (parasitic, bacterial) and hematomas from trauma. These can usually be distinguished from malignant lesions by patient age, presenting symptoms, and radiographic appearance and often do not require biopsy.

DIAGNOSIS

Definitive diagnosis of hepatoblastoma can be made by biopsy but is highly suggested by elevation in AFP. The presentations of hepatoblastoma and hepatocellular carcinoma are so similar (including elevations in AFP) that biopsy may be necessary to distinguish them, even though the patient's age may suggest which is more likely. In adults with hepatocellular carcinoma, biopsy is not routinely performed due to the potential for tumor spill. Therefore, in older children with risk factors for hepatocellular carcinoma, such as cirrhosis or a history of viral hepatitis, biopsy may be excluded. The decision regarding biopsy in these older children should be made by a multidisciplinary team.

TREATMENT

Treatment strategy for hepatoblastoma is based upon the pretreatment extent of tumor (PRETEXT system). This system characterizes whether or not the tumor can be safely resected while preserving an adequate liver remnant. Complete surgical resection is the basis for cure. If patients are able to undergo initial complete resection, adjuvant chemotherapy improves survival and is routinely given. However, more than one-half of patients present with either an unresectable primary tumor or metastatic disease. In these patients, the appropriate treatment strategy is biopsy followed by neoadjuvant chemotherapy. Chemotherapy regimens vary between different pediatric oncology study groups. After initiation of chemotherapy, periodic reassessment is made to determine if the tumor has become resectable. The greatest effect on tumor reduction is seen in the initial two cycles of chemotherapy and consideration regarding potential liver transplantation should be made at that time.

Complete hepatectomy with liver transplantation is an option for children with hepatoblastoma localized to the liver which cannot otherwise be resected with preservation of an adequate hepatic remnant after neoadjuvant therapy. This occurs in children with very large unifocal tumors involving all segments of the liver, and in those children in which centrally located tumors involve either the porta hepatis or the confluence of the hepatic veins. Transplantation is also used in children with multifocal disease. Overall, survival is comparable to those in whom resection is accomplished without transplantation.

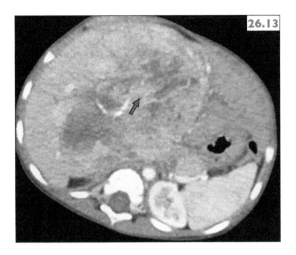

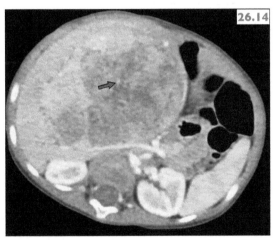

26.13, 26.14 Hepatoblastoma involving both lobes of the liver (arrow).

Wilms tumor

DEFINITION AND EPIDEMIOLOGY

Wilms tumor (also known as a nephroblastoma) is the most common renal malignancy in children (**26.15–26.17**), representing 6% of all pediatric malignancies. Most children present between 1 and 4 years of age with a mean age of 3 years. Children with Beckwith–Weidemann and Denys–Drash syndromes are at increased risk, but most cases are sporadic.

CLINICAL PRESENTATION AND DIAGNOSIS

Most children present with an asymptomatic abdominal mass but hematuria occurs in 20% of patients at presentation. While definitive diagnosis is made by histology, Wilms tumors have a sufficiently characteristic appearance on imaging studies so that therapeutic plans can be made without biopsy. CT scan typically shows a large mass arising from the kidney with preserved renal tissue partially encircling it ('claw sign'). Nephroblastoma may extend into the renal vein, inferior vena cava, and even into the right atrium. This intravenous extension should be sought preoperatively with ultrasound as it may be indication for preresection chemotherapy. Routine preoperative biopsy should be avoided as this upstages the tumor, requiring the intensification of chemotherapy and abdominal radiation. Wilms tumor occurs bilaterally in approximately 10% of patients. Renal preservation in concert with oncologic control is thus more complicated in this subset of children.

TREATMENT

The treatment of Wilms tumor is multimodality and has been well-defined through the National Wilms Tumor Study (and its successor the Children's Oncology Group) in North America and the International Society of Paediatric Oncology in Europe. Overall prognosis for children with Wilms tumor is excellent when treated with multimodality therapy. The most important determinants of prognosis are diffuse anaplastic histology and tumor stage. Anaplasia is a marker for resistance to chemotherapy and is associated with worse outcomes for all stages. Loss of heterozygosity at 1p and 16q has recently been identified as a marker for increased risk in children with tumors without anaplasia. The question of whether children whose tumors have loss of heterozygosity benefit from intensification of therapy is currently being investigated.

There is a significant difference in approach to the treatment of Wilms tumor between North America and Europe with regards to the timing of surgical resection. The American approach favors upfront resection, if possible, to provide immediate local control and accurate staging. This strategy may potentially diminish the required chemotherapy. The European strategy treats with chemotherapy presumptively without biopsy or initial resection in most cases. This strategy simplifies resection as there is often a dramatic response to chemotherapy. Both approaches yield similar overall results, and there is an ongoing debate about the comparative strengths and weaknesses.

The goal of operation is complete excision usually via nephrectomy while avoiding spillage of the tumor. Regional lymph nodes are sampled for staging purposes. Almost all patients receive either adjuvant (North American approach) or neoadjuvant (European approach) chemotherapy. The regimens for favorable histology tumor are well-defined and typically include vincristine and dactinomycin with doxorubicin added for higher-stage disease. Treatment of children with anaplastic tumors is less well defined and is currently the focus of clinical trials. Abdominal radiation therapy is used to enhance local control in children with tumor spill, positive resection margins, or lymph node metastases. Whole lung radiation is used to treat pulmonary metastases.

Children with Wilms tumor have been reported as being at increased risk for small bowel intussusception. This scenario presents as an early postoperative bowel obstruction and is typically diagnosed via CT scan or ultrasound.

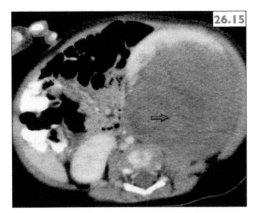

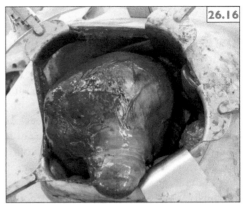

26.15 Axial CT image of left-sided Wilms tumor. The normal renal parenchyma is splayed over the mass anteriorly ('claw sign') (arrow).

26.16 Resection of Wilms tumor. The tumor is very large and the preserved lower pole of the kidney has a darker violet hue.

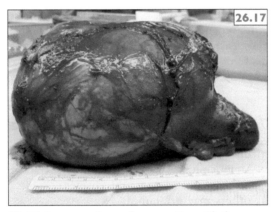

26.17 Intact specimen after resection with the normal lower pole of kidney at the right.

Neuroblastoma

DEFINITION AND ETIOLOGY

Neuroblastoma is a tumor that originates from the neural crest cells (**26.18, 26.19**). These tumors arise in the adrenal medulla or from the sympathetic chain. They may therefore occur anywhere from the neck to the pelvis. Neuroblastomas are unusual in that there are widely divergent outcomes which depend on the biology of the tumor. For example, an infant with metastatic disease to the liver and skin (stage 4S) may require minimal therapy as the tumor will mature and regress. In contrast, a 4-year-old child with metastatic disease is likely to succumb to the disease despite intense myeloablative therapy with stem-cell transplantation. Given this diverse clinical behavior, treatment and prognosis are driven by stratification of risk, and it is difficult to draw generalities for neuroblastoma as a whole. Factors considered in risk stratification are: tumor stage, patient age, amplification of MYCN, DNA ploidy, and histology.

CLINICAL PRESENTATION

Several aspects of presentation with neuroblastoma are of particular interest as one considers GI disease. Many children with neuroblastoma may present with a large abdominal mass, but others may present with extensive liver metastases despite a small primary tumor. Infants with 4S disease may present with extensive liver metastases that result in abdominal compartment syndrome. Neuroblastomas can produce vasoactive intestinal peptide which causes intractable, watery, and explosive diarrhea. Tumors which present in this fashion are often low risk. Pelvic neuroblastomas may present with fecal incontinence due to growth through neural foramina and spinal compromise. Alternatively, pelvic neuroblastoma may result in large bowel obstruction due to extrinsic compression. Children with advanced neuroblastoma often have protein-calorie malnutrition, but the diagnosis is usually suggested by other signs and symptoms. Anemia is common if there is metastasis to the bone marrow.

PATHOPHYSIOLOGY

Tumor stage takes into account not only the presence of distant metastatic disease and lymph node involvement but also whether the tumor can be resected. Abdominal neuroblastomas are often quite large and are prone to encase the visceral vessels. Older staging schemas used extension across the midline as a marker for resectability, while newer systems use CT evidence of vascular encasement and tumor extension. Younger children fare better than the older children. MYCN is a proto-oncogene which mediates a pathway that inhibits p53, a tumor suppressor protein. Amplification of MYCN to greater than 10 copies is a strong poor prognostic indicator independent of stage and patient age. DNA ploidy greater than 1 also correlates with worse outcomes. Histologic classification of neuroblastoma is based on the work by Shimada and is based upon the amount of associated stroma. These risk factors are used to assign children into low-, intermediate-, and high-risk groups. The details of the specific factors for treatment of each of these strata are beyond the scope of this chapter.

DIAGNOSIS AND TREATMENT

Cross-sectional imaging is usually suggestive of the diagnosis. Typically, neuroblastomas have some calcification within the tumor. Additionally, the propensity for growth through the neural foramina and into the spinal canal is characteristic of neuroblastomas and is not commonly seen with other pediatric tumors. Definitive diagnosis is by biopsy. The importance of complete surgical resection is dependent upon the risk strata to which the patient belongs. In general, surgical resections of neuroblastomas should be done in a manner to avoid resection or compromise of adjacent organs. Chemotherapy decisions are influenced by the risk stratum and degree of tumor resection. Therapy varies from expectant observation to myeloablative therapy with tandem stem-cell transplant depending upon the risk factors discussed above. Radiation therapy is used when there is residual disease after surgery and chemotherapy.

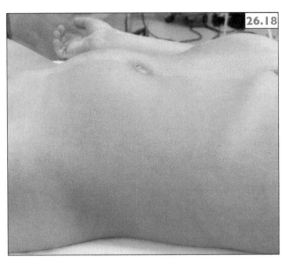

26.18 Abdomen of a 4-year-old boy with large pelvic neuroblastoma. Obvious fullness in the lower abdomen is due to the tumor which is easily palpable on abdominal examination and fills the pelvis on rectal examination.

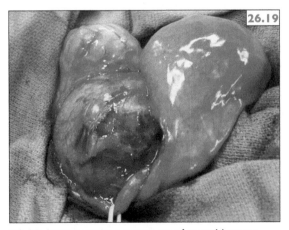

26.19 Intraoperative appearance of neuroblastoma in the same child as **26.18**. Tumor is left center. The chronically obstructed bladder is to the right with the right ureter encircled with the yellow vessel loop. Sigmoid colon is at the top of the photograph.

Rhabdomyosarcoma

DEFINITION AND ETIOLOGY

Rhabdomyosarcoma is a malignant tumor arising from the mesenchyme; hence it can develop in virtually any location including the periorbital tissues, extremities, extrahepatic bile ducts, retroperitineum, and genitourinary organs. There are two histologic subtypes: embryonal and alveolar. Embryonal is more common and has a more favorable prognosis. Other important prognostic factors are: age, anatomic site, tumor size, nodal status, and metastases. Extent of surgical resection is also an important postoperative prognostic variable.

CLINICAL PRESENTATION AND DIAGNOSIS

Rhabdomyosarcoma may occur in the biliary tree, typically in pre-school children. These children present with direct hyper-bilirubinemia due to biliary obstruction. Chemotherapy and radiation are effective and surgical resection of the biliary tree is not usually required. Perineal rhabdomyosarcoma presents with a palpable perineal mass, constipation, or pain with bowel movements. These lesions are problematic from a surgical standpoint as resection risks destruction of the continence mechanism. Typically biopsies are followed by chemotherapy. Residual tumor is then typically resected. Local control of these lesions is challenging as the lifelong morbidity of perineal resection must be weighed against the implications of possible compromised fertility and pelvic growth arrest from radiation. Finally, bladder and prostate rhabdomyosarcomas may be present with constipation or colonic obstruction.

These pelvic tumors can be very large at presentation such that the tumor fills the pelvis. A diverting colostomy may be required while cytoreductive chemotherapy is given. The major goal of surgery for genitourinary rhabdomysarcoma is complete resection with preservation of bladder function. Typically these genitourinary tumors are not amenable to this type of resection at presentation and so neoadjuvant therapy is commonly used.

TREATMENT

Rhabdomyosarcoma is typically treated with a combination of surgical resection and chemotherapy. Chemotherapy is often used in a neoadjuvant fashion to avoid the need for morbid surgical resections. The backbone of the regimen is often vincristine, actinomycin-D, and cyclophosphamide (VAC). Ifosfamide and etoposide may be added to VAC. The goal of surgical resection is to achieve complete excision with margins of normal tissues. Radiation therapy is used as an adjunct in children with gross or microscopic residual disease after resection.

Conclusion

- Abdominal tumors are the most common non-neurologic solid tumors in children.
- Pediatric GI tract tumors are rare.
- Most pediatric solid malignancies are treated with multiple therapeutic modalities.
- Cross-sectional imaging is essential in the diagnosis and therapeutic planning as well as in post-treatment surveillance.

Bowel Obstruction

Anne C. Kim, Saleem Islam

- **Introduction**

NEONATE

- **Duodenal atresia/web/annular pancreas**
- **Jejunoileal atresia**
- **Malrotation/midgut volvulus**
- **Meconium ileus**
- **Meconium plug syndrome**
- **Hirschsprung disease**

INFANT

- **Intussusception**
- **Duplications**

CHILD

- **Ruptured appendicitis/Meckel diverticulitis**
- **Intestinal malignancies (lymphomas)**

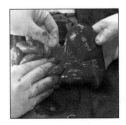
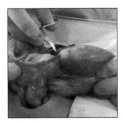
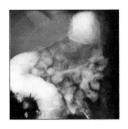

Introduction

Depending on the age of the pediatric patient, causes of intestinal obstruction may be related to congenital or acquired processes. Thus the discussion is divided into the general categories of neonate, infant, and child causes.

NEONATE

Duodenal atresia/web/ annular pancreas

Duodenal atresia occurs with an incidence of 1 in 7500 births and represents 50% of intestinal atresias seen. Duodenal atresia is associated with Down syndrome in approximately 30% of patients, with 20% of these neonates having an associated congenital heart defect. Other anomalies associated with duodenal atresia include annular pancreas, malrotation, esophageal atresia, and imperforate anus, as well as vertebral and renal anomalies. When diagnosed prenatally, ultrasound reveals polyhydramnios (33%) and often signs of duodenal obstruction (16%). Because of the presence of polyhydramnios, there is a tendency for these neonates to be born prematurely (46%). At birth, there is meconium-staining of the amniotic fluid due to the persistent *in utero* vomiting of the fetus.

The obstruction usually occurs near and just beyond the ampulla (**27.1**), with resultant bile-staining of any emesis, although it is certainly possible to have nonbilious emesis if the obstruction is proximal to the ampulla. The diagnosis can be confirmed with the use of a plain abdominal radiograph with the injection of 10–20 ml of air through a naso/orogastric tube. This should yield a 'double bubble' sign which reflects a distended stomach and duodenum proximal to the obstruction, separated by the pylorus. There will be no distal bowel gas in an atresia, but if there is a stenosis, web, or windsock deformity, a small amount of gas may pass distally. In cases where this classic radiographic finding is not present, an upper gastrointestinal (GI) fluoroscopy study may be needed to confirm the diagnosis or presence of a web.

It is important to differentiate the bilious emesis from an atresia as opposed to malrotation with midgut volvulus. Thus, the presence of scattered amounts of distal air should prompt further evaluation with an urgent upper GI fluoroscopic study. Such a study will delineate the anatomy with respect to the ampulla and help guide surgical treatment.

Regardless of the exact nature of the obstruction, surgical bypass is generally achieved by creation of a duodenoduo-denostomy. The use of a transverse incision in the bowel proximal to the obstruction anastomosed to a longitudinal incision in the distal bowel, results in the classically described diamond-shaped anastomosis that tends to hold the anastomosis open. It is important to confirm the patency of the anastomosis with

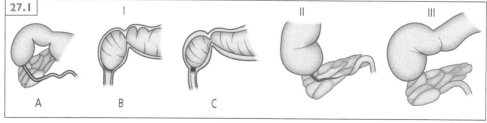

27.1 Types of duodenal atresia. Type I is shown in A–C, while types II and III are noted as being connected by a cord, or have no connection at all.

air injection or passage of a catheter to ensure that the obstruction has been effectively bypassed prior to the completion of the anastomosis. Postoperatively, feeding will be initiated once there are reliable signs of return of bowel function, such as a decrease in nasogastric tube output and bowel movements.

Jejunoileal atresia

In contrast to duodenal atresia, the formation of the more distal atresias is caused by vascular accidents that cause a disruption of the vascular supply to those portions of the intestine. Jejunoileal atresias, as a whole, are just slightly less common than duodenal atresia, comprising 46% of a large series. They are noted in 16% of gastroschisis cases and 2% of omphalocoele cases. In addition, a jejunoileal atresia may occur from the volvulus of a portion of bowel related to inspissated meconium, which should prompt consideration of cystic fibrosis as a possible related diagnosis.

Jejunoileal atresias are characterized into four types (**27.2**):
- Type I: diaphragm of tissue between the proximal and distal segments (23%).
- Type II: fibrous cord between blind-ending proximal and distal segments (27%).
- Type IIIa: separation of the blind ends with a V-shaped mesenteric defect (18%) (**27.3**).
- Type IIIb: 'apple-peel' or 'Christmas tree' deformity resulting from an extensive mesenteric defect leading to the retrograde blood flow to the distal ileum from the ileocolic artery, around which the bowel is twisted (7%).
- Type IV: multiple atresias or sausage chain of links (24%).

Prenatally, there is a variable amount of polyhydramnios, dependent on how distal the obstruction is located. Preterm delivery

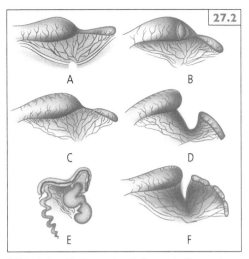

27.2 Jejunoileal atresias. A: Stenosis; B: type I or web; C: type II; D: type IIIa; E: IIIb; F: IV (chain of links). Type IIIb depicts the distal bowel perfused by retrograde blood supply via the ileocolic vessel.

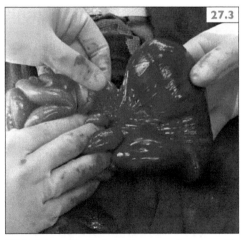

27.3 A type IIIa ileal atresia, as can be seen with the small V-shaped mesenteric defect and the massively dilated proximal ileum.

occurs in these infants 44% of the time. These neonates may pass meconium as it is common to have meconium distal to the obstruction. Abdominal radiographs will show dilation of the bowel proximal to the malformation, with no air distal to it. In order to characterize fully the obstruction, a constrast enema should be obtained, which will reveal a small caliber microcolon. This finding will differentiate a more distal colonic atresia although it may be difficult to differentiate this entity from a meconium ileus.

Treatment will depend on the intra-operative assessment of the entire bowel for multiple atresias *versus* a single affected portion. The dilated proximal portion should be resected or tapered to create an end-to-end anastomosis in order to allow for the best bowel function afterward. Nasogastric decompression is continued postoperatively until the drainage becomes less bilious and there are further signs of bowel function.

Malrotation/midgut volvulus

Malrotation is the condition of having imperfect rotation and fixation of the intestines to the retroperitoneum, resulting in a configuration and bands of tissue that may predispose to the development of midgut volvulus. Because the bowel rotates around the superior mesenteric artery during normal development and is fixed in a fashion that allows for a long area of fixation from the ligament of Treitz in the left upper quadrant down to the cecum in the right lower quadrant, a normally rotated bowel has very little opportunity to twist. In malrotation, the bowel can more easily rotate around this axis of the superior mesenteric artery and cause rapid strangulation of the entire midgut. In addition, abnormal bands of tissue between the cecum to the retroperitoneum cross the duodenum and may cause varying degrees of partial obstruction.

The most common sign of midgut volvulus is bilious emesis, especially in a neonate who was previously healthy. Over one-quarter of patients diagnosed with malrotation are less than 1 week old; over two-thirds of these are less than 3 weeks old, and 86% are less than 6 months of age. Thus, bilious emesis in the neonate is a surgical emergency unless proven otherwise. Clinical findings may be minimal, as a patient will not develop abdominal pain unless they are developing peritonitis.

Work-up of a suspected midgut volvulus must be performed in an urgent manner and must include an upper GI barium series, which is 95% sensitive and 86% specific for malrotation. The key feature of this study is the characterization of the position of the ligament of Treitz, which should be slightly to the left of the vertebrae. A corkscrew appearance of the small intestine on the barium study is associated with a midgut volvulus, as is an obstruction at the distal duodenum.

If there is any suggestion of volvulus on imaging, emergent laparotomy is indicated, often through a transverse, supraumbilical incision. Because the volvulus is generally clockwise, the bowel should be rotated counterclockwise and the bowel should be observed for improvement in its color. Following this procedure, the mesentery should be stretched out and any adhesive bands should be divided to allow it to lie flat. The duodenum is allowed to drain straight down in the right abdomen. The small bowel is placed in the right abdomen and the colon in the left. Any necrotic bowel should be resected, with creation of a primary anastomosis. If the bowel appears of questionable viability with regards to perfusion, a second exploration should be planned, especially if the at-risk portion of bowel is extensive. These children are at risk of adhesive obstruction in the future.

Meconium ileus

Approximately 13–17% of neonates born with cystic fibrosis (1:2000 live births) are at risk of developing an obstruction due to the thick nature of meconium. These neonates present with abdominal distention and failure to pass meconium. They may also have an abdominal mass if there was *in utero* perforation, which often calcifies and can be seen on radiographic imaging.

In an uncomplicated case of meconium ileus, abdominal radiographs will show dilated, air-filled loops proximally and it may be initially difficult to distinguish from ileal atresia or total colonic aganglionosis. The initial diagnosis and potential treatment would be with a water-soluble contrast enema, which would ideally reveal a microcolon with contrast reflux into the terminal ileum. The hyperosmolar nature of this contrast would help loosen the viscid meconium and facilitate its evacuation.

Operative intervention for meconium ileus is required in approximately 40–50% of neonates who fail radiologic therapy. Surgery generally involves either the creation of a temporary ileostomy or the placement of a T-tube catheter into the dilated, obstructed ileum to allow for irrigation with pancreatic enzymes or other agents, such as N-acetylcysteine to solubilize the meconium. Once bowel function returns, the nasogastric decompression is stopped and feeds are slowly initiated with rapid introduction of pancreatic enzymes.

Complicated cases of meconium ileus may require operative intervention if the antenatal perforation does not heal and there are ongoing signs of peritonitis. The neonate should receive resuscitation and have any electrolyte imbalance addressed, as well as receive antibiotics. Necrotic tissue should be debrided and any obstruction should be relieved during the course of this operation, with full awareness that the peritonitis may lead to friability of the tissue and ongoing problems with bleeding.

The adolescent form of this kind of obstruction is called distal intestinal obstruction syndrome or meconium ileus equivalent, and is managed in a different way than the neonatal process.

Meconium plug syndrome

Obstruction may occur from a long, white meconium plug, often due to a colonic dysmotility seen in premature neonates or infants of diabetic mothers. Generally speaking, these neonates have abdominal distention and will pass minimal meconium. Abdominal radiographs will reveal dilated bowel loops, and a contrast enema will reveal a large meconium plug and may result in the passage of this plug, followed by spontaneous stooling. The failure of the neonate to have a more normal stooling pattern following this study should prompt further work-up with the sweat chloride test and suction rectal biopsy to rule out cystic fibrosis or Hirschsprung disease, respectively.

Hirschsprung disease

The basis of this disorder is a lack of ganglion cells in the muscle layers lining the intestinal tract. As a result, normal peristalsis does not occur in the aganglionic segment, causing a functional obstruction at the level of the aganglionic bowel. On a histologic level, the affected segment contains no ganglion cells and demonstrates hypertrophic nerve roots that stain darkly positive for acetylcholinesterase because of an amplification process caused by the lack of nerve cells for the propagation of neurotransmission. As a rule, such a segment ends at the well-described 'transition zone' that starts 1–2 cm above the dentate line, which itself contains no ganglion cells and no nerves. Most often, the rectosigmoid colon is affected, but the extent of aganglionosis can continue more

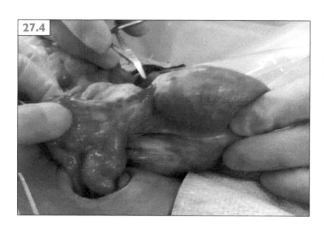

27.4

27.4 A type I atresia of the colon associated with a gastroschisis. Note the absence of any mesenteric defect.

proximally, with 'long-segment' (transition point seen in the ascending colon) or total colonic aganglionosis occurring 1–10% of the time. The incidence is 1 in 5000 live births, with a male predominance and evidence of heritability, particularly in patients with long-segment/total colonic aganglionosis.

Suspicion of Hirschsprung disease is raised in any full-term neonate who fails to pass meconium within the first 24 hours of life. However, it is possible for Hirschsprung to present later in life, with ongoing constipation problems.

The diagnosis is suggested by contrast enema revealing a dilated normal bowel proximal to a diminutive, diseased distal bowel. However, this picture may also be seen in small left colon syndrome (mimicking a transition zone in the transverse colon), distal ileal atresia (mimicking total colonic aganglionosis), or colonic atresia (mimicking a short-segment aganglionosis) (**27.4**). The definitive diagnosis is made by rectal biopsy that determines whether there are ganglion cells and hypertrophic nerves present in the muscularis layers. The biopsy can be performed with use of a suction device that pulls up a piece of the rectum into the biopsy chamber and is cut off by a guillotine-type action initiated by a trigger. This method, effective in neonates and infants, is generally not effective in larger children, who require an open rectal biopsy. In either situation, it is imperative that the biopsy be taken at least 2 cm above the dentate line in order to assure that that the transition zone is not biopsied.

Treatment consists of two components: 1) assuring an appropriate level of resection; and 2) pull-through of the normal bowel to restore intestinal continuity. The level of resection is confirmed by a full-thickness biopsy to ensure the presence of ganglion cells. Depending on the dilation of the proximal bowel, the size of the child at the time of resection, and whether or not enterocolitis is present, a colostomy may need to be created and staged pull-through performed.

Finally, enterocolitis may occur preoperatively or result from stasis or any constipating pathology postoperatively. Hirschsprung-associated enterocolitis is recognized by severe abdominal distention, explosive expulsion of flatus or feces upon rectal examination, and other systemic signs of infection. In its milder forms, it may be treated on an outpatient basis, but it may become a life-threatening problem that may require hospitalization, fluid resuscitation, broad spectrum intravenous antibiotics, and serial rectal irrigation.

Anorectal malformations are also an important cause of neonatal bowel obstruction, and are covered in Chapter 51.

INFANT

Intussusception

Intussusception is an intermittently obstructing process in which the intestine is enfolded on itself and continues to propagate at this point through peristalsis, such that a sleeve of intestine is doubled on itself. The initial intussuscipiens may be formed by hypertrophied lymphoid tissue leading to ileocolic intussusception, the most common form. Alternatively, a polyp or small bowel tumor (such as that seen in Peutz–Jeghers syndrome) or a portion of a persistent omphalomesenteric remnant may form the lead point for a small bowel–small bowel intussusception. Interestingly, this latter entity may also be seen following resection of a retro-peritoneal tumor.

The diagnosis is suggested by a history of intermittent, severe abdominal pain causing the child to cry out or draw up their knees with a frequency related to the recurrence of peristalsis as it tries to move beyond the point of obstruction. On examination, the classic finding is an abdominal mass in the right upper abdomen. Abdominal radiographs may be helpful if they show no air in the cecum on left lateral decubitus view, but the definitive diagnosis and potential treatment is made by air contrast enema.

Duplications

Duplications refer to lesions that are cystic or tubular in nature which represent a range of malformations that may result from abnormal twinning, unusual recanalization of the alimentary tract, or even some abnormality of the development of the notochord and enteral diverticula during the separation of the notochord from the endoderm. Duplications can occur throughout the alimentary tract, but they are most common in the intestine, specifically the ileum (**27.5**).

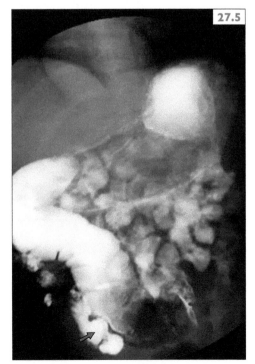

27.5 Intestinal duplication noted on barium imaging (arrow) in a child with abdominal pain.

The presentation of these may be quite variable. They may be identified prenatally, or may be found due to pain or the finding of a mobile abdominal mass. Smaller, cystic duplications can serve as the lead point for an intussusception. Larger duplications may cause compression of the surrounding bowel resulting in obstruction. They may contain ectopic gastric mucosa, which may become symptomatic if it develops ulceration or bleeding, as in peptic ulcer disease. Diagnosis in such a situation may be aided by a technetium–pertechnetate scan. Otherwise, a computed tomography (CT) scan may help to elucidate this entity as the cause of obstruction, although the definitive diagnosis may not be made until the time of abdominal exploration.

Interestingly, in contrast with Meckel diverticula, duplication cysts occur on the mesenteric side of the intestine and may even be within the mesentery completely. If tubular, these cysts often share a common wall with the adjacent intestine, necessitating resection or marsupialization if the duplication is extremely long, as resection would possibly result in short bowel syndrome.

CHILD

Ruptured appendicitis/ Meckel diverticulitis

As one of the most common pathologies seen in children, ruptured appendicitis will cause an ileus. However, it is also possible that there will be an adhesive bowel obstruction as a result of the inflammation that occurs, and this finding may result in the need for earlier interval appendectomy. Similarly, inflammation of a Meckel diverticulum may cause a bowel obstruction in a similar fashion. Diagnosis is suggested by history and by the rational use of abdominal radiograph and CT scan if necessary. Treatment is typically nonoperative initially, with use of gastric decompression and intravenous antibiotics, with eventual appendectomy or resection of the Meckel diverticulum.

Intestinal malignancies (lymphomas)

Intra-abdominal lymphomas often present with bowel obstruction from the sheer size of the mass. These malignancies are generally Burkitt lymphomas, although there may be other B-cell lymphoma types. Physical examination may reveal a large abdominal mass and some tenderness if there is any obstructive component. Diagnosis is made by CT scan. Treatment consists of resection of the affected component, followed by chemotherapy based on the pathology from this specimen.

Necrotizing Enterocolitis

Jose Greenspon, Elizabeth A. Fialkowski, Brad W. Warner

DEFINITION AND EPIDEMIOLOGY

Necrotizing enterocolitis (NEC) is the most common gastrointestinal (GI) emergency of the premature neonate. NEC is an acute inflammatory state of the intestine which affects all layers of the intestinal wall (**28.1**). This inflammation can range from a mild, focal area of involvement of the small intestine and/or colon (**28.2**) to diffuse and extensive ischemia of the entire small and large bowel (**28.3**) resulting in necrosis and perforation, and in some cases, death. NEC occurs in 2–5% of all premature neonates, although about 90% of cases occur in infants that are less than 36 weeks gestation.

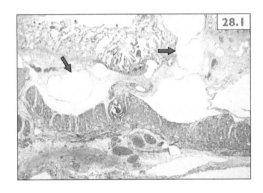

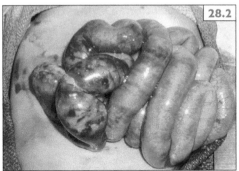

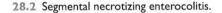

28.1 Severe necrotizing enterocolitis with intramural gas (arrows) as well as mucosal and submucosal necrosis.

28.2 Segmental necrotizing enterocolitis.

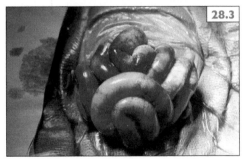

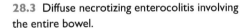

28.3 Diffuse necrotizing enterocolitis involving the entire bowel.

The estimated incidence of NEC ranges from 0.5 to 5 per 1000 live births. The time frame in which NEC develops appears to be inversely proportional to infant gestational age, as infants that are less than 30 weeks gestation develop NEC, on average, at around day of life 20, while infants who are 31–33 weeks develop NEC at around 14 days. This time frame is further reduced to approximately 6 days in infants who are greater than 34 weeks gestation.

Risk factors for NEC identified from epidemiologic studies include hypoxia in the early postnatal period, congenital heart disease, and respiratory distress. Additionally there is evidence that NEC may be related to infectious causes as evidenced by clusters of NEC cases within neonatal intensive care units. The most consistent risk factors, however, remain prematurity and low birth weight.

CLINICAL PRESENTATION AND PATHOPHYSIOLOGY

Characteristically, NEC causes inflammation of the intestinal wall resulting in epithelial barrier disruption. During this period there is also bacterial overgrowth which then invades the disrupted mucosal barrier layer. In its most severe form, NEC results in full-thickness intestinal wall destruction, with necrosis and perforation. This can rapidly result in overwhelming septic shock and death. The Bell criteria for NEC utilize the patient's signs, symptoms, and radiographic findings and stage the patients into suspected, definite, or severe disease (*Table 28.1*).

The underlying cause of NEC has not been identified; however, it is most likely multifactorial. To this end, research regarding intestinal maturity in the preterm neonate, altered intestinal microbial colonization, and immature circulatory regulation of the premature intestine is being actively pursued. Additionally, while rapid advancement of formula feedings has been associated with the development of NEC, it has not been found to be absolutely causative. Breast milk has been shown to be protective against the development of NEC, and premature infants have a reduced risk of NEC when fed with human breast milk.

Table 28.1 Bell Stages of necrotizing enterocolitis

	I. Suspected disease	II. Definite disease	III. Advanced disease
Systemic signs	Temperature instability, lethargy, apnea, bradycardia		Hemodynamic instability hypoxia, multiorgan dysfunction thrombocytopenia
Gastrointestinal signs	Poor feeding, emesis, abdominal distension, fecal occult blood		Abdominal wall crepitus, edema
Abdominal radiographic findings	Distension with mild ileus	Significant bowel distension, small bowel thickening, pneumatosis intestinalis, persistent bowel loops, portal venous gas.	Pneumoperitoneum

Adapted from Bell MJ *et al.* Neonatal necrotizing enterocolitis: therapeutic decisions based on clinical staging. *Ann Surg* 1978;**198**: 1–7.

Maternal risk factors felt to increase the incidence of NEC development in the preterm neonate include placental insufficiency and maternal cocaine use, both of which may contribute to the development of NEC by predisposing the neonatal gut to relative oxygen deprivation. In addition, there are mounting data to suggest that transfusion of packed red blood cells to premature, very low birth weight infants may be related to the development of NEC. The reasons for this are unclear and further research, looking at whether this is a causative phenomenon versus an indicator of severe illness, needs to be pursued.

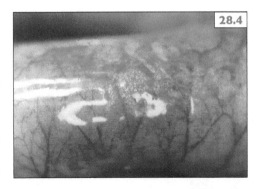

DIFFERENTIAL DIAGNOSIS

Because the presentation of NEC can be quite variable, it is not uncommon for NEC to mimic many other conditions. Amongst these, the most common is sepsis, which frequently manifests in the neonate as distention, emesis, and temperature instability, as well as altered white blood cell count. A generalized ileus from other conditions may also present as abdominal distention and emesis such as severe enterocolitis associated with Hirschsprung disease.

Another important consideration within the continuum of NEC is focal intestinal perforation (FIP). FIP often presents as an incidental finding of pneumoperitoneum, but without associated pneumatosis intestinalis. These neonates often lack systemic signs of shock or sepsis. FIP more commonly affects low birth weight and premature neonates and is often associated with indomethacin or dexamethasone use.

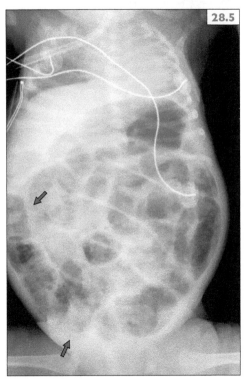

28.4, 28.5 Pneumatosis intestinalis.
28.4: Pneumatosis intestinalis seen grossly as gas within the intestinal wall; **28.5**: pneumatosis intestinalis outlining the intestinal wall (arrows) as well as bubbly appearance overlying the loops in the right lower quadrant.

DIAGNOSIS

The diagnosis of NEC is often established by the findings on plain abdominal radiography. These include 'pneumatosis intestinalis' (**28.4, 28.5**), which is air within the bowel wall, and 'portal venous gas' (**28.6**), which is air within the portal venous system in the liver. Additionally, the identification of a dilated bowel loop whose appearance

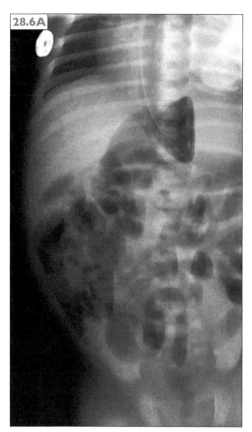

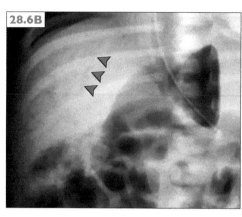

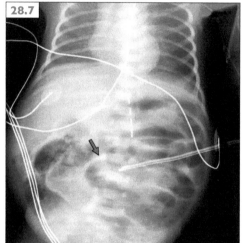

28.6 Portal venous gas (A) seen in the magnified region of the abdominal radiograph (arrowheads) (B). Also seen is pneumatosis intestinalis.

28.7 Thickened bowel loops (arrow).

and position remain unchanged on serial abdominal radiographs ('fixed loop') as well as thickened loops of bowel (**28.7**) may also raise suspicion of NEC.

When NEC has progressed to perforation, free intraperitoneal air can be identified in several ways. It can be seen as a relative lucency overlying the liver on a plain supine abdominal radiograph (**28.8**), as well as the 'Rigler's sign' (**28.9**), also known as the 'double-wall sign', which is when both sides of the intestinal wall can be seen because free air on both sides separates a given loop from adjacent loops of bowel. On a left lateral decubitus film, the pneumoperitoneum can be seen as air subjacent to the liver (**28.10**), and in a cross table lateral with the patient in a supine position, the free air can be seen anteriorly (**28.11**).

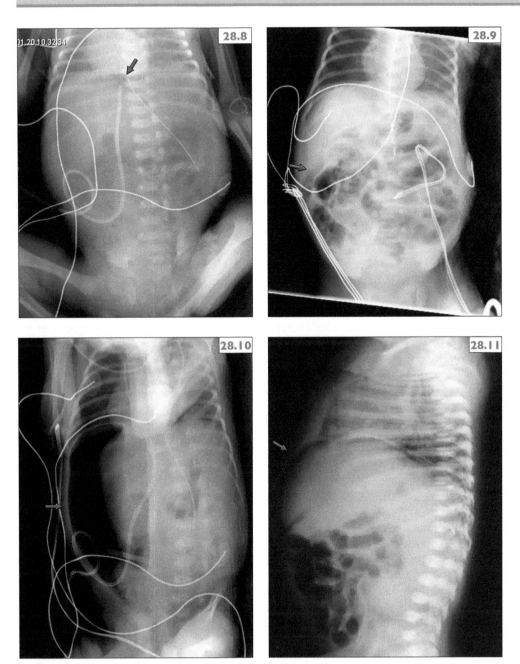

28.8–28.11 Radiography of perforation. **28.8**: The liver typically appears radiopaque relative to the gas-filled bowel. The area over the liver appears more radiolucent in this radiograph, concerning for perforation (arrow); **28.9**: air is seen outlining the outside of the bowel loop, referred to as a Rigler's sign (arrow); **28.10**: air is seen overlying the liver in the left lateral decubitus view (arrow); **28.11**: the cross table lateral view shows the pneumoperitoneum anteriorly (arrow).

TREATMENT

The majority of patients with NEC are treated medically with bowel rest, naso- or orogastric tube decompression, broad-spectrum intravenous antibiotics, fluid resuscitation, and careful monitoring for further deterioration. Often, progression of injury in NEC results in rapid deterioration manifested by sudden increase in ventilatory support and an increase in inotropic requirement. Serial physical examination, radiography, and laboratory evaluation are used for surveillance. Early identification of patients who are failing medical therapy is of extreme importance so that those who are in the earlier stages of NEC can be watched more carefully and initiation of gut rest can begin promptly.

Few data exist regarding optimal antibiotic regimens and duration of therapy, although broad-spectrum coverage based on resistance patterns within an individual neonatal intensive care unit is recommended. Additionally, in severely ill patients who remain refractory to broad-spectrum coverage, addition of antifungal agents should be considered. Also, patients who develop profound thrombocytopenia and are coagulopathic consistent with disseminated intravascular coagulation should be treated with platelet and plasma transfusions as appropriate.

While a majority of patients with NEC respond to nonsurgical management, up to 30% will require surgical intervention. The most clear-cut indication for an operation is evidence of intestinal perforation – most frequently diagnosed as the presence of free intraperitoneal air on a plain abdominal radiograph. A relative indication is rapid and/or progressive clinical decline despite escalation of medical support. This clinical decline can manifest as worsening acidosis, increased abdominal distention, thrombocytopenia, bowel obstruction on an abdominal radiograph, or the development of abdominal wall discoloration or erythema which can be associated with bowel necrosis and perforation.

The choice of surgical technique has been the subject of much debate over the past several decades. Often, the clinical stability and gestational age of the patient help guide the decision of whether to perform a traditional laparotomy with bowel resection versus placement of a peritoneal drain. In several studies, patients who had a peritoneal drain placed because they were too unstable to undergo an abdominal exploration had a reported mortality of approximately 50%. However, recent prospective randomized studies in both Europe and the United States have shown that peritoneal drainage and laparotomy carry a similar 90-day mortality, as well as need for total parenteral nutrition (TPN) and length of hospital stay at 90 days when the neonate's birth weight is in the 1000–1500 g range.

The technique of peritoneal drainage involves making a small incision on the lower abdomen (**28.12**), away from the liver edge, irrigation of the peritoneal cavity with warmed saline, and placement of an intraperitoneal Penrose drain. This is secured to the patient's skin with a suture and left in place until the drainage of the intestinal contents has stopped. This often takes several days. At this point the drain is slowly removed.

For neonates who are felt to be candidates for laparotomy, a transverse incision is made in the abdomen through which the patient's bowel is carefully eviscerated (**28.13**). The findings during laparotomy range from an isolated perforation (**28.14, 28.15**), which most often occurs in the ileum, with otherwise normal bowel, to total intestinal involvement (defined as NEC-totalis). In NEC-totalis, or pan-intestinal necrosis (**28.16**), careful evaluation of remaining normal bowel must be undertaken in order to evaluate whether the injury is survivable. More often than not, focal areas of necrosis are identified with intervening normal bowel. In this scenario,

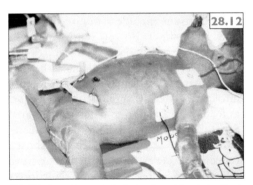

28.12 A peritoneal drain is placed for intestinal perforation.

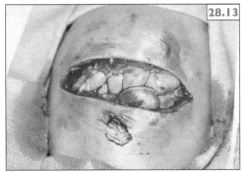

28.13 A transverse abdominal incision performed for necrotizing enterocolitis (NEC). At exploration, this patient was found to have severe NEC with liquefaction of the bowel.

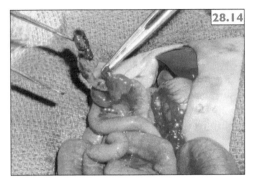

28.14 Focal intestinal perforation.

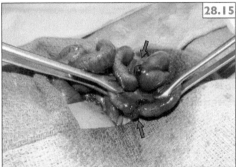

28.15 Segmental areas of necrotizing enterocolitis with otherwise normal bowel (arrows).

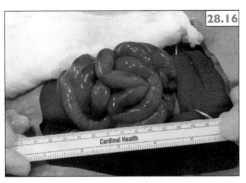

28.16 Necrotizing enterocolitis totalis.

necrotic areas can be resected. Options for the remaining bowel include reanastomosis versus ostomy formation (**28.17**). In a small fraction of patients, such as those with pan-intestinal necrosis or in patients with areas of marginal viability, a second-look laparotomy is warranted in order to preserve optimal bowel length.

Postoperatively, the patients are kept *nil per os* and continued on broad-spectrum intravenous antibiotics as well as TPN. During this period, patients are carefully evaluated for clinical improvement. Once bowel function has returned, as evidenced by production of stool, enteral feeds are reinitiated with extreme caution to ensure patients will tolerate this new stress to their intestinal tract. Closure of the ostomy is often delayed for several weeks to months to allow for patient growth and to diminish the risk of further injury to the bowel secondary to immature scar formation.

Complications

While the most serious complication of NEC is perforation and necrosis, other complications include stricture formation (**28.18**), short bowel syndrome, and neurodevelopmental delay. Strictures may develop in up to 30% of patients with NEC. These patients will manifest with feeding intolerance after either reinitiation of feeds or as feeds are increased to a determined goal. Stricture formation can be further evaluated with a contrast enema which will show a transition zone at the area of the stricture. If a stricture is present, surgical resection or stricturoplasty is indicated in order to alleviate the obstruction.

Short bowel syndrome occurs after an extensive resection, leaving inadequate bowel length to allow for nutritional absorption. These patients become reliant on long-term TPN and are at risk of developing central venous catheter infections, cholestatic liver disease and in the worst cases, cirrhosis. These patients may ultimately require bowel lengthening procedures or small bowel transplantation.

Finally, long-term neurodevelopmental complications affect up to 50% of patients with NEC.

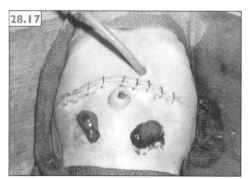

28.17 After segmental removal of the affected bowel, an ostomy and mucous fistula have been created.

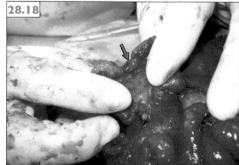

28.18 Colonic stricture (arrow) in an infant with necrotizing enterocolitis managed medically and not able to tolerate feedings.

CHAPTER 29

Nutrition Overview

Katie McDonald

- **Introduction**
- **Routes of administration**
- **Specific routes of EN**
- **Method of nutrient delivery**
- **Choice of formula**
- **Parenteral nutrition**
- **Nutrition management**

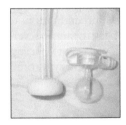
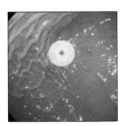
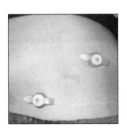
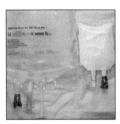

Introduction

Specialized nutrition support (SNS) refers to the provision of nutrients with a therapeutic intent by oral, enteral, parenteral, or a combination of these routes. Optimal pediatric care and the delivery of appropriate SNS requires the application of evidence-based practice guidelines to assist clinicians in the development of nutrition care plans for their patients. A comprehensive nutrition care plan includes individual nutrient requirements, intake goals, and objectives for nutritional care as well as the route of nutrition administration. All aspects of SNS should be guided by standardized policies and procedures, monitored carefully over time for adequacy and appropriateness, and adjusted as needed with changes in a patient's condition.

Age-appropriate growth is a primary indicator of nutrition status in children. Careful, ongoing monitoring and evaluation using standardized growth charts allows for prompt intervention when any deviation from the expected growth rates is detected. A child who will not or cannot safely ingest adequate nutrients to maintain normal growth should receive alternative forms of SNS.

Routes of administration

The route selected for delivery of nutrition must be determined by the patient's medical condition and disease process. The gastrointestinal (GI) tract is the preferred mode of nutrient delivery whenever possible, as use of the GI tract promotes mucosal growth and function, reducing bacterial translocation and improving nutrient utilization with fewer hepatobiliary and infectious complications.

Oral nutrition is taken by mouth. Enteral nutrition (EN) via gastric or intestinal direct access supplies nutrients distal to the oral cavity via a tube, catheter, or stoma. Indications for EN include a functional gut with sufficient length and absorptive capacity with a prolonged period of either nothing by mouth (*nil per os* or NPO) or suboptimal oral nutrition. Specific indications for EN may include: 1) insufficient oral intake due to primary or secondary anorexia; 2) increased caloric needs and/or malabsorption; 3) oral motor dysfunction; 4) functional or structural abnormality of the GI tract; 5) primary therapy for metabolic disease or inflammatory bowel disease; and 6) traumatic injury, burns, respiratory failure, or surgery. The goal of EN should be to meet estimated nutrient requirements in the safest and most timely manner. Risks of EN complications are minimized with vigilant and continuous surveillance of EN including physical examination, recording of anthropometrics, and potential laboratory monitoring.

When EN is deemed appropriate, a specific enteral access route must be determined. The patient's underlying disease state; GI anatomy including surgical history, gastric and intestinal motility and function; risk of aspiration; and estimated duration of therapy should be factored into the selection of a specific enteral access device and whether it should be placed endoscopically or surgically.

Gastric feeds are more physiologic than direct intestinal feeds and allow a more normal digestive process and hormonal response to feeds. Bolus feeds and a higher rate of feeding volume infusion are possible with the stomach acting as a reservoir. Gastric feeds permit a more flexible feeding schedule, which is especially important for the ambulatory EN patient. Contraindications to gastric feeds may include gastroparesis, severe gastroesophageal reflux, persistent or severe emesis, aspiration risk, dumping syndrome, or pancreatitis.

Specific routes of EN

Enteral access devices for short-term use in hospitalized patients are usually inserted via nasal or oral routes. Nasogastric (NG) feeds are used for short-term EN for the patient with normal gastric function, little or no gastroesophageal reflux, and low risk of aspiration. The smallest diameter tube should be placed in this setting while considering the size of the patient as well as the rate and viscosity of enteral product to be infused. Typically, tube length is determined by measuring the distance between the tip of the patient's nose to the earlobe and the earlobe to the xiphoid process.

Orogastric (OG) feeds are used in premature or small infants who are often obligate nose breathers, in order to avoid obstructing the nasal passages. OG feeds may be used in patients with choanal atresia or basilar skull fractures who require EN.

For the critically ill child, there are insufficient data to recommend gastric versus transpyloric feedings. Transpyloric feeding may improve caloric intake when compared to gastric feeds in such a clinical setting. Postpyloric feeding may be considered in children who have failed a trial of gastric feeding or who are at high risk of aspiration.

Nasojejunal (NJ) feeds may be placed for short-term management of patients who cannot tolerate NG feeds due to gastric motility disturbances, such as gastroparesis, or for patients at risk of aspiration (**29.1**).

Patients with persistent dysphagia or chronic conditions requiring EN should have a long-term enteral access device placed.

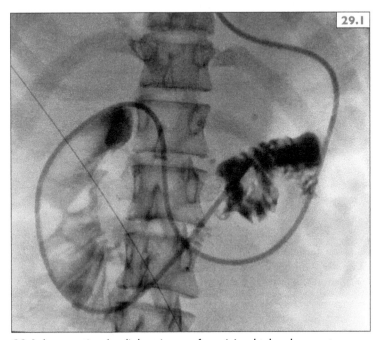

29.1 Interventional radiology image of nasojejunal tube placement.

Gastric feeding devices (for example, gastric tubes) can be placed directly into the stomach by surgical, interventional radiology, or endoscopic techniques (**29.2–29.4**). Gastric feeds can be given as a bolus, continuous drip, or as a combination of the two methods. Testing (endoscopy, pH/impedance monitor) may be needed to determine if a fundoplication or other antireflux procedure is required before placement of a gastric feeding device. Complications of gastric feeding devices are rare and include localized cellulitis, inflammatory tissue (granulation tissue), and a gastric tube tip or bumper that has accidentally undergone excessive traction leading to the tube being lodged in the surrounding tissue but not in the stomach ('buried bumper syndrome') (**29.5**).

Jejunal (intestinal) feeds bypass the stomach which can be helpful in clinical scenarios such as gastroparesis, but they also bypass gastric acid digestive and bactericidal processes (**29.6–29.8**). Because there is

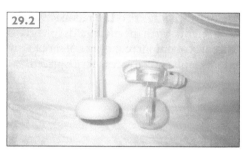

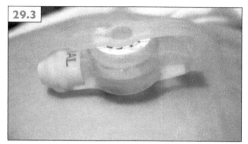

29.2, 29.3 Gastric devices can have a long stem such as a gastric tube (**29.2**) or short stem such as a gastric button (**29.3**), in place through a gastrostomy.

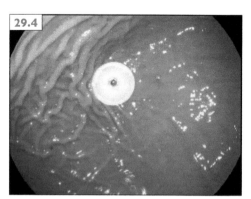

29.4 Mucosal view of the stomach showing a percutaneous gastrostomy tube.

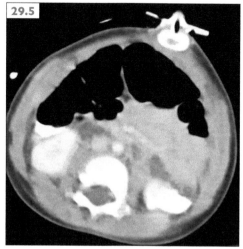

29.5 CT image of the abdomen showing the tip of a gastrostomy tube lodged in abdominal tissue, but not in the stomach lumen, consistent with 'buried bumper' syndrome.

no gastric reservoir available, jejunal feeds require continuous drip infusions over a long duration. Hyperosmolar formula products might not be well tolerated using this route as they may lead to dumping syndrome. In the critical care setting, pediatric patients receiving jejunal feeds may be able to advance to caloric feeding goals more quickly compared to adults.

As an example, specially trained providers, such as interventional radiologists, can efficiently place NJ tubes. Radiologic confirmation of NJ tube placement is required prior to initiation of feeds. Jejunal tubes, placed through a pre-existing gastrostomy site (ex. gastrojejunal tube, 29.9) or directly into the small intestine, may become dislodged or can migrate back into the stomach. Because jejunal tubes are usually long and small in diameter, they have an increased incidence of clogging; administration of certain medications and inadequate or improper flushing are a major cause for clogging.

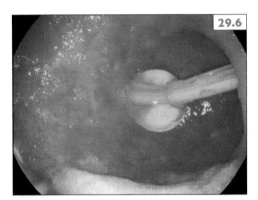

29.6 Endoscopic view of a gastrojejunal tube as it enters the stomach.

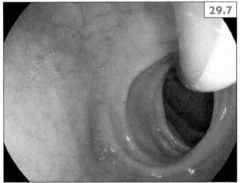

29.7 Endoscopic view of a gastrojejunal tube as it enters the jejunum.

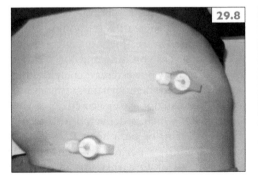

29.8 Nutrition delivery in a medically complex child with cerebral palsy requiring both gastrostomy (right side of image) and separate jejunostomy tube (left side of image) placement. (Courtesy of Practical Gastroenterology [2006]. Shugar Publishing, Westhampton Beach, New York.)

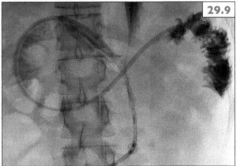

29.9 Interventional radiology image of gastrojejunal tube placement.

Method of nutrient delivery

Enteral feeds can be administered as continuous or intermittent drip feedings, boluses, or a combination of continuous drip and bolus feeding techniques. Considerations in deciding the feeding schedule include the location of the enteral access device (gastric or jejunal), the clinical condition of the patient, and feeding tolerance history.

Bolus feeds can be given in a relatively rapid manner through the gastric route which provides both near-normal physiologic access to nutrition as well as flexibility in the patient's schedule to receive nutrition. Continuous feeds are mandatory in patients with jejunal access and are frequently also used in patients with NG or gastrostomy access. Continuous feeding may be considered for the critically ill child with hemodynamic instability, abdominal distension or discomfort, or vomiting with bolus feedings. Patients with malabsorption or short bowel syndrome may experience improved absorption with continuous infusion of feeds. Nocturnal continuous feeds may be used as an adjunct to an oral diet in patients who are unable to ingest adequate calories and nutrients during daytime hours.

For patients starting on continuous drip feedings, EN may be initiated with full strength formula at 0.5–1 ml/kg/h (typically not higher than 25–30 ml/h) and by advancing the same volume increase every 4–6 hours to eventually achieve a final energy requirement and volume goal. Once the goal feedings are tolerated, the duration of the continuous feeds may be shortened gradually so that the full EN volume is delivered in less than 24 hours, if indicated. Continuous feeds require an infusion pump for a consistent rate of formula delivery.

Combination feeds of both bolus and continuous feeds are also a consideration depending on the clinical scenario.

Choice of formula

Important criteria for appropriate EN formula selection include the age of the child, prior feeding history, medical condition, and the type of enteral access (gastric or jejunal). For infants under 1 year of age, human milk or infant formulas are used for EN. Pediatric-specific formulas are indicated for children aged 1–10 years. Adult EN products can be used for children older than 10 years of age or adolescents. Most patients will tolerate age-appropriate polymeric formulas. Protein hydrolysate formulas or L-amino acid formulas are used in specific clinical scenarios such as allergic GI disease or feeding intolerance.

Parenteral nutrition

Parenteral nutrition (PN), the delivery of nutrients intravenously through a central catheter, should be used when the GI tract is not functional, cannot be accessed, or caloric needs are greater than those which can be met through the GI tract (**29.10, 29.11**). Specific conditions that may benefit from PN include: 1) GI obstruction; 2) enterocolitis (such as necrotizing enterocolitis); 3) prolonged ileus; 4) digestive fistula; 5) peritonitis; 6) bowel ischemia; 7) pancreatitis (although jejunal feeds are used in treatment of pancreatitis as well); 8) severe vomiting and/or diarrhea; 9) inflammatory bowel disease complications; and 10) extreme hemodynamic instability.

PN is usually categorized as either central PN which is delivered into a large diameter vein, or peripheral PN which is delivered into a peripheral vein (usually in the hand or forearm). Because of the concentration of osmolarity-generating components, most nutritionally adequate PN formulations require central access to avoid thrombophlebitis. Peripheral PN should only be used for a limited time and only when the osmolarity does not exceed 850 mOsm/l.

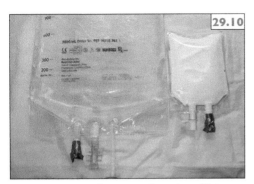

29.10 Example of parenteral nutrition. This source of nutrition will require central venous access.

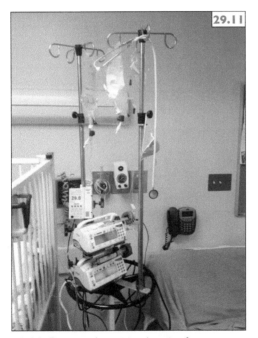

29.11 Parenteral nutrition hanging from a patient's bedside.

Nutrition management

Specific nutrition management for various clinical conditions is described elsewhere in this book. However, it is important to involve a registered dietician in the management of patients with complex nutrition issues to prevent worsening malnutrition, obesity, or the complications of refeeding syndrome (such as hypophosphatemia and other electrolyte abnormalities).

Anthropometrics, including weight, height, and body mass index, are essential in determining initial and follow-up dietary goals of patients. Specific laboratory data will be needed in nutrition management, including serum electrolytes, magnesium, calcium, phosphorus, and triglyceride levels. Other laboratory parameters, such as zinc, iron, or vitamin B12 levels, will be necessary to monitor depending on the clinical scenario. Assessment of a patient's overall nutrition state can be followed with laboratory tests such as a serum albumin, prealbumin, or retinol binding protein.

PANCREAS

CHAPTER 30

Congenital Anomalies of the Pancreas

Kathy D. Chen, Sohail Z. Husain

- **Introduction**
- **Ductal abnormalities**
- **Defects in pancreatic migration**
- **Defects leading to reduced pancreatic volume**

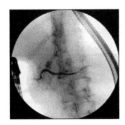
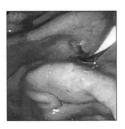
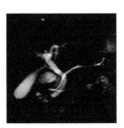
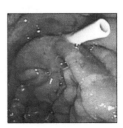

Introduction

Understanding how congenital abnormalities of the pancreas come about requires that we recognize the complex development of the pancreas. Early in gestation, the pancreas arises from the foregut around week 5–6. Two buds, a dorsal and a ventral, develop from the endodermal lining of the primitive duodenum. The buds elongate, rotate around the duodenum, and migrate towards one another. The ventral pancreatic bud migrates dorsally, forming what will become the inferior head and uncinate process of the pancreas. In most cases, the main pancreatic duct (of Wirsung) is formed by fusion of the entire length of ventral duct as well as a portion of the distal dorsal duct. This fused duct then enters the duodenum at the major papilla. The common bile duct also drains into this system. The proximal portion of the dorsal duct forms the accessory duct (of Santorini), which enters the duodenum by way of the minor papilla. Most pediatric pancreatic abnormalities result from alterations of this development (**30.1**).

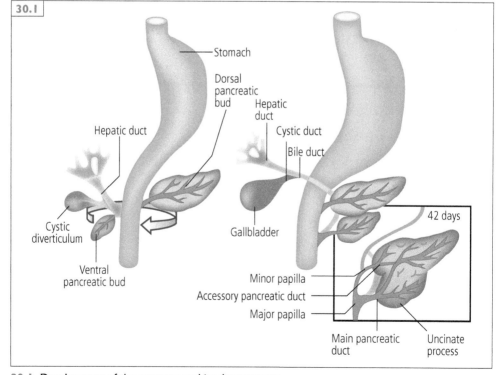

30.1 Development of the pancreas and its duct systems.

Ductal abnormalities

Pancreas divisum

Pancreas divisum (PD) is the most common congenital anomaly of the pancreas. It is caused by a failure of the ventral ductal system to fuse with the distal dorsal ductal system. Based on sheer autopsy data, PD occurs in roughly 10% of the general population. The result in most cases, called complete (or classic) PD, is that the entire dorsal pancreas (the superior head, body, and tail) drains through the minor papilla. Variations such as incomplete PD occur when a small ductal branch connect the two ducts.

The association of PD and recurrent acute or chronic pancreatitis is controversial. More than 95% of patients with PD do not develop pancreatitis. In the less than 5% who have pancreatitis, the cause is thought to be related to obstruction of flow from the minor papilla, which in patients with PD drains the bulk of the pancreas. However, the vast majority of patients with pancreatitis do *not* have PD. Nonetheless, some reports demonstrate an increased prevalence of PD in patients with pancreatitis. Thus, while PD may be considered a predisposing factor, it is likely that additional other factors are present to cause pancreatitis.

A diagnosis of PD is made either by endoscopic retrograde cholangiopancreatography (ERCP) (**30.2**) or magnetic resonance cholangiopancreatography (MRCP) (**30.3**). Secretin stimulation prior to MRCP (S-MRCP) can improve visualization. Ultrasound is not sensitive enough to capture this ductal anomaly.

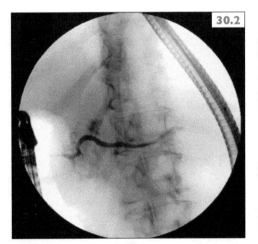

30.2 Endoscopic retrograde cholangiopancreatography of dorsal duct pancreatogram via minor papilla, showing no communication with the ventral pancreatic duct in pancreas divisum. (Courtesy of Jeffrey Tokar, MD; Foxchase Cancer Center, Philadelphia.)

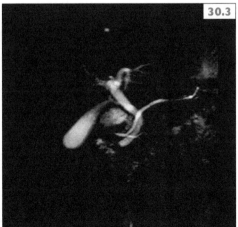

30.3 MRI of pancreas divisum. (Courtesy of Jeffrey Tokar, MD; Foxchase Cancer Center, Philadelphia.)

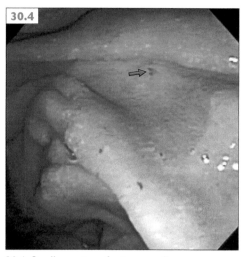

30.4 Small opening of minor papilla seen on endoscopy of pancreas divisum. (Courtesy of Jeffrey Tokar, MD; Foxchase Cancer Center, Philadelphia.)

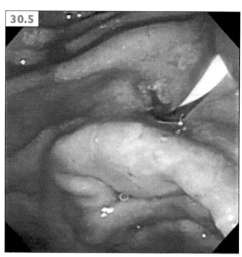

30.5 Wire guide placed in minor papilla. (Courtesy of Jeffrey Tokar, MD; Foxchase Cancer Center, Philadelphia.)

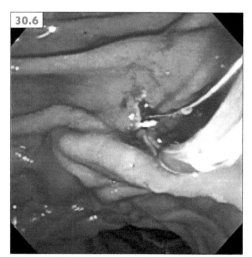

30.6 Minor papillotomy being performed. (Courtesy of Jeffrey Tokar, MD; Foxchase Cancer Center, Philadelphia.)

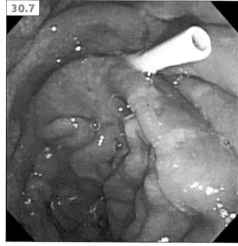

30.7 Prophylactic stent in minor papilla. (Courtesy of Jeffrey Tokar, MD; Foxchase Cancer Center, Philadelphia.)

Management of PD is generally conservative. Intervention may become necessary if PD is associated with debilitating pancreatitis. The goals for therapy are primarily to relieve the presumed obstruction. Options include endoscopic dilation, papillotomy, and sphincterotomy of the minor papilla, with or without stent placement (**30.4–30.7**), or surgical sphincterotomy, combined with major papilla sphincteroplasty. There is a greater likelihood of symptom relief for PD-associated acute recurrent pancreatitis (82%) than for chronic pancreatitis (56%).

Anomalous pancreatobiliary union

Anomalous pancreatobiliary union (APBU), also known as anomalous pancreatobiliary junction, is a rare congenital abnormality with a prevalence of 3 in 10,000 persons in one population-based series from Japan. Whereas the common bile duct and the main pancreatic duct normally meet within the duodenal wall, in patients with APBU the two ducts join outside the duodenum, and they converge into a long common channel 8–20 mm in length. APBU may result from failure of the embryologic ducts to migrate fully in the duodenum. Most (70%) are associated with congenital bile duct dilation and choledochal cysts or biliary cysts. There is regurgitation of pancreatic juice into the biliary tree (pancreatobiliary reflux) and of bile into the pancreatic duct (biliopancreatic reflux). A diagnosis of APBU is usually made by ERCP or MRCP, during an evaluation for biliary cysts. Because of an increased risk of cholangiocarcinoma, surgical resection with cyst excision and cholecystectomy is recommended.

Defects in pancreatic migration

Ectopic pancreas (pancreatic rest)

The next major classification of congenital anomalies are the disorders of migration. These defects result during the progression of embryologic development, as the progenitor tissue makes its way to its final destination. Ectopic pancreas, or a pancreatic rest, is pancreatic tissue that lacks anatomic or vascular continuity with the pancreas. Estimates are that pancreatic rests occur in up to 14% of the general population. The majority of ectopic pancreatic tissue is found in the foregut, with 75% in the stomach, particulary the prepyloric gastric antrum (**30.8**). Other reported locations are at the gallbladder, bile ducts, the minor and major papillae, and within a Meckel diverticulum. Typically, these lesions are discovered incidentally during endoscopy, surgery, radiographic contrast studies, or at autopsy. They most commonly consist of exocrine cells, although endocrine pancreatic tissue and a combination of exocrine and endocrine cells have also been reported. Asymptomatic rests can be followed conservatively. Clinically

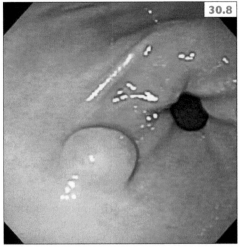

30.8 Endoscopy of pancreatic rest found incidentally in the gastric antrum.

significant findings are present in fewer than one-half of occurrences and include epigastric pain, dyspepsia, and gastrointestinal (GI) bleeding. Complications are rare and include stenosis, ulceration, and intussusception. When symptomatic, rests may require resection by endoscopic snare or band ligation, but surgical resection is indicated if the muscularis propria is involved.

Annular pancreas

Annular pancreas is a rare congenital anomaly in which a segment of the head of the pancreas either partially or completely encircles the second part of the duodenum. Annular pancreas has a prevalence of about 1 in 2,000 persons and can occur either as an isolated finding or with other congenital abnormalities such as Down syndrome, esophageal and duodenal atresia, imperforate anus, and Meckel diverticulum.

The development of annular pancreas is not completely understood. Three main hypotheses prevail. The first is that there is an adhesion of the right ventral portion of the early pancreas to the duodenal wall, which then leads to an incomplete rotation during development and causes constriction of pancreatic tissue around the duodenum (Lecco's theory). The second hypothesis is the mere persistence and subsequent enlargement of the left ventral portion of the pancreas (Baldwin's theory). The third hypothesis is that there is abnormal hypertrophy of both ventral and dorsal buds that fuse before rotation and thereby encircle the duodenum. Reports of familial annular pancreas support a genetic basis for this disease. Mice with loss of function mutations in the gene for Indian Hedgehog (IHH), a transcription factor that promotes foregut growth and differentiation, have increased ventral pancreatic mass and complete annular pancreas, demonstrating a link between this anomaly and early signaling pathways in pancreatic development.

Annular pancreas presents differently based on age of presentation. Whereas one-half to two-thirds of adult cases of annular pancreas remain asymptomatic and are found incidentally, the majority of children with annular pancreas develop gastric outlet obstruction within the first few days of life. The most common pediatric presentation is a neonatal small bowel obstruction just proximal to the ampulla of Vater. Newborns can present with feeding intolerance, bilious vomiting, and abdominal distention. Polyhydramnios is a feature if complete duodenal obstruction is present *in utero*. Overall, annular pancreas obstructs the duodenum in 10% of cases. In contrast to children, adults who are symptomatic present with abdominal pain, nausea, postprandial fullness, vomiting, upper GI bleeding from peptic ulceration, acute or chronic pancreatitis, and, rarely, biliary obstruction.

Children with annular pancreas have a higher association with other congenital abnormalities, the most common being Down syndrome and congenital heart disease. Associated GI malformations include intestinal malrotation, duodenal web, stenosis and atresia, tracheoesophageal fistula, imperforate anus, Meckel diverticulum, and Hirschsprung disease.

A diagnosis of annular pancreas is suspected based on prenatal ultrasound or plain abdominal radiographs shortly after birth that demonstrate a classic 'double bubble' sign (**30.9**). Although nonspecific, this finding is highly suggestive of duodenal obstruction. In this very young age group, surgical correction is immediately indicated, and confirmation of annular pancreas is made during laparotomy. In older children or adults, the diagnosis is usually made with an upper GI series or abdominal computed tomography (CT) scan showing duodenal narrowing and a filling defect across the second portion of the duodenum, along with proximal dilatation (**30.10**). ERCP can be helpful to further delineate the accessory duct and C-loop encircling the duodenum, thus confirming a diagnosis. Endoscopic ultrasound and MRCP can also aid in the diagnosis.

Treatment aims to bypass the obstruction without transecting the pancreatic tissue.

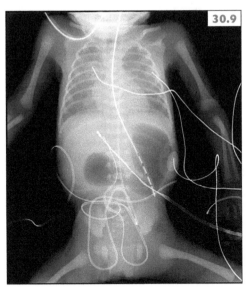

30.9 Classic 'double-bubble' sign on abdominal X-ray in a neonate with vomiting, feeding intolerance, and abdominal distention, all signs of gastric outlet obstruction. The patient was found to have annular pancreas at surgery.

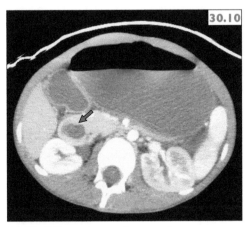

30.10 CT scan image of an annular pancreas (arrow).

In children, the treatment of choice is a duodenal bypass. Resection of the annulus is usually avoided because of the risk of pancreatitis, pancreatic fistula formation, or an incomplete relief of the obstruction.

The prognosis of patients with annular pancreas depends on the age of onset of symptoms. Infants have a higher mortality, due to the associated congenital abnormalities.

Defects leading to reduced pancreatic volume

Pancreatic agenesis or pancreatic hypoplasia

Both pancreatic agenesis and hypoplasia (OMIM #260370) are rare findings which are described in case reports and have been described alone or in association with other congenital abnormalities. The syndrome results from a more global defect in pancreatic development. Some cases are linked to homozygous or compound heterozygous mutations in the pancreatic and duodenal homeobox (PDX1) gene, also known as insulin promoter factor-1. Patients have both exocrine and endocrine deficiencies. Infants present with neonatal insulin-dependent diabetes mellitus, intrauterine growth retardation, subsequent failure to thrive from pancreatic insufficiency, and they require pancreatic enzyme replacement therapy. Imaging with ultrasound or CT scan can reveal absence of pancreatic tissue.

Other congenital defects of volume present with pancreatic insufficiency. These syndromes show fatty or fibrous replacement of the pancreas and are described in more detail in Chapter 31, Exocrine Pancreatic Insufficiency.

CHAPTER 31

Exocrine Pancreatic Insufficiency

Aliye Uc

- **Introduction**
- **Cystic fibrosis**
- **Shwachman–Diamond syndrome**
- **Pearson marrow–pancreas syndrome**
- **Johanson–Blizzard syndrome**
- **Isolated enzyme deficiencies**

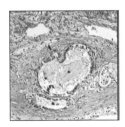
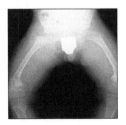
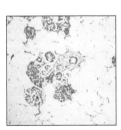
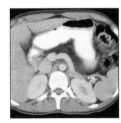

Introduction

Exocrine pancreatic insufficiency (EPI) is a term used to define patients who have lost a significant amount (usually more than 95%) of pancreatic exocrine function, and therefore their ability to digest and assimilate nutrients normally. The causes of EPI in childhood are listed in *Table 31.1*. Cystic fibrosis (CF) is by far the most common form of EPI in children. Chronic pancreatitis, another cause of EPI, will be covered in detail in Chapter 32.

Cystic fibrosis

DEFINITION AND EPIDEMIOLOGY

CF is the most common life-threatening autosomal recessive disease in the Caucasian population (~1 in 2,500 births). CF is caused by a mutation in the gene that encodes the cystic fibrosis transmembrane conductance regulator (CFTR) protein. CFTR is expressed in many epithelial cells (sweat duct, airway, pancreatic duct, intestine, biliary tree, vas deferens) and functions as an apical membrane anion channel (mainly involved in chloride and bicarbonate secretion). Patients with CF suffer primarily from progressive lung disease that causes significant morbidity and mortality. The pancreas is frequently involved in CF. Approximately 50–65% of people with CF have overt EPI at birth, and 20–30% of pancreatic sufficient patients become insufficient during the first few months to years of life.

CLINICAL PRESENTATION

EPI presents primarily as fat malabsorption defined by a fecal fat greater than 7% of oral fat intake in a 3–5 day fat balance study. Fat malabsorption, steatorrhea (bulky, foul-smelling stools), and malnutrition are the hallmarks of CF patients with EPI.

Insufficient secretion of pancreatic enzymes (proteases, amylase, lipase, colipase) leads to maldigestion and malabsorption. Patients with EPI suffer from poor weight gain or weight loss, diarrhea, steatorrhea, bloating, and flatulence. Although the etiology of malnutrition is multifactorial (inadequate intake, increased losses, lung disease, increased energy needs), EPI seems to have a major impact on growth, nutrition, and lung disease outcome. In severe cases, the fat malabsorption can lead to deficiencies of fat-soluble vitamins A, D, E, and K. Routine vitamin supplementation has made clinically evident vitamin deficiency now uncommon.

Nevertheless, vitamin K and D deficiencies may still occur. Patients with CF are chronically depleted of vitamin D despite the inclusion of extra vitamin D in their regimen of fat-soluble vitamin supplementation. Recent studies suggest that the vitamin D bioavailability might be impaired in patients with CF. It appears that vitamin D has important functions in CF outside the bones, including pulmonary function, innate immunity, and regulation of insulin, which are all pertinent to CF. Therefore it is important to maintain adequate levels of vitamin in D in these patients.

Patients with EPI can ultimately develop impaired glucose tolerance and spontaneous hyperglycemia. CF-related diabetes is associated with a rapid decline in pulmonary function, higher morbidity, and greater mortality from CF.

DIAGNOSIS
Sweat chloride

An adequate sweat specimen can be collected for sweat chloride (Cl^-) in infants starting at 2 weeks of age, ideally weighing at least 2 kg. Sweat Cl^- reference ranges for children are shown in *Table 31.2*. Children with intermediate results should undergo repeat sweat Cl^- testing and further evaluation, including a detailed clinical assessment and *CFTR* gene mutation analysis.

DNA analysis

For children with intermediate sweat Cl⁻ values, deoxyribonucleic acid (DNA) analysis can help establish the diagnosis of CF. Genetic testing for CF is not straightforward. Although more than 1900 *CFTR* mutations have been identified, the functional importance is known only for a small number of mutations. The DNA analysis for *CFTR* mutations should be done in consultation with a CF specialist.

Pancreatic function tests

The pancreatic function tests (PFTs) are classified as direct and indirect. Direct PFTs involve the stimulation of pancreas with pancreatic secretagogues followed by collection of duodenal fluid and analysis of its contents (i.e. enzymes, chloride, bicarbonate). Direct PFTs are more sensitive and specific than indirect tests, but they are invasive and difficult to perform. Shortening the sampling times and failing to correct for intestinal losses have led to misclassification of pancreatic sufficient patients as insufficient. Indirect tests are widely available and easier to perform but have low sensitivity and specificity.

Indirect tests
Fecal fat excretion

This test involves a 72-hour stool collection and calculation of coefficient of fat absorption (CFA: grams of fat ingested – grams of fat excreted)/ (grams of fat ingested) ×100). In children younger than 6 months of age, a fecal fat greater than 15% of fat intake is considered abnormal although this value is 7% for children over 6 months of age. When performed correctly, CFA is very useful to determine the degree of fat malabsorption and to evaluate response to enzyme therapy. Fecal fat excretion does not discriminate among hepatobiliary, intestinal mucosal, or pancreatic causes of fat malabsorption. The lack of accuracy and reproducibility limits its use. In general the stool collection is not well accepted by patients and parents.

Fecal elastase-1

The measurement of fecal trypsin and chymotrypsin tests may be inaccurate due to intraluminal degradation and cross-reactivity with ingested enzymes. Fecal elastase-1 (FE-1) is resistant to degradation; therefore, it is the preferred stool enzyme test to diagnose EPI. FE-1 is a widely available, easy

---

Table 31.1 Etiologies of pancreatic insufficiency in childhood

Cystic fibrosis (most common)

Shwachman–Diamond syndrome

Chronic pancreatitis

Pearson marrow–pancreas syndrome

Johanson–Blizzard syndrome

Isolated enzyme deficiencies (lipase, colipase, trypsinogen, amylase, enterokinase)

Table 31.2 Sweat chloride test for cystic fibrosis (CF)

Age	Cl⁻ (mmol/l)	Indication
<6 months		
	≤29	CF unlikely
	30–59	Intermediate risk
	≥60	Indicative of CF
>6 months		
	≤39	CF unlikely
	40–59	Intermediate risk
	≥60	Indicative of CF

to use, and is a relatively inexpensive enzyme-linked immunosorbent assay (ELISA)-based method to measure the exocrine pancreatic function. A FE-1 value of less than 100 µg/g is considered diagnostic of EPI. Intermediate values of FE-1 (100–200 µg/g) may be due to loss of pancreatic function, but are not severe enough to call EPI. The sensitivity of FE-1 to diagnose moderate and severe EPI is close to 100%, but in patients with mild loss of pancreatic function, the test sensitivity is approximately 25%. Thus, the value of FE-1 to determine patients with mild EPI or borderline normal pancreatic function is limited. FE-1 may be falsely low when the stool is diluted (i.e. infectious diarrhea, severe enteropathies, short bowel syndrome, stool collected from an ileostomy).

Serum immunoreactive trypsinogen

The serum immunoreactive trypsinogen (IRT) test measures trypsinogen (probably trypsinogen I or cationic trypsinogen) in the serum. In healthy individuals, only small amounts of trypsinogen should be present in serum. The elevation of IRT is an indication that the enzyme escapes to the blood stream from a damaged pancreas. Indeed, IRT is elevated in babies with CF at birth and declines as the EPI develops over time. IRT is currently used as a newborn screening (NBS) test for CF in the United States. Usually, after an abnormal IRT value is identified, most NBS programs perform DNA testing to identify known *CFTR* gene mutations (IRT/DNA strategy), while other programs repeat the IRT measurement in a second blood sample obtained from the infant at age approximately 2 weeks (IRT/IRT strategy). Both strategies provide ~90–95% sensitivity and identify newborns at risk for CF. Although it is useful as a screening test for CF, IRT should not be used for the diagnosis of EPI.

Direct tests
Pancreatic stimulation tests

Although the indirect tests are useful to diagnose EPI, they cannot accurately measure the pancreatic acinar cell reserve and ductal cell function. The direct tests involve the collection of pancreatic fluid secreted into the intestine and measurement of enzymes (pancreatic acinar function), and fluid volume and electrolytes (pancreatic ductal function). In patients with exocrine pancreatic involvement, fluid volume, chloride and bicarbonate concentrations and total enzyme output are low and the response to pancreatic secretagogues (cholecystokinin and secretin) is abnormal. However, there is no standardized methodology for pancreatic stimulation tests. The invasive and complex nature of these tests (placement of a nasoduodenal catheter, IV cannulation, sedation, and radiation exposure) limits their routine clinical use. Pancreatic stimulation tests are not routinely used for the assessment of exocrine pancreatic function in children.

Imaging studies

In patients with CF, ultrasonography, computed tomography (CT), and magnetic resonance imaging (MRI) usually show an atrophied pancreas with fatty replacement. Areas of calcifications may also be present (**31.1**). These findings are nonspecific for CF.

PATHOPHYSIOLOGY

Pancreatic lesions in CF vary considerably in severity and, in general, are more severe with increasing age. The early lesions are deposits of periodic acid Schiff (PAS)-positive material within some acini and ductules with associated flattening of the epithelium. Pancreatic lesions then progress to include degeneration of acinar cells and lack of zymogen granules, dilatation of acini and ducts filled with inspissated PAS-positive material, and ductular proliferation. When severely affected, the characteristic morphologic features of the CF pancreas include marked acinar atrophy, fibrosis, and fatty replacement (**31.2**). These morphological changes reflect the progressive nature of the pancreatic disease process.

While sufficient exocrine pancreatic function is present and pancreatic enzyme supplementation is not needed, the pancreas of CF patients with pancreatic sufficiency is never normal. The pancreas in CF is destroyed by acidic, dehydrated, and protein-rich secretions, which then plug the lumen and trigger an inflammatory response.

TREATMENT
Pancreatic enzyme replacement therapy
Currently, there are six Food and Drug Administration (FDA)-approved pancreatic enzyme replacement therapy (PERT) preparations in the United States. They are all of porcine origin. To avoid the activation of pancreatic enzyme preparations by gastric acid and pepsin and prolong their contact with the intestine, the delayed-release forms have been developed. One formulation contains a proton pump inhibitor, to inhibit

stomach acid, thus increasing efficacy of the pancreatic enzymes. H2-receptor antagonists or proton pump inhibitors may be added to the medical regimen to provide the same effect. Patients with CF and other forms of pancreatic insufficiency need the pancreatic enzymes to treat their malnutrition, growth delay, diarrhea, and steatorrhea, but this replacement therapy does not provide full symptom relief in all patients.

PERT is based on the unit of lipase per meal. Children <4 years of age require approximately 1,000 lipase units/kg per meal while approximately 500 lipase units/kg per meal is used for children >4 years of age. For snacks, half of the dose is recommended. Infants may be given 2,000–4,000 units per 120 ml of infant formula or per breast feeding. The daily dose for most patients is <10,000 units of lipase/kg per day or 6,000 units of lipase/kg per meal to minimize incidence of fibrosing colonopathy. For children who cannot swallow capsules, delayed-release capsules containing enteric

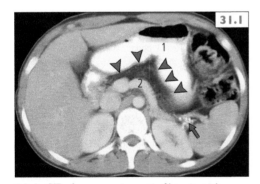

31.1 CT of pancreas in cystic fibrosis with fatty replacement of the parenchyma. Note the fatty attenuation of pancreas (arrowheads) lying between the stomach (1) and the splenic vein (2) and the calcifications (arrow) at the pancreatic tail. (Courtesy of Simon C. Kao, MD; University of Iowa.)

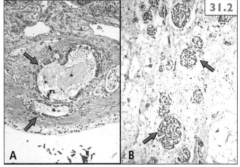

31.2 Pancreas from a 12-year-old male with cystic fibrosis who died from lung complications of the disease, showing almost complete acinar atrophy with fibrosis and fatty replacement (A, B). Ducts are dilated with eosinophilic material and mucus (A, arrows). Pancreatic islets are relatively spared (B, arrows). (Courtesy of David K. Meyerholz, MD and Marcus Nashelsky, MD; University of Iowa.)

coated microspheres or microtablets may be opened and the contents sprinkled on soft food with a low pH that does not require chewing (applesauce, gelatins, pureed apricot, banana, or sweet potatoes). Foods having a pH > 7.3, such as milk, custard, or ice cream, should be avoided as a vehicle for the sprinkled enzymes because the protective enteric coating can dissolve.

Optimizing nutrition

Children with CF and poor nutritional status are more prone to lung infections than those with good nutritional status, and children with normal pancreatic function have a better pulmonary prognosis than those with EPI. Therefore, the growth of children with CF should be closely monitored and the nutritional issues should be aggressively managed. Consultation with a dietician with expertise in CF is recommended.

Breastfeeding is recommended for infants with CF until 12 months of age. For older children, a balanced diet enhanced with high-fat snacks and supplements is necessary to meet the high-energy needs. Children with EPI need a 20–50% increase over the recommended daily allowance. For children who are unable to gain weight with oral intake or if the oral intake is limited, nutritional supplementation can be maintained with a nasogastric tube or gastrostomy feedings.

Vitamin supplementation

Because patients with EPI are prone to fat malabsorption that may lead to deficiencies of the fat-soluble vitamins A, D, E, and K, all patients with CF should receive supplementation of these vitamins (*Table 31.3*). Vitamin levels should be checked yearly for monitoring.

Table 31.3 Fat-soluble vitamin supplementation for patients with cystic fibrosis and pancreatic insufficiency

Vitamin	Age group	Daily intake	Monitoring parameters
A	< 3 years	1,500 IU/d	Serum retinol, abnormal if <20 µg/dl (0.7 µmol/l)
	1–3 years	5,000 IU/d	
	4–8 years	5,000 to 10,000 IU/d	
	>8 years–adults	10,000 IU/d	
D	<1 year	400 IU/d	Serum 25(OH)D in late autumn or winter, abnormal if <30 ng/ml, supplementation may be increased to correct the deficiency
	>1 year	400–800 IU/d	
E	0–12 months	40–50 IU/d	Serum alpha-tocopherol abnormal if <300 µg/l
	1–3 years	80–150 IU/d	
	4–8 years	100–200 IU/d	
	>8 years–adults	200–400 IU/d	
K	0–18 years	0.3–0.5 mg/d	Serum prothrombin time
	Adults	2.5–5 mg/week	

Shwachman–Diamond syndrome

DEFINITION AND EPIDEMIOLOGY

Shwachman–Diamond syndrome (SDS) is the second most common form of EPI in children. It is estimated to occur in one in 76,000 births.

CLINICAL PRESENTATION AND DIAGNOSIS

Patients with SDS usually present in infancy with symptoms of EPI (diarrhea, steatorrhea, bloating, flatulence, malnutrition), neutropenia (absolute neutrophil count <1,500 neutrophils/mm³ for ≥3 measurements taken over a period of ≥3 months), skeletal defects, and short stature. Neutropenia (persistent or intermittent) is present in almost all affected children, often before the diagnosis of

SDS is made. Other cytopenias may also be present. Skeletal defects are characterized by delayed appearance of secondary ossification centers, causing bone age to appear to be delayed; variable widening and irregularity of the metaphyses in early childhood (i.e. metaphyseal chondrodysplasia), followed by progressive thickening and irregularity of the growth plates; and generalized osteopenia (31.3). SDS is inherited in an autosomal recessive manner, but *de novo* mutations have been reported. In approximately 90% of affected patients, mutations can be detected in the Shwachman–Bodian–Diamond syndrome (SBDS) gene located on chromosome 7. A negative test for SBDS gene mutations does not exclude the diagnosis, because approximately 10% of patients clinically diagnosed with SDS lack these mutations. If the pancreatic tissue is available, histopathology will show few acinar cells and

31.3 Metaphyseal chondrodysplasia, Shwachman–Diamond type. Note the symmetric shortening of both femora and irregular metaphyseal lucent and sclerotic changes at hip and knee regions. (Courtesy of Simon C. Kao, MD; University of Iowa.)

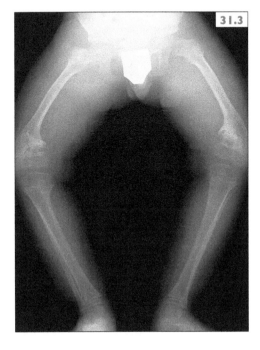

extensive fatty infiltration (**31.4**). Contrary to CF, pancreatic ducts are not involved in SDS. Abdominal ultrasonography, CT, or MRI will reveal a small and fatty pancreas.

Diagnosis of SDS is usually made by characteristic clinical findings. Genetic testing may be used to confirm the diagnosis.

TREATMENT

Treatment should be directed towards the manifestations of the disease. EPI is treated with pancreatic enzymes and fat-soluble vitamins as described in the previous section. Blood and/or platelet transfusions may be needed for hematological complications. Granulocyte-colony stimulation factor may be considered for recurrent infections and severe neutropenia ($<500/mm^3$). Patients with SDS may later be candidates for hematopoietic stem cell transplantation for the treatment of severe pancytopenia or development of complications (myelodysplastic syndrome, acute myelogenic leukemia).

PROGNOSIS

Poor growth does not usually improve despite adequate pancreatic replacement therapy. Pancreatic insufficiency is often transient, and steatorrhea may spontaneously improve over time. Recurrent suppurative infections (otitis media, pneumonia, osteomyelitis, dermatitis, sepsis) are common and a frequent cause of death.

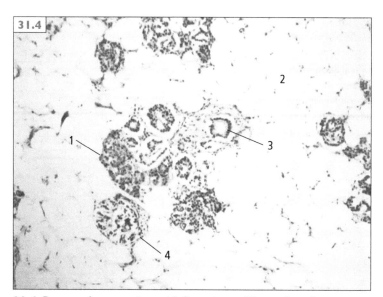

31.4 Pancreas from a patient with Shwachman–Diamond syndrome showing reduced number of acinar cells and extensive fatty infiltration. Pancreatic ducts are not involved. 1: Pancreatic acini; 2: fatty stroma; 3: pancreatic duct; 4: islet of Langerhans. (Courtesy of Peter R. Durie, MD; University of Toronto, Canada.)

Pearson marrow–pancreas syndrome

DEFINITION AND EPIDEMIOLOGY
This is a rare multisystem disorder involving the hematopoietic system, pancreas, liver, and kidneys, caused by defects in oxidative phosphorylation due to sporadic mutations in mitochondrial DNA.

CLINICAL PRESENTATION AND DIAGNOSIS
Patients typically present in infancy with severe, transfusion-dependent, hypoplastic macrocytic anemia; a variable degree of neutropenia and thrombocytopenia; and normal or reduced bone marrow cellularity with vacuolated precursors. Other features are exocrine and endocrine pancreas dysfunction, hyperlipidemia, liver steatosis, proximal tubular insufficiency, higher urinary excretion of lactate and organic acids, metabolic acidosis, failure to thrive, and skin lesions.

Pearson marrow–pancreas syndrome is distinguished from SDS by the presence of sideroblastic anemia, bone marrow changes (cell vacuolization and ringed sideroblasts), pancreatic fibrosis rather than lipomatosis, and the absence of bone lesions. Diagnosis is confirmed by Southern blot analysis that detects mitochondrial DNA rearrangements.

TREATMENT AND PROGNOSIS
There is no specific treatment available and patients usually succumb to death in infancy or early childhood due to metabolic disorders and/or infections.

Johanson–Blizzard syndrome

This rare autosomal recessive disorder is characterized by EPI and multiple congenital anomalies (aplasia or hypoplasia of the alae nasi, congenital deafness, microcephaly, midline ectodermal scalp defects, absence of permanent teeth, cardiac and urogenital malformations, imperforate anus), hypothyroidism, and developmental delay. Diabetes may develop over time. In contrast to SDS, children with Johanson–Blizzard syndrome do not have bone marrow and skeletal abnormalities. New studies have shown mutation in the ubiquitin E3 ligase *UBR1* gene in these patients and possibly intrauterine destruction of the pancreas.

Isolated enzyme deficiencies

The isolated deficiencies of trypsinogen (protein malabsorption), lipase and colipase (fat malabsorption), and enterokinase are very rare. Enterokinase is an intestinal brush border enzyme that activates pancreatic proteases (trypsinogen, chymotrypsinogen); therefore, its deficiency will lead to protein malabsorption. Patients with deficiencies of trypsinogen or enterokinase present with failure to thrive, hypoproteinemia, and edema. Isolated amylase deficiency is developmental, clinically transient, and resolves by 2–3 years of age.

Pancreatitis – Acute and Chronic

Mark Bartlett, Tara Holm, Sarah Jane Schwarzenberg

- **Introduction**
- **Acute pancreatitis**
- **Chronic pancreatitis**

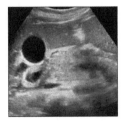 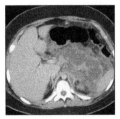 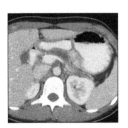 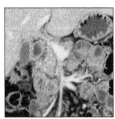

Introduction

Inflammation of the pancreas parenchyma is classified as either acute or chronic. While both are less common in children than in adults, these diseases are associated with significant morbidity and mortality. Acute pancreatitis may occur as an isolated illness or may be a complication of many other childhood illnesses. It is usually a completely reversible injury. Chronic pancreatitis is a progressive disease involving changes in the structure and histology of the organ. Unfortunately, the changes from chronic pancreatitis are often irreversible.

Acute pancreatitis

EPIDEMIOLOGY

There are no population-based studies of the incidence of acute pancreatitis in children. Incidence figures of 13–15 per 100,000 children have been suggested using data from North American referral centers. There has been an increase in the diagnosis of acute pancreatitis in children over the last 10 years in both North America and Australia, although this may reflect increasing awareness resulting in increased amylase and lipase testing in children or increased referral to tertiary pediatric centers.

CLINICAL PRESENTATION

Children usually present with a combination of abdominal pain and nausea and vomiting. Pain may be localized to the midepigastric area, or the right or left upper quadrants. Young children may present with irritability alone or periumbilical pain, delaying their diagnosis. A review of 215 children evaluated for acute pancreatitis at a single center showed that the three most common findings at presentation were abdominal tenderness or irritability, nausea or vomiting, and tenderness in the epigastrium on palpation. In this study, children less than 2 years of age demonstrated these three features less frequently. Pain may radiate to the back, but in children this symptom occurs in less than 10% of cases. In some cases, acute pancreatitis may be accompanied by cardiovascular collapse, ileus, abdominal distention, fever, jaundice, ascites, and/or pleural effusion.

As pancreatitis may accompany many other serious childhood illnesses, a classic presentation may not be apparent in the child with burns, leukemia, or Henoch–Schönlein purpura, for example. Children on mechanical ventilation for other illness at the time of onset of acute pancreatitis may not be able to communicate their state. Thus, a high index of suspicion is important.

ETIOLOGY/PATHOPHYSIOLOGY

The etiologies of acute pancreatitis are diverse and can be divided into the following categories: anatomic abnormalities, trauma, metabolic disorders, biliary disease, systemic illnesses, and drugs (*Table 32.1*). A significant percentage of cases in children remain idiopathic even after extensive evaluation.

Of anatomic variants, the most common causes are choledochal cyst and pancreas divisum. Other structural findings, such as anomalous junction of the biliary and pancreatic ducts, ampulla obstruction, and annular pancreas, have all been implicated as a cause of acute pancreatitis. Trauma has been estimated to account for 10–40% of pediatric cases and can be from blunt accidental injury or from abuse. The metabolic derangements most often associated with acute pancreatitis are diabetic ketoacidosis, hypercalcemia, and hypertriglyceridemia, but some inborn errors of metabolism can also result in acute pancreatitis. Biliary obstruction, both gallstones and sludge, is responsible for around 10% of cases in most reviews and almost 30% in a study of Korean children. Obesity is a risk factor for gallstones, and the incidence of biliary pancreatitis may rise with the pediatric obesity epidemic.

Table 32.1 Etiologies of acute pancreatitis

Anatomic
- Pancreas divisum
- Annular pancreas
- Obstructed ampulla
- Anomalies of biliary and pancreatic ducts
- Cyst
- Diverticulum

Biliary
- Choledochal cyst
- Cholelithiasis
- Sludge in bile ducts

Genetic
- *PRSS1* mutations
- *CFTR* mutations

Medications
- Azathioprine
- L-Asparaginase
- Metronidazole
- Mercaptopurine
- Pentamidine
- Prednisone
- Tetracyclines
- Valproic acid

Metabolic
- Glycogen storage diseases
- Hypercalcemia
- Hyperlipidemia
- Organic acidemias

Systemic diseases
- Diabetic ketoacidosis
- Hemolytic uremic syndrome
- Henoch–Schönlein purpura
- Inflammatory bowel disease
- Sepsis
- Sickle-cell disease

Trauma
- Accidental
- Nonaccidental/abuse
- Burns

Idiopathic

Systemic illness from infections is associated with pancreatitis. Sometimes the infection itself involves the pancreas (mumps and varicella virus, among others). Systemic inflammatory response from many causes, including burns, systemic lupus erythematosus, hemolytic uremic syndrome, or Henoch–Schönlein purpura, is also associated with acute pancreatitis. Lastly, many drugs have been implicated in pancreatitis, most notably valproate (valproic acid), mercaptopurine, L-asparaginase, and prednisone.

DIFFERENTIAL DIAGNOSIS

- Intestinal obstruction/ischemia, including volvulus and intussusception.
- Peptic ulcer, severe esophagitis, gastritis, and duodenitis.
- Acute cholecystitis or choledocholithiasis.
- Diabetic ketoacidosis.
- Mesenteric infarction.
- Ruptured ectopic pregnancy.
- Hepatitis.
- Gastroenteritis.
- Peritonitis.
- Pneumonia.

DIAGNOSIS

Diagnosis of acute pancreatitis requires at least two of these three features: first, a clinical picture consistent with acute pancreatitis; second, elevation of amylase or lipase to at least three times normal level; and third, radiographic changes on ultrasound or computed tomography (CT) consistent with acute pancreatitis. The diagnosis of acute pancreatitis can be challenging since there is no single test used for confirmation. In some patients the enzymes remain normal but the radiographic findings are highly suggestive and used for diagnosis. Younger or nonverbal children may only have irritability, making imaging more important.

When pancreatitis is suspected based on symptoms and labs, ultrasonography (US) is still the initial imaging modality used at most centers. There are no large studies to validate the use of US or to document exactly which features are most diagnostic in children. Diffuse or focal enlargement of the pancreas is thought to be a feature of acute pancreatitis, but may be absent in up to one-half of the cases. Pancreatic duct diameter may be the most suggestive feature of pancreatitis since the mean diameter is significantly larger than that seen in healthy controls. Other US findings reported to be significant include altered echogenicity, gallstones, biliary sludge, or fluid collections in or around the pancreas (**32.1**).

Because of its associated radiation exposure, CT is not recommended for diagnosis of acute pancreatitis unless the pancreas cannot be visualized on US and the diagnosis is unclear. CT can be useful later during the clinical course if pancreatic necrosis is suspected (**32.2**). A recent development has been the increased use of endoscopic ultrasound (EUS) in children. It has high diagnostic accuracy and a much lower complication rate than endoscopic retrograde cholangiopancreatography (ERCP) for imaging the pancreas and bile ducts. Magnetic resonance imaging (MRI) and magnetic resonance cholangio-pancreatography (MRCP) are also imaging techniques that may be of more use in the future. At present, the necessity to remain still for the length of the study is a challenge for children in significant pain.

TREATMENT

The medical management of acute pancreatitis in children is bowel rest, fluids, and pain control. Early resuscitation with intravenous fluids is essential as acute pancreatitis can occasionally be life-threatening from significant third spacing and cardiovascular collapse. Early nutritional support is important for healing in pancreatitis. Parenteral nutrition was long considered the standard of care during pancreatitis; more recently several studies have shown better outcomes with early jejunal feedings. When children are diagnosed with

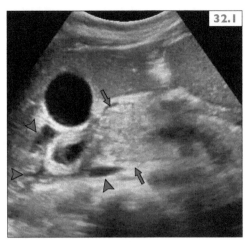

32.1 Ultrasound image demonstrating an enlarged pancreatic head (arrows) with surrounding edema (arrowheads) in a teenage patient with early acute pancreatitis.

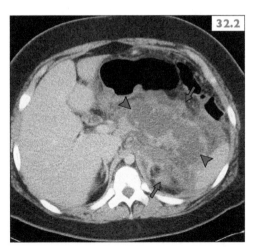

32.2 Noncontrast axial CT image demonstrating massive enlargement of the pancreas with intrapancreatic low attenuation and fluid from necrosis (arrowheads), diffuse peripancreatic fat stranding, and ill-defined fluid (arrows) in a teenage patient with acute necrotizing pancreatitis.

acute pancreatitis, it is important to assess severity and watch closely for complications with close attention paid to monitoring vital signs and watching for hypotension. Ranson's Criteria, used in adults, have not been validated in children under age 18 years. Several recent studies have compared a variety of scoring systems for predicting severity. The factors most associated with poor outcome are younger age and low weight; however, a CT scan index has recently been shown to be more sensitive than using clinical indices. It is difficult to recommend CT solely as a scoring method, given the known risk of unnecessary radiation exposure. If CT is used for identifying pancreatitis after trauma, the findings may not be evident at the time of presentation, but accuracy improves if the scan is delayed until at least 3 days after the injury.

Patients can suffer from respiratory failure from adult respiratory distress syndrome that develops from a combination of fluids leaking into the lung alveoli and generalized inflammation. Other life-threatening complications of acute pancreatitis include an infected and necrotic pancreas with multi-organ failure. This complication is rare in children, with pancreatic necrosis occurring in less than 1% of cases. Systemic complications include septic shock, pulmonary edema, coagulopathy, as well as metabolic derange-ments including hypocalcemia and hyper-glycemia.

One complication of acute pancreatitis that requires unique management is pan-creatic pseudocyst. A pseudocyst is a cystic cavity without epithelial lining that forms after injury to the pancreatic parenchyma (**32.3**). If asymptomatic, these fluid collections can be followed with intermittent ultrasound and often will resolve spontaneously. One series in children suggests that about 1/3 of pseudocysts will resolve spontaneously. Drainage is required if the pseudocyst is causing pain, compressing adjacent bowel or biliary duct (**32.4**), or if it is infected or bleeding. Current approaches to pancreatic pseudocyst drainage are as follows: open surgery, percutaneous catheter drainage, or endoscopic drainage. The last method has been described in numerous case reports and is becoming the preferred approach now that EUS is being used more skillfully for pediatric patients. Endoscopic drainage can be either transmural into the stomach or transpapillary into the duodenum. Deciding when and how to drain a pseudocyst depends some on the specific case and expertise available at a given institution (**32.5**).

Two additional indications for surgery in the management of acute pancreatitis are the debridement of infected or necrotic pancreatic tissue and cholecystectomy in cases where gallstones or biliary sludge are the cause. In cases where surgical debridement is necessary, there is controversy in the adult literature regarding timing. Some advocate deferring for at least 2 weeks so the infection can be controlled and the necrotic tissue is more easily demarcated from the healthy organ. The American College of Gastroenterology practice guidelines, however, emphasize the importance of prompt intervention. These guidelines also highlight the emerging use of endoscopy for necrosectomy often supplanting the need for surgery.

The management of biliary pancreatitis often includes cholecystectomy, done prefer-ably after resolution of acute pancreatitis. Children with sludge alone can be started on ursodeoxycholic acid, rather than having cholecystectomy.

PROGNOSIS

Mortality is low in children with acute pancreatitis and is usually related to the underlying disease, rather than the pan-creatitis itself. Acute pancreatitis is generally fully reversible with no long-term sequelae. Approximately 10–20% of children develop a pseudocyst, usually when the etiology of the pancreatitis is traumatic.

32.3 Transverse ultrasound image of a large pseudocyst anterior to the body of the pancreas.

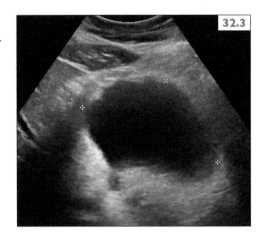

32.4 Axial contrast-enhanced CT image of a young child with a very large post-traumatic pancreatic pseudocyst (arrows) with mass effect displacing the pancreas (arrowheads) posteriorly.

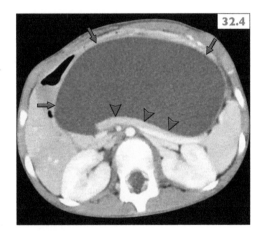

32.5 Fat-suppressed fluid-sensitive MRI demonstrates a pseudocyst with a drain to the stomach. The drain is not visible. There is gas, fluid, and debris within the partially decompressed pseudocyst (arrowheads). There is mild surrounding residual free fluid.

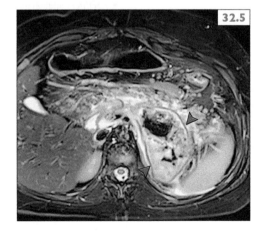

Chronic pancreatitis

DEFINITION AND EPIDEMIOLOGY

Chronic pancreatitis is persistent, destructive pancreatic inflammation with histologic and functional change that is often irreversible. It is often associated with daily or near-daily pain.

There is limited information in the pediatric literature regarding chronic pancreatitis. Population-based incidence information is not available, but adult incidence values were 4.05/100,000 individuals in Olmsted County, Minnesota, USA. In this study, individuals ages 0–34 years had an incidence rate of 0.5/100,000, with increased age associated with increasing incidence. Chronic pancreatitis is a rare condition in childhood. However, children with chronic pancreatitis are often heavy utilizers of the healthcare system. A multi-center effort has been launched to survey,

---

Table 32.2 Etiologies of chronic pancreatitis

Anatomic
- Pancreas divisum
- Annular pancreas
- Anomalous biliary or pancreatic ducts
- Obstructed ampulla
- Cyst

Autoimmune

Genetic
- *PRSS1* mutation
- *CFTR* mutations
- *SPINK1* mutation (modifier)

Medications
- Azathiprine
- L-Asparaginase
- Mercaptopurine
- Metronidazole
- Pentamidine
- Prednisone
- Tetracyclines
- Valproic acid

Systemic disease
- Diabetes
- Inflammatory bowel disease

Idiopathic

define, and document better cases of recurrent and chronic pancreatitis in children. In the future we may know more about the incidence of this condition.

CLINICAL PRESENTATION

The clinical picture of chronic pancreatitis is of intermittent episodes of pancreatitis. The most common presenting symptoms are abdominal pain and vomiting. Pain may be intermittent or constant. It is usually epigastric or mid-abdomen and may radiate to the back. Some patients have low-grade fever, but temperature >38°C should prompt concern for superimposed infection. Food frequently stimulates onset of pain.

Early in the course, patients may have significant amylase and lipase elevations during each episode, but after many such episodes, they may experience pain without enzyme elevation (so-called 'burning out' of the pancreas). Pain usually resolves after an exacerbation, but in severe cases there may be low-grade continuous pain, particularly with meals. Of course, care must be taken to insure that other gastrointestinal disease does not coexist with chronic pancreatitis. This may lead to endoscopic procedures to exclude gastritis, esophagitis, or peptic ulcer disease. Constipation may be a complication of narcotic treatment of pancreatitis, and pain from constipation must be considered in children whose episode of exacerbation is not resolving. Because of the difficulty diagnosing chronic pancreatitis, and because it is often treated with narcotics, symptom complaints may occasionally be falsified by parent or child.

ETIOLOGY AND PATHOPHYSIOLOGY

Whereas chronic pancreatitis in adults is linked to alcohol consumption in over two-thirds of cases, pediatric cases are more often linked to anatomic or genetic conditions (*Table 32.2*). In a study examining the cause of recurrent pancreatitis in 36 children seen at a single center in North America over 9 years, the etiologies were determined to be gallstones (3/36), pancreas divisum (2/36), metabolic disorder (1/36), medication-related (1/36), genetic condition (23/36), and idiopathic (6/36). A study of 42 Chinese children with chronic pancreatitis found idiopathic chronic pancreatitis in 31/42, anatomic abnormalities in 8/42, and 1 child each with hyperlipidemia, trauma, and choledochal cyst as the etiologies of the pancreatitis. Genetic causes of pancreatitis were not reported, but genetic testing was not performed in this group of children. A study of 32 children with recurrent or chronic pancreatitis found 15/32 had at least one genetic mutation associated with chronic pancreatitis, compared to no such mutations in a group of healthy controls.

Genetic conditions include three well described categories of hereditary mutations that put children at risk for chronic pancreatitis: the cationic trypsinogen gene, serine protease 1 (*PRSS1*), the serine protease inhibitor Kazal type 1 (*SPINK1*), and the cystic fibrosis transmembrane conductance regulator (*CFTR*). *PRSS1* mutations are associated with hereditary pancreatitis, a form of chronic pancreatitis with autosomal dominance inheritance with incomplete penetration. Gene frequency is difficult to assess in this rare disease but has been estimated at 0.3/100,000 in France. While the median age at presentation with chronic pancreatitis with *PRSS1* mutations is 10 years of age, clinical presentation has been reported from infancy well into adulthood. One study recorded a 9 year delay from first episode of pain to diagnosis of hereditary pancreatitis. Many children recall repeated bouts of undiagnosed abdominal pain preceding the episode that resulted in diagnosis.

Over 1900 mutations in the *CFTR* gene have been described. Of those mutations, the presence of functionally severe mutations at both *CFTR* alleles is associated with classic cystic fibrosis (CF). *CFTR* genotypes associated with mild CF phenotype (pancreatic sufficiency, mild lung disease) confer risk of developing pancreatitis. In addition, carriage of a single mutant allele of *CFTR* is over-represented in populations of 'idiopathic' chronic pancreatitis. In this case, the abnormal *CFTR* allele may be only one factor contributing to the development of chronic pancreatitis.

SPINK1 mutation alone may be inadequate to cause chronic pancreatitis, but it has been shown to be a potentiating factor in chronic pancreatitis associated with alcohol and tropical chronic pancreatitis.

In a study of recurrent pancreatitis in North America, genetic mutations were divided among mutations in *PRSS1* (29%), *CFTR* (48%) and *SPINK1* (27%). Several children had more than one mutation. In a Korean population, only *SPINK1* and *PRSS1* mutations were seen, highlighting differences in the etiologies of chronic pancreatitis in different populations. Recommendations around genetic testing in children with recurrent pancreatitis are evolving; however, most experts advocate testing for genes predisposing to chronic pancreatitis in any child who has two or more episodes of acute pancreatitis or who presents with established chronic pancreatitis. Other recommendations are to test even if there are other explanations for pancreatitis such as drugs, infection, or structural anomalies. In the aforementioned study of chronic pancreatitis in Korea, four of the six children with pancreas divisum had at least one chronic pancreatitis-associated genetic mutation.

Autoimmune pancreatitis has been reported occasionally in children, although the prevalence is unknown. It is a lympho-plasmacytic sclerosing pancreatitis with elevated levels of immunoglobulin (Ig) G4 in pancreatic parenchyma and (usually) in serum. It is characterized by obstructive jaundice resulting from enlargement of the pancreatic head or mural thickening of the bile duct. It may mimic a pancreatic mass lesion.

DIFFERENTIAL DIAGNOSIS

- Peptic ulcer disease.
- Inflammatory bowel disease.
- Cholecystitis or choledocholithiasis.
- Mesenteric ischemia.
- Intestinal obstruction.
- Irritable bowel syndrome.
- Postherpetic neuralgia or radiculopathy.
- Abdominal wall pain.
- Gastroparesis.
- Nephrolithiasis.
- Somatization disorders.

DIAGNOSIS

The diagnosis of chronic pancreatitis is made using a combination of clinical, functional, anatomic, and histologic findings. In the setting of appropriate clinical presentation, functional tests can aid in diagnosis of chronic pancreatitis but the organ has to have significant injury before its function becomes limited. Evidence of normal function does not rule out chronic pancreatitis. Reduction in fecal elastase-1 levels correlates well with moderate to severe chronic pancreatitis and indicates pancreatic exocrine insufficiency. A more sensitive test of exocrine pancreatic function is secretin-stimulated pancreatic function testing, in which duodenal fluid is collected during endoscopy after secretin stimulation and bicarbonate and pancreatic enzyme levels are measured. Bicarbonate levels less than 80 mmol/l in the duodenal fluid after secretin stimulation are considered evidence of pancreatic insufficiency. This direct pancreatic function testing is more costly and invasive, and there is still no consensus protocol used by different centers. Loss of endocrine pancreatic function is generally a late finding in chronic pancreatitis and typically occurs after exocrine insufficiency. Exocrine insufficiency alone is not diagnostic of chronic pancreatitis, since in some diseases, such as Shwachman–Diamond syndrome, there is enzyme insufficiency without destruction of the organ itself.

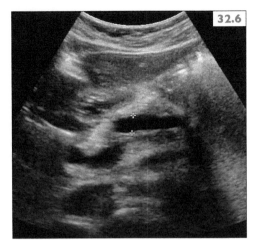

32.6 Chronic pancreatitis. Ultrasound image with an enlarged pancreatic duct (+) with a paucity of surrounding pancreatic tissue.

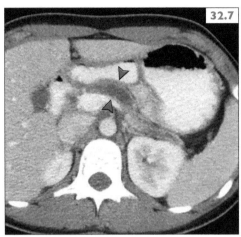

32.7 Axial CT image demonstrating severe pancreatic atrophy and an enlarged pancreatic duct (arrowheads).

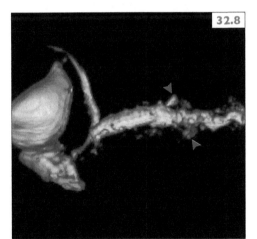

32.8 MRI 3D maximal intensity projection image with an enlarged pancreatic duct and multiple abnormally dilated pancreatic duct side branches (arrowheads).

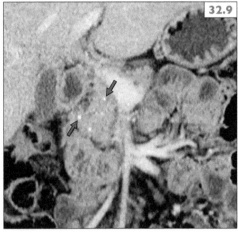

32.9 Coronal CT image demonstrating multiple punctuate calcifications in the pancreatic head (arrows).

As with acute pancreatitis, a variety of imaging techniques are used to help with diagnosis in chronic pancreatitis. Those most commonly used include CT, MRI, MRCP, EUS, and ERCP (**32.6–32.9**). The MRCP protocols in recent years have greatly improved imaging of the pancreatic ducts. Secretin administered prior to the studies renders over 90% of main ducts visible. MRCP also allows the visualization of the ducts in their physiologic state, whereas an ERCP images the ducts while under pressure. EUS is commonly used as a diagnostic tool for chronic pancreatitis in adults, but not without significant controversy. While EUS may prove helpful for diagnosis of chronic pancreatitis in children, specific criteria have not been developed and no validation studies have been performed. ERCP provides excellent images but in the era of MRCP and EUS, ERCP has little place as a diagnostic modality alone, and should be reserved for cases that might benefit from intervention. The disadvantage of ERCP is that it can cause significant morbidity including a risk of pancreatitis and bleeding if sphincterotomy is performed.

TREATMENT

Targeted treatment for chronic pancreatitis based on a known cause is possible for a limited number of etiologies. Withdrawing offending drugs or surgically removing a choledochal cyst may improve or completely relieve chronic pancreatitis. For many causes of chronic pancreatitis, there is no specific treatment, and therapy must be directed toward reduction in exacerbations and relief of pain and malnutrition.

Pain relief is difficult and complex in chronic pancreatitis. Combinations of over-the-counter analgesics, including aceta-minophen (paracetamol) or nonsteroidal anti-inflammatory drugs are the first line of therapy, but many patients require weak opioids (e.g. tramadol) or narcotics for pain relief and optimal function. The lowest dose that provides relief should be used since the pain in chronic pancreatitis can be quite severe and dependence on narcotics is a risk. Concomitant therapy with antianxiety medications or antidepressants may be helpful, and nonmedical management strategies, such as cognitive behavioral therapy, should be pursued early in the course of the disease to establish the child's locus of control and comfort with these therapies. Withholding pain relief because of fear of addiction or to 'build character' is inappropriate. If the provider is uncomfortable with managing the child's pain, consultation with a pediatric pain management program is essential.

Many therapies have been trialed to reduce exacerbations in chronic pancreatitis. Low doses of oral pancreatic enzymes reduce exacerbations and improve pain relief through negative feedback inhibition of pancreatic secretion. Randomized trials of this therapy have demonstrated an effect only with nonenteric-coated enzymes. Enteric-coated products have not been shown to have the same effect on pain. No trials have been performed in children, but treatment is low risk. With the return of a nonenteric-coated enzyme product to the United States market, a trial of this therapy is recommended in chronic pancreatitis.

Cocktails of antioxidant micronutrients have a long history in the management of chronic pancreatitis in adults, but no large multi-center studies have been done. Many different combinations have been trialed. Because of the differences in etiology between pediatric and adult chronic pancreatitis it is hard, on the basis of the previous studies, to recommend antioxidant therapy in children.

Endoscopic management of pain has included pancreatic duct decompression via ERCP, with duct dilatation and stent placement, as well as removal of obstructing pancreatic stones. In adults, pain relief occurs in the majority of patients, but may recur with time. In one study of children, 46 pediatric patients with chronic pancreatitis received therapeutic ERCP, for a total of 110 procedures. Of these procedures, 17.3% were associated with complications, including mild/moderate pancreatitis and mild cholangitis. In long-term follow-up (mean 61.4 months), 24 of 42 patients had complete pain relief and 5 of 42 underwent surgery for recurrent pain. Thus, ERCP may improve pain in some children with chronic pancreatitis. Importantly, this treatment is dependent on a very skilled and experienced ERCP endoscopist.

Patients with continued exacerbations of chronic pancreatitis and chronic pain unresponsive to therapies described above are often referred for surgical management of their disease. Surgical procedures to relieve pain associated with chronic pancreatitis include drainage procedures and partial or total pancreatic resection. Lateral pancreaticojejunostomy (LPJ, or Puestow procedure) is a drainage procedure that relieves ductal strictures, allows stone removal, and preserves pancreatic function. A report of four children treated with LPJ and followed for 2–6 years demonstrated good pain relief although one child became diabetic. Duodenum-preserving pancreatic head resection (DPPHR, or modified Frey procedure) involves both drainage and partial pancreatic resection. One center reported this operation in six pediatric patients; 4/6 were pain-free without narcotics at 46 months and none had developed diabetes. In another study, 11 children underwent either LPJ or DPPHR; 8/11 had good results with an average follow-up of 4.6 years. These numbers illustrate the very limited data on pediatric drainage and partial pancreatic resection studies as well as the relatively short follow-up periods for these reports. Such procedures in adults have shown pain recurrence rates of 30–50%, but, again, direct comparison to pediatrics is challenging and basing pediatric treatment decisions on adult data is not recommended.

Recent reports suggest complete pancreatectomy with auto-transplantation of islet cells (TPIAT), if performed before complete loss of endocrine pancreatic tissue, can preserve endocrine function in a large number of children and significantly improve their quality of life. In Minnesota USA, 53 children have had TPIAT since 1977. The 1-year, 5-year, and 10-year survival rates are 98%, 98%, and 79%, respectively. At a cross-sectional analysis at 3 years, 55% were insulin independent, 25% had partial islet function, and 20% were fully insulin dependent. Younger children experienced better outcomes. Quality of life in children (physical and emotional components) significantly improved after surgery. Children with previous surgical pancreatic drainage and/or resection had lower islet yields. Future research to identify better those children at risk of developing chronic pain is important to permit early use of TPIAT in the appropriate population.

PROGNOSIS

No long-term natural history studies of children with chronic pancreatitis exist. Limited studies of this type have been done in adults with diseases that also present in children. In a French study, the clinical courses of 200 patients with *PRSS1* mutations were examined. Exocrine insufficiency occurred in 34% (median age of occurrence 29 years of age) and diabetes mellitus occurred in 26% (median age of occurrence 38 years of age). In general, pediatricians will not see the more severe long-term consequences of hereditary pancreatitis.

Children who develop exocrine insufficiency will need to be managed by clinicians familiar with pancreatic enzyme therapy and vitamin supplementation and monitoring. Chronic pancreatitis of any etiology is associated with increased risk for adenocarcinoma of the pancreas. Individuals with *PRSS1* mutations are at particular risk, with their rates of this cancer approaching 50% in some studies.

CHAPTER 33

Other Pancreatic Disorders

Kathy D. Chen, Sohail Z. Husain

- **Trauma**
- **Neoplasms**

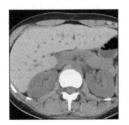
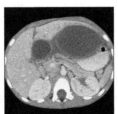
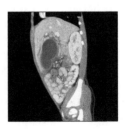

Trauma

ETIOLOGY, EPIDEMIOLOGY, AND CLINICAL PRESENTATION

Trauma to the pancreas is most commonly due to blunt abdominal trauma. Children are more vulnerable to blunt force than adults. They have a relatively smaller torso with a shorter anterior–posterior diameter, which reduces the area over which the force of injury can be dispersed. Further, children also have relatively less overlying protective fat and weaker abdominal muscles.

Motor vehicle accidents, auto–pedestrian injuries, and falls are the three most common causes of blunt abdominal injury in children. Other significant causes include injuries related to bicycles, all-terrain vehicles, and child maltreatment. Abdominal trauma typically occurs in one of two scenarios: 1) either as an isolated injury caused by a direct blow to the upper abdomen; or 2) multi-system trauma caused by a high-energy mechanism (e.g. motor vehicle or fall from a large height).

Pancreatic injury is less common after blunt abdominal trauma than liver or spleen injury. Nonetheless, pancreatic trauma should always be considered because inflammatory complications may not develop until days to weeks after the traumatic event. Blunt abdominal trauma, and pancreatic trauma in particular, may not be readily apparent on initial evaluation.

DIAGNOSIS

A careful clinical history that elicits the mechanism of injury, along with a thorough abdominal examination, should alert the clinician to the possibility of abdominal involvement. Serial physical examinations need to be conducted since abdominal injury can be obscured by other concurrent injuries. Additionally, young patients may not be able to articulate the causative events or localize their pain sensation. Thus, clinicians should maintain a high index of suspicion for blunt trauma. An important physical finding is abdominal wall bruising, which can indicate potential underlying injury.

In children with mild to moderate blunt abdominal trauma, abnormal laboratory findings may serve as the first clue to underlying injury. A complete blood count (CBC) should be performed to assess hemodynamic stability. Other baseline laboratory tests include preoperative tests (prothrombin time, partial thromboplastin time, type and cross), serum electrolytes, glucose, urinalysis, amylase, lipase, and hepatic transaminases, including alanine aminotransferase (ALT) and aspartate aminotransferase (AST).

Whereas elevated transaminases are a sensitive and specific indicator of liver injury, pancreatic enzymes are less sensitive for pancreatic injury. In a prospective study of trauma patients who had serial measurements of amylase and lipase, elevations in these serum pancreatic enzymes did not correlate with the extent of pancreatic injury, since there were other nonpancreatic, gastrointestinal sources for the rise. Nonetheless, measuring amylase and lipase in children with blunt abdominal trauma may serve as a marker for the presence of pancreatic trauma.

A contrast-enhanced abdominal computed tomography (CT) scan is the preferred imaging modality to assess for pancreatic injuries. Ultrasound can be used for follow-up examinations due to wide availability, but overlying intestinal gas from an ileus during the acute phase may obstruct visualization. Magnetic resonance imaging (MRI) or magnetic resonance cholangiopancreatography (MRCP) can better characterize pancreatic ductal anatomy or fluid collections, if applicable.

Pancreatic injuries can be classified into three categories that are based on the extent and character of involvement at presentation.

Injury without ductal disruption

Most patients with pancreatic trauma fall into this group. The injury is usually a simple contusion or hematoma with minimal parenchymal disruption. The diagnosis is suspected from an elevated serum amylase and lipase and confirmed by CT, which shows swelling and hemorrhage in and around the pancreas without evidence of transection or other major parenchymal or ductal disruption. Treatment is conservative management, including bowel rest, intravenous hydration, and parenteral nutrition. In a case series of 43 children with pancreatic injury after blunt trauma, all 18 of the children who had mild pancreatic injury were managed nonoperatively, and none developed complications.

Injury with ductal disruption

Pancreatic trauma with ductal disruption can be difficult to recognize on CT scan (**33.1**), and an endoscopic retrograde cholangiopancreatogram (ERCP) or MRCP may be needed to delineate the diagnosis. If recognized early, distal duct disruption can be treated by distal pancreatectomy. Proximal ductal disruption can be managed by bowel rest and supportive care. Proximal ductal stenting is also an option. If this injury is missed at an early stage or the patient presents with delayed findings, conservative management with bowel rest and total parenteral nutrition is indicated. However,

the clinical course may be prolonged over weeks or months.

Pseudocyst

Patients with delayed presentation of pancreatic trauma or those whose injuries were missed on initial presentation can develop a pancreatic pseudocyst, which is a fluid collection within the pancreas surrounded by a thick, fibrotic, nonepithelial lining (**33.2, 33.3**). Pseudocysts develop in up to one-half of children with ductal disruption who are initially treated nonoperatively and up to 10% of those who undergo surgery. Children develop pseudocysts after trauma more commonly than adults. They present with complaints of epigastric pain, vomiting, early satiety, a palpable abdominal mass, peritonitis, and elevated lipase or amylase. CT or ultrasound confirms the diagnosis. Treatment is conservative with bowel rest, parenteral nutrition, pain control, and monitoring with serial ultrasounds. Some pseudocysts resolve spontaneously by 4–6 weeks, while others require external or internal drainage. Endoscopic cystgastrostomy and endoscopic ultrasound-guided drainage are emerging as treatment options for children with these fluid collections.

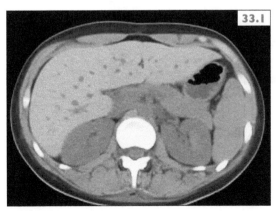

33.1 CT scan showing transected pancreas following trauma from child abuse. The patient required partial pancreatectomy.

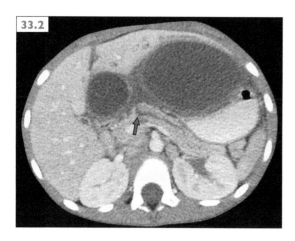

33.2 CT scan showing transection of the large pancreatic duct with surrounding pseudocysts (arrow). The child presented 4 weeks after the initial injury, which was due to abuse.

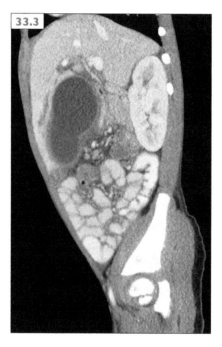

33.3 Lateral view showing displacement of abdominal organs from the large size of a pseudocyst.

PROGNOSIS

Prognosis of pediatric pancreatic trauma depends on the presence or absence of associated injuries, and mortality depends on how many structures are involved. Isolated pancreatic injury causes less than 20% mortality. Mortality increases however, if other gastrointestinal organs are involved, and mortality can increase up to 50% if the major blood vessels are injured.

Neoplasms

Pancreatic neoplasms in children are rare and have a wide range of histopathologic diversity. In an Italian registry dedicated to pediatric pancreatic tumors, only 21 cases were identified from 2000–2009. A similar United States series found only 27 cases from 1986 to 2010. Pediatric neoplasms can be classified by their ability to secrete neurohormones; thus, the terms neuroendocrine and non-neuroendocrine are used (*Table 33.1*).

Neuroendocrine pancreatic tumors

The endocrine pancreatic tumors include insulinomas (50% of cases), gastrinomas (30%), VIPomas (15%), and glucagonomas (only reported in adults). Islet cell tumors as a group account for 20% of all malignant pancreatic tumors in children and 5% in adults.

Insulinomas are composed of insulin-secreting beta cells, and they are the most common endocrine pancreatic tumor in both children and adults. The major clinical feature is hypoglycemia, which is often provoked by fasting. The two peak ages of presentation are during infancy and puberty, and there is a female predominance. More than 90% of these tumors are benign and 80% are solitary. Insulinomas are associated with MEN-1 (multiple endocrine neoplasia) or Wermer syndrome; in these cases, however, there are multiple tumors. Ultrasound, CT scan, or MRI can detect insulinomas that are greater than 2 cm in diameter, and endoscopic ultrasound may detect smaller tumors. Medical management of symptoms includes monitoring for hypoglycemia, frequent feedings, and the use of diazoxide or a somatostatin analog, octreotide, to decrease insulin release. The outcome is excellent when the tumor can be identified and surgically resected.

Gastrinomas cause Zollinger–Ellison syndrome (ZES). They produce high circulating levels of serum gastrin, which causes the proliferation of gastric parietal cells and leads to excessive gastric acid secretion. The most common clinical symptom is abdominal pain from dyspepsia or peptic ulcers. Diarrhea can develop due to gastric hypersecretion. A diagnosis is established by the finding of high fasting serum gastrin levels or, in equivocal cases, a rapid rise in serum gastrin upon secretin stimulation. In addition to standard imaging modalities, somatostatin receptor scintigraphy can further aid in localizing tumor burden. The primary medical management of gastrinomas is acid suppression using high-dose proton pump inhibitors. Since up to 65% of gastrinomas are malignant, early surgical resection is indicated.

VIPomas are so-named because they secrete vasoactive intestinal polypeptide (VIP), a neurohormone that induces intestinal and pancreatic fluid and electrolyte secretion. Affected patients develop a watery, secretory diarrhea, along with dehydration, hypochlorhydria, hypokalemia, and metabolic acidosis. In addition to the above clinical and biochemical disturbances, a diagnosis of VIPoma is established by an elevated serum VIP level and increased urinary catecholamines. Although most adult cases originate in the pancreas, VIPomas in children are also found in other locations,

Table 33.1 Terminology used in pancreatic tumors

Neuroendocrine pancreatic tumors
- Insulinoma
- Gastrinoma
- Vasoactive intestinal polypeptide (VIP)oma
- Glucagonoma

Non-neuroendocrine pancreatic tumors
- Pancreatoblastoma
- Ductal adenocarcinoma
- Solid-cystic papillary tumor

including the liver, retroperitoneum, and mediastinum. CT scan and somatostatin receptor scintigraphy can assist in localizing the tumor. Treatment consists of correction of the metabolic derangements and surgical resection. Approximately one-half of VIPomas are malignant.

Non-neuroendocrine pancreatic tumors

In children, the non-neuroendocrine pancreatic tumors are less common than the neuroendocrine tumors. Such non-neuroendocrine tumors include pancreatoblastoma, ductal adenocarcinoma, and solid-cystic papillary tumors. Pancreatoblastoma accounts for 0.5% of epithelial tumors of the pancreas. Boys are affected twice as often as girls, and there is a higher incidence in children from east Asia. The mean age of presentation is 4 years. Typically, affected patients present with a large, palpable abdominal mass, and they have nonspecific symptoms such as epigastric pain, anorexia, vomiting, diarrhea, and weight loss. Obstructive jaundice may also be present. Serum alpha-fetoprotein is elevated in one-quarter to one-half of all patients, and this tumor may secrete adrenocorticotropic hormone. There is an association between pancreatoblastoma and Beckwith–Wiedemann syndrome. On imaging, a large, well-defined, often multilobular solitary mass

within the pancreas can be seen displacing the rest of the pancreas. Any region of the pancreas can be involved, and the mass can be seen on ultrasound, CT, or MRI. Treatment is surgical resection; chemotherapy is used if the tumor is invasive or metastases are present.

Pancreatic ductal adenocarcinoma is a major cause of cancer in adults; however, it rarely presents in childhood. The main symptoms are pain and weight loss, and more than one-half of patients have obstructive jaundice. The most common area of involvement is the head of the pancreas. Although small in size, the tumor commonly causes dilatation of both the pancreatic duct and the common bile duct. Treatment is surgical resection with or without pancreaticoduodenectomy. Invasive disease requires chemotherapy.

Solid-cystic papillary tumor is also known as solid pseudopapillary tumor or Frantz's tumor. It is found in greater proportions among females and Asian and African ethnic groups. The mean age of presentation is 26 years, and one-fifth of all cases occur in children. Patients typically present with a palpable abdominal mass. Ultrasound and CT scan demonstrate a large, well-defined solid lesion in the head of the pancreas. Treatment is surgical resection, and children have a better prognosis than adults due to a lower likelihood of metastasis and local invasion.

CHAPTER 34

Choledochal Malformation

Mark Davenport

DEFINITION

Choledochal malformation (CM) is a generic term which includes different patterns of bile duct dilatation other than those associated primarily with obstruction. The older term was choledochal cyst, but this rather implies a spherical, globular appearance only seen in one subtype of CM.

Normally the pancreatic duct and bile duct open independently into the ampulla of Vater, each with a separate sphincter to control secretion. This arrangement limits any intermixing of pancreatic secretions and bile and therefore premature activation of pancreatic enzymes. Most CMs are associated with an abnormal junction with the main pancreatic duct short of the ampulla and is termed the common channel.

CLINICAL PRESENTATION

CM may present with a number of different symptoms in children including:

- Conjugated jaundice (cholestasis) – due to bile flow obstruction and showing pale white stools and dark urine.
- Acute pancreatitis – secondary to obstruction of the common channel and rare in infants and toddlers.
- Antenatally detected hepatic or subhepatic cyst – about 15% will be detectable and usually are associated with a Type 1c malformation; some will have early-onset jaundice and present similarly to cystic biliary atresia, while others may be completely asymptomatic.
- Palpable right upper quadrant mass (<5%).
- Cholangitis (<5%) – usually found in association with biliary stones and obstruction:
- Cirrhosis (<2%) – found in association with other symptoms and signs of hepatic fibrosis.
- Perforation (<5%) – either into the retroperitoneal compartment with vague abdominal pain and tenderness or more acute features of peritonitis if spillage occurs into the peritoneal cavity.

CMs are associated with malignancy but this typically occurs after several decades and is very rare in children. The peak age of CM-associated cholangiocarcinoma is 40–50 years of age.

EPIDEMIOLOGY AND ETIOLOGY

There is a marked female predominance (4:1) and a much higher incidence of CM in Asia, particularly Japan, China, and Taiwan.

The cause of CM is not known although there are two broad theories of origin. The older theory suggests that there is a congenital distal bile duct stenosis and thus proximal expansion follows with a higher intraluminal pressure driving the dilatation. Alternatively, the common channel, that is present in most CMs, allows free reflux of pancreatic secretions into the bile duct where these secretions may damage its epithelial lining and structure causing dilatation. This theory is known as the Babbitt hypothesis, after the American radiologist who first observed the reflux. This latter hypothesis implies a dynamic postnatal process arising from a congenital anomaly.

Recent studies have related the pressure in the choledochus to a lack of epithelial integrity and histologic damage, suggesting that in most cases the dilatation arises as a result of a sustained high intrabiliary pressure due to a distal stenotic segment. Although reflux is observed, this finding actually is associated with lower pressures and normal appearing epithelial lining.

Classification

The Kings College Hospital classification of CM (**34.1**) is a modification of the older Todani classification. The three commonest variants are Type 1c (cystic CM), Type 1f (fusiform CM), and Type 4 (intra- and

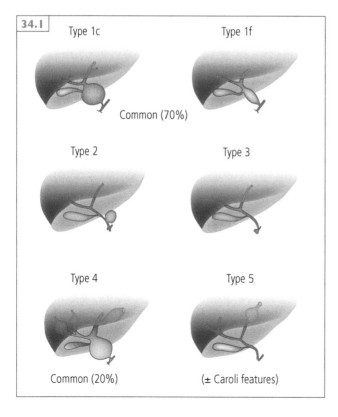

34.1

Type 1c

Type 1f

Common (70%)

Type 2

Type 3

Type 4

Type 5

Common (20%)

(± Caroli features)

34.1 Kings College Hospital classification of choledochal malformation.

extra-hepatic dilatation). Currently the most frequently seen are Type 1f, Type 1c, and Type 4. Fusiform malformations (**34.2**) are generally smaller and have a less distinct caliber change than the classic cystic malformation which usually has a clear and distinct cut-off both proximally and distally (**34.3, 34.4**). The Type 4 CM appears to be a later stage of the other two common CMs and again seems to be the one with the highest sustained intrabiliary pressure (**34.5**). Effective extrahepatic surgery allows free drainage of dilated intrahepatic ducts, and the ducts may shrink in size and even normalize after a couple of years.

There are two distinct variants of Type 5 (intrahepatic) CM. The least common is an isolated cystic dilatation, within the right lobe

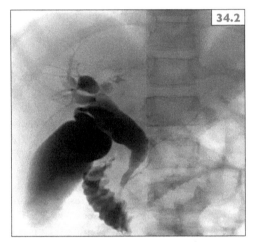

34.2 Fusiform choledochal malformation (Type 1f) in 9-year-old girl with a history of pancreatitis.

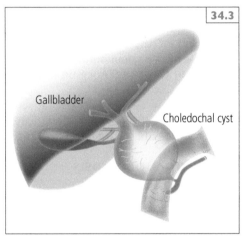

34.3 Schematic illustration of cystic choledochal malformation (Type 1c).

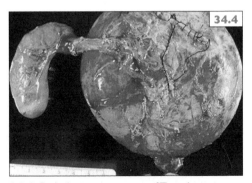

34.4 Pathologic appearance of Type 1c choledochal malformation. Note the sharp cut-off of the distal cystic component and the relatively normal size and appearance of the gallbladder.

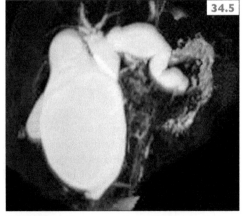

34.5 Magnetic retrograde cholangiopancreatography showing intra- and extrahepatic dilatation (Type 4) in a 3-year-old girl with recurrent abdominal pain and jaundice.

and is probably of congenital origin. Unless there is any obstruction to bile flow and/or stone formation, then a Type 5 CM can be simply observed. The more common type of Type 5 CM is usually termed Caroli syndrome and is one of the fibropolycystic diseases of the liver. Unlike all the other CM variants it has a clear genetic etiology and relationship with renal pathology. It is characterized by bilobar, multiple saccular dilatations of the bile ducts, and early-onset intrinsic liver fibrosis probably with normal intrabiliary pressure and no common channel (**34.6**). Mutations of the autosomally recessive *PKHD1* gene are commonly identified with this type of CM and fibrocystin is its gene product.

A common channel in the absence of significant choledochal dilatation is sometimes described as a *forme-fruste* variant.

DIFFERENTIAL DIAGNOSIS

- Early-onset jaundice:
  - Cystic biliary atresia.
  - Biliary stricture.
  - Spontaneous biliary perforation and formation of biliary pseudocyst.
- Late-onset jaundice:
  - Gallstones.
  - Biliary stricture/stenosis.
  - Chronic pancreatitis.
- Acute pancreatitis:
  - Pancreas divisum, pancreatic duct strictures.
  - Gallstones.
  - Drugs, trauma.

DIAGNOSIS

Liver biochemistry may show elevated conjugated bilirubin, γ-glutamyl transpeptidase, and aspartate transaminases levels. Elevated serum plasma amylase and aspartate and alanine transaminase suggest on-going pancreatic inflammation.

Biliary ultrasound should identify the degree of bile duct dilatation (cystic is usually larger than fusiform dilatation)

and any evidence of intrahepatic bile duct dilatation. Magnetic retrograde cholangiopancreatography (MRCP) is the key investigation tool in determining the anatomy and relationship with the pancreatic duct (**34.7**).

There may be cases where there are stones or a distal biliary stenosis and it is not clear if there is an underlying CM. Endoscopic retrograde cholangiopancreatography (ERCP) may then be needed to define diagnosis and relieve jaundice by duct clearance of stones or stent placement.

TREATMENT

Surgery excision and reconstruction is indicated in most cases unless there are contraindications to anaesthesia and the CM is asymptomatic. The surgical aim is to excise the gallbladder and the entire extrahepatic biliary system down to the junction with the pancreatic duct and up to the common hepatic duct and bifurcation. It is then important to visualize the intrahepatic duct system using a video-endoscope to clear any residual debris and deal with any residual duct stenosis in the higher order ducts (**34.8**). Similarly, it is not enough just to detach the bile duct from the common channel without first ensuring it too is clear of debris and drains effectively (**34.9**). The reconstruction usually involves creation of a long Roux loop passed behind the colon to anastomose with the transected bile duct. In many centers, the surgery can be carried out in a quasi-laparoscopic manner, though it is very much a technique for the advanced practitioner.

It is possible to achieve long-term survival with their native livers in almost all children. A small proportion may present with advanced cirrhosis and be at risk, but even here biliary decompression is very worthwhile.

Malignancy is a possible complication in the longer term, but its true prevalence is not known following the change of surgical practice in the 1980s from simply internally draining cysts to actual resection and bile duct reconstruction.

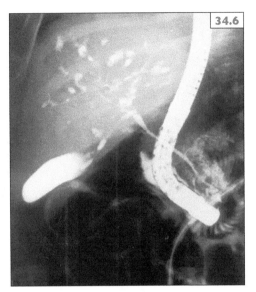

34.6 Endoscopic retrograde cholangiopancreatography image of a child with Caroli's syndrome. (Reproduced with permission from Keane F, Hadzic N, Wilkinson ML, *et al*. Neonatal presentation of Caroli's disease. *Arch Dis Child* 1997; **77**: F145–6; King's College Hospital, London.)

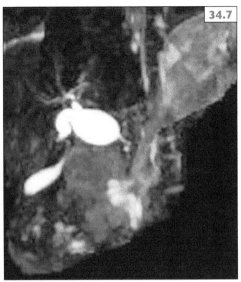

34.7 Magnetic retrograde cholangiopancreatography showing Type Ic choledochal malformation.

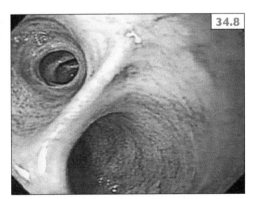

34.8 Endoscopic view of intrahepatic bile ducts acquired intraoperatively. Branching ducts are smooth-walled without evidence of stenosis or stone formation.

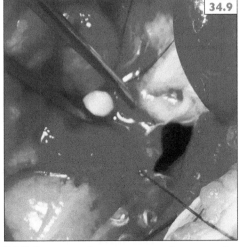

34.9 Intraoperative appearance of a pancreatic stone removed from the common channel of a child with a history of recurrent pancreatitis and choledochal malformation.

Biliary Atresia

Mark Davenport

DEFINITION AND EPIDEMIOLOGY

Biliary atresia (BA) is an obliterative cholangiopathy affecting the extra- and intrahepatic bile ducts which presents in the first few weeks after birth with jaundice, pale stools, and dark urine. Biliary atresia is the most common cause of liver transplantation in children.

There is a variable incidence across the world, ranging from about 1 in 15–20,000 live births in the United Kingdom, Europe, and North America to about 1 in 5–10,000 live births in Taiwan, China, and Japan demonstrating a higher incidence in Asia and the Pacific region. Familial clusterings are very rare. There is no observed seasonal variation, and both genders are affected equally.

CLINICAL PRESENTATION

Infants with BA will present with conjugated jaundice that persists beyond 14 days of age, pale stools, and dark urine. Malnutrition and bleeding (even intracranial hemorrhage) due to fat malabsorption and vitamin K deficient coagulopathy are also possible presentations. Liver fibrosis and cirrhosis (e.g. ascites, hepatosplenomegaly) occur earlier in BA relative to other neonatal cholestatic liver diseases such as Alagille syndrome. Beyond 100 days of life, liver fibrosis and cirrhosis are invariably present.

ETIOLOGY AND PATHOPHYSIOLOGY

The etiology of BA is essentially unknown, although two broad mechanisms have been suggested including a congenital and a perinatal form. The congenital form may involve primary failure of bile duct development as seen in those with syndromic BA (typically biliary atresia with splenic malformations such as polysplenia [or asplenia], situs inversus, preduodenal portal vein, absence of vena cava) or those with cystic BA, where the cyst may be seen on antenatal ultrasound. Alternatively there may be perinatal destruction of formed bile ducts, as may be seen in cytomegalovirus (CMV) immunoglobulin M-positive associated BA.

The variation in phenotypes suggests the involvement of multiple factors including genetic, metabolic, environmental, and immunologic abnormalities. CMV infection, abnormal bile acids, and innate neonatal immunity are only a few specific examples of potentially influencing factors. Regardless of the mechanism involved, this necroinflammatory process will eventually result in liver fibrosis and cirrhosis. If untreated, portal hypertension, liver failure, and death will result within the first 2 years of life.

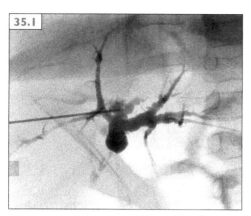

35.1 Acquired biliary atresia in an infant born with gastroschisis, who initially passed normal colored stool then developed cholestatic conjugated jaundice and pale stool. Ultrasound showed dilated intrahepatic bile ducts and a percutaneous transhepatic cholangiogram (PTC) was performed. The PTC shows clear demarcation and atresia of the common hepatic duct. There was no bile in the gallbladder at operation and an hepaticojejunostomy was performed which relieved the jaundice completely.

DIFFERENTIAL DIAGNOSIS

- Medical:
  - Neonatal hepatitis.
  - Giant cell hepatitis.
  - Alpha-1 antitrypsin deficiency.
  - Alagille syndrome (due to bile duct paucity).
  - Progressive familial intrahepatic cholestasis (Type 1, 2, and 3).
- Surgical:
  - Choledochal malformation.
  - Acquired biliary atresia/stenosis (e.g. following neonatal duodenal atresia surgery) (**35.1**).
  - Inspissated bile syndrome (**35.2**).
  Spontaneous bile duct perforation.

DIAGNOSIS

Ultrasound (US) examination is an important part of the diagnostic work-up as this can exclude other possible surgical diagnoses such as choledochal malformation. An atrophic or nonemptying gallbladder may be suggestive of BA. A more controversial US finding is the 'triangular cord sign' which represents a solid proximal biliary remnant anterior to the bifurcation of the portal vein. Maternal prenatal US may show evidence of cystic BA although a cystic choledochal malformation would deserve consideration.

Work-up should also include confirmation of biochemical conjugated hyperbilirubinemia

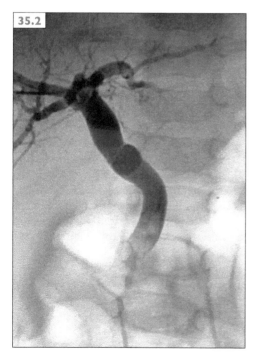

35.2 Inspissated bile syndrome in a preterm infant born at 28 weeks who developed necrotizing enterocolitis. This required an ileostomy and parenteral nutrition. Conjugated jaundice and pale stools became obvious at 5 weeks of age. Ultrasound showed a dilated common bile duct and intrahepatic ducts. A percutaneous transhepatic cholangiogram was performed and showed a dilated duct filled with inspissated bile. This was cleared with saline lavage and the jaundice resolved.

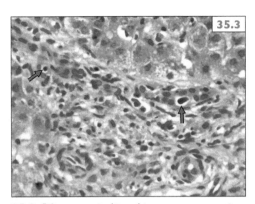

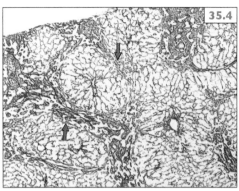

35.3 Biliary atresia. Liver biopsy at presentation, age 27 days. Expansion of large interlobular portal tract by edema and a mixed infiltrate of leucocytes. Fibrosis is not apparent. The lumen of two bile ducts contain khaki-colored bile plugs (arrows). (Courtesy of Dr. Alex Knisley; Kings College Hospital, London.)

35.4 Biliary atresia. Expanded connective tissue (silver salt impregnated stain) (arrow), consistent with bridging hepatic fibrosis with centrilobular sparing in a 65-day-old infant. (Reticulin, 40×.) (Courtesy of Dr. Alex Knisley; Kings College Hospital, London.)

and elevated gamma-glutamyl transferase (GGT) with exclusion of medical causes (e.g. Alagille syndrome, neonatal hepatitis, familial cholestasis). Surgical causes other than BA are rare. Liver biopsy should show bile duct proliferation (**35.3**) and, with time, fibrosis and ultimately cirrhosis (**35.4**). In the United Kingdom, the United States, and most of Europe. percutaneous liver biopsy is the usual method of preoperative diagnosis. In some centers, evaluating duodenal contents for bile using a nasoduodenal tube has been used in the evaluation of cholestasis when BA is suspected. Radioisotope hepatobiliary scans can also help detect the presence/absence of intestinal bile, although these tests may not differentiate BA from other causes of severe cholestasis. In cases of suspected BA, an intraoperative cholangiogram provides a definitive diagnosis leading to surgical intervention.

TREATMENT

The preferred treatment of infants with BA is radical surgical excision of the extrahepatic bile ducts and Roux loop reconstruction or Kasai portoenterostomy (KPE) (**35.5**).

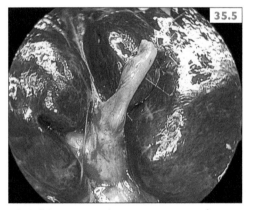

35.5 Biliary atresia. Laparoscopic view of an infant aged 40 days with biliary atresia. The gallbladder has been mobilized from its bed and is atrophic and contains no bile.

The purpose of this surgery is to restore bile flow, and its success improves if performed before 60 days of age. Liver transplantation is reserved for those patients where the KPE option fails as well as infants who clinically present very late with obvious cirrhosis. Although corticosteroids and ursodeoxycholic acid have been studied as potential adjuvant therapies, there are few published data to support their routine use.

Postoperative complications include ascending cholangitis and portal hypertension. These complications are due to the liver fibrotic process seen in BA regardless of the integrity of the KPE. Cholangitis, characterized by fever and worsening jaundice, is more likely to occur in the setting of BA than with choledochal malformations. Portal hypertension is due to liver fibrosis and may result in varices and ascites. Again, it is the fibrotic process or perhaps the abbreviation of this process via KPE that determines variceal formation rather than age at surgery.

PROGNOSIS

The overall survival to adulthood in BA has improved over the past 35 years from 10% to 90%. Surgery remains the most effective therapy although pharmacologic treatments to reduce the liver fibrotic process early in the disease are needed. This heterogenous group of diseases resulting in the obliterative cholangiopathy, known collectively as BA, has many factors that influence prognosis. Although age at KPE may be useful to some degree in predicting outcome, other factors, such as the presence of CMV, associated congenital anomalies, or surgical center experience, may also have a major impact on case outcome. Clearance of jaundice should be achieved in 50% of patients and in large centers with high KPE case loads. This should allow about 40% of patients to reach adolescence with their native livers. There is still a 10% mortality associated with BA principally due to deaths on transplant waiting lists and uncorrectable associated anomalies.

CHAPTER 36

Pediatric Autoimmune Liver Diseases

Samra S. Blanchard, William Twaddell

- **Introduction**
- **Autoimmune hepatitis**
- **Overlap syndrome**
- ***De novo* AIH after liver transplantation**

 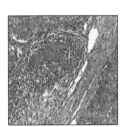 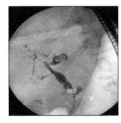

Introduction

Autoimmune liver disease in childhood is a rare chronic progressive liver disease that includes autoimmune hepatitis (AIH), autoimmune sclerosing cholangitis (ASC), overlap syndrome (combination of the AIH and ASC) and *de novo* autoimmune hepatitis after liver transplantation. The clinical presentation of autoimmune liver disease is nonspecific and can be similar in clinical presentation to other liver disorders.

Autoimmune hepatitis

DEFINITION AND EPIDEMIOLOGY

AIH is a chronic disease of unknown etiology which presents as a progressive inflammatory liver disease characterized by elevated serum liver enzymes and immunoglobulin (Ig) G with presence of autoantibodies. Two types of AIH have been described, depending on the type of circulating autoantibodies. Type 1 or classic AIH commonly seen in adults but present in children, is characterized by the presence of smooth muscle antibody (SMA) and/or antinuclear antibody (ANA). AIH type 2 is positive for antiliver–kidney microsomal type 1 antibody (anti-LKM-1) and/or antiliver cytosol type 1(anti-LC1) and is mainly seen in the younger pediatric population.

The exact prevalence in children is unknown but AIH-1 accounts for two-thirds of cases and presents between 10 and 20 years of age, whereas AIH-2 presents in younger ages including infancy. In both forms of AIH, females represent 75% of cases. ASC has the same prevalence as AIH-1 in childhood but both genders are equally affected.

CLINICAL PRESENTATION

AIH can present with a variety of clinical patterns. The most common presentation is acute hepatitis when patients have malaise, nausea, vomiting, abdominal pain, and often will progress to jaundice. Asymptomatic patients are usually diagnosed incidentally during routine blood work. In a small number of cases, patients present with acute liver failure with poor synthetic function and significant jaundice. Acute liver failure is more common in AIH-2. One-half of the patients may demonstrate an insidious onset that, by the time they present, have hepatic cirrhosis and portal hypertension. A subgroup of these patients present with complications of portal hypertension as their first symptom with hematemesis from esophageal varices. Rarely, patients are diagnosed during evaluation and management of another autoimmune disease such as thyroiditis, diabetes, celiac disease, or lupus.

DIAGNOSIS

Physical examination varies from normal findings to the presence of jaundice, hepatomegaly, splenomegaly, cachexia, and cutaneous stigmata of chronic liver disease (spider angioma, palmar erythema, sclera icterus).

Laboratory values reveal elevated transaminases, possible conjugated hyperbilirubinemia, elevated IgG or total protein levels, with presence of ANA, SMA, or anti-LKM-1 antibodies.

Liver biopsy is necessary to make the diagnosis. The typical histology is interface hepatitis which includes a dense mononuclear and plasma cell infiltration of the portal and periportal areas expanding into the liver lobule and periphery of the lobule with erosion of the limiting plate (**36.1**).

The diagnosis of AIH requires the presence of autoantibodies, IgG elevation, pertinent histology, and exclusion of viral hepatitis.

Overlap syndrome

Some patients within the spectrum of autoimmune liver diseases present with characteristics of both AIH and cholestatic liver disease like sclerosing cholangitis. ASC in children is a term used to designate a group of children with primary sclerosing cholangitis (PSC) who also have findings of AIH. The presentation of ASC is similar to AIH. Patients with ASC can have cholestatic symptoms like pruritus or fever due to cholangitis. Inflammatory bowel disease is present in 45% of children with ASC compared to 20% in AIH. Children with ASC should be screened for inflammatory bowel disease even if they are asymptomatic. Clinical and laboratory findings are similar to AIH but 75% of patients with ASC have positive atypical perinuclear antineutrophil cytoplasmic antibody (pANCA) compared to 45% in AIH. Histology is similar to AIH with occasional periductal inflammation seen in PSC (**36.2**). The diagnosis is usually made with typical multifocal stricturing and dilation of intra- and/or extrahepatic bile ducts on cholangiography (MRCP or ERCP) (**36.3**) in the setting of positive antibodies.

36.1 Portal, interface and lobular lymphoplasmacytic inflammation (arrowhead) with hepatocellular loss (arrow) in autoimmune hepatitis.

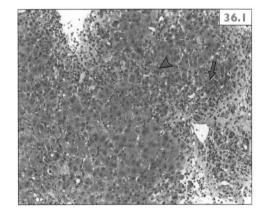

36.2 Portal tract showing a damaged bile duct and granuloma formation (arrow) in a case of autoimmune sclerosing cholangitis–autoimmune hepatitis overlap syndrome. There is an inflammatory infiltrate of lymphocytes and numerous plasma cells, with focal interface hepatitis (arrowhead).

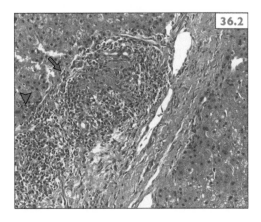

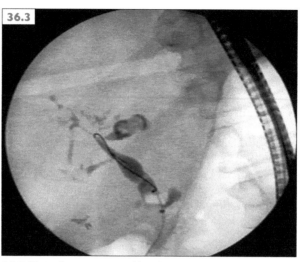

36.3 Typical stricturing and beading appearance of overlap syndrome on endoscopic retrograde cholangiopancreatography. (Courtesy of Eric Goldberg, MD; University of Maryland Medical Center.)

TREATMENT

AIH is usually responsive to immunosuppressive therapy and treatment should be started quickly after exclusion of other etiologies. The goal of treatment is to control inflammation, induce remission, and prolong survival. Remission is defined as normalization of liver enzymes and IgG levels, decreased titers of autoantibodies, and histologic resolution of inflammation.

Retrospective studies have shown a good long-term outcome to treatment with transplant-free survival rate of 90% over 5–10 years. In ASC, treatment is effective in controlling parenchymal inflammation, but less effective in preventing progressive bile duct disease and the 7-year transplant-free survival rate is 85%.

Standard treatment of AIH consists of prednisone and azathioprine or 6-mercaptopurine. Prednisone is usually started at a dose of 2 mg/kg/day (up to 60 mg/day) and gradually decreased over a period of 6–8 weeks depending on the improvement of liver enzymes. Patients are often maintained on a low daily dose of prednisone (2.5–5 mg/day).

Relapse during treatment can occur in 40% of patients which may require either an increase of steroid dose or addition of steroid-sparing agent. The use of azathioprine varies according to the protocols used in different institutions. The starting dose of azathioprine is 0.5 mg/kg/day, increased to 2–2.5 mg/kg/day in the absence of side-effects. It is important to remember that azathioprine is hepatotoxic and can suppress bone marrow function. Measurement of thiopurine methyltransferase activity level prior to initiating azathioprine therapy is recommended to predict drug metabolism and toxicity. Liver function tests and complete metabolic panel should be checked periodically while on these medications. Measurement of the azathioprine metabolites may be useful to monitor for toxicity and adherence to treatment although there is no defined therapeutic level of 6-thioguanine that is required to achieve and sustain remission in AIH.

Up to 10% of patients receiving standard treatment do not achieve remission. In this group of patients, mycophenolate mofetil and calcineurin inhibitors can be used as an alternative immunosuppressant. The optimal duration of immunosuppressive therapy for AIH is unknown.

ASC responds to the same treatment regimen but bile duct disease can persist despite treatment. Ursodeoxycholic acid (UDCA) is usually added to immuno-suppressive treatment at the dose of 13–15 mg/kg/day; however, the efficacy of UDCA in treating bile duct disease remains to be established. Long-term high-dose UDCA (25–30 mg/kg/day) has been reported to be associated with higher rates of serious adverse events in adult patients. Antibiotics have been used in several adult case series to treat PSC. In pediatric patients with inflammatory bowel disease and PSC, small group series showed improved liver function and improved clinical symptoms with the use of vancomycin although this antibiotic has not been evaluated in large patient studies.

Liver transplantation

Liver transplantation is indicated in patients who present with fulminant liver failure and those who develop end-stage liver disease despite medical management. Approximately 10% of children with AIH and 20% of those with ASC will require liver transplantation. After liver transplantation, disease recurrence has been described in 20% of AIH patients and in 70% of ASC patients. These patients may require more maintenance immunosuppression compared to other transplant patients to prevent disease recurrence.

De novo AIH after liver transplantation

Post-transplant *de novo* AIH was initially described in 1998 among patients who underwent liver transplantation for disorders other than AIH. Clinical and histologic findings are similar to AIH with increased IgG levels and positive autoantibodies. The treatment is also similar to AIH with use of steroids and azathioprine therapy and reduction of the calcineurin inhibitor over time, if possible.

CHAPTER 37

Viral Hepatitis

Robert Baker

- **Introduction**
- **Hepatotropic viruses**
- **Nonhepatotropic viruses that may cause hepatitis**
- **Conclusion**

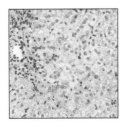
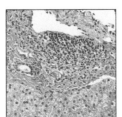
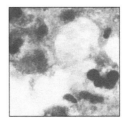

Introduction

There are a number of ways to categorize viruses that cause hepatitis in children. Some viruses affect mainly the liver, and are known as the 'hepatotropic viruses'. These are named by letters of the alphabet, starting with A and going to G (there is no F). Although the hepatotropic viruses predominantly cause hepatitis, they can involve other organ systems such as lymphoid tissue, the gastrointestinal tract, or the skin. Other viruses may affect the liver but also affect other parts of the body. For instance, Epstein–Barr virus (EBV) affects mainly lymphoid tissue but can lead to hepatitis, and rubella causes congenital anomalies and skin rash, but also can cause hepatitis. Additionally, not

Table 37.1 Causes and differential diagnosis of infectious hepatitis in children

Hepatotropic viruses
Hepatitis A virus
Hepatitis B virus
Hepatitis C virus
Hepatitis D virus
Hepatitis E virus
Hepatitis non-A–E viruses

Systemic viral infection that may include hepatitis
Adenovirus
Arbovirus
Coxsackievirus
Cytomegalovirus
Enterovirus
Epstein–Barr virus
'Exotic' viruses (e.g. yellow fever)
Herpes simplex virus (HHV-1, HHV-2)
Human immunodeficiency virus
Paramyxovirus
Rubella
Varicella zoster

Nonviral liver infections
Amebiasis
Bacterial sepsis
Brucellosis
Fitz–Hugh–Curtis syndrome (complication of pelvic inflammatory disease)
Histoplasmosis
Leptospirosis
Tuberculosis

all cases of infectious hepatitis in children are due to viruses. While not covered in this chapter, a number of nonviral organisms can invade the liver causing hepatitis. Viral and nonviral causes of infectious hepatitis in the pediatric age group are summarized in *Table 37.1*.

Other ways to group viruses causing hepatitis in children is to divide them by how the virus is transmitted, whether it causes chronic disease or only acute hepatitis, whether there is a vaccine or other preventative measures, and whether treatment is available (*Table 37.2*).

Table 37.2 Characteristics of viral hepatitis

Hepatotropic viruses

Virus	Type	Transmission	Time	Vaccine	Treatment	Comment
HAV	DNA	Fecal–oral	Acute	Yes	No	Rarely has long-term sequelae
HBV	DNA	Blood	Acute, chronic	Yes	Yes	
HCV	RNA	Blood	Acute, chronic	No	Yes	Most frequent reason for transplant
HDV	RNA	Blood	Chronic	No	No	Only in conjunction with HBV
HEV	RNA	Fecal–oral	Acute	Yes	No	Vaccine not commercially available
HGV		Blood	?	No	No	Scant evidence that it causes disease

Nonhepatotropic viruses that may cause hepatitis

Virus	Type	Transmission	Time	Vaccine	Treatment	Comment
EBV	DNA	Respiratory Blood Transplant	Acute, chronic	No	No	Steroids may reduce symptoms
CMV	DNA	Respiratory Transplacental	Acute, chronic	No	Yes	
Rubella	DNA	Respiratory Transplacental		Yes	No	
Herpes 1, 2	DNA		Chronic	Yes	Yes	
Parvovirus B19	DNA	Respiratory Transplacental	Acute, chronic (?)	No	No	Fifth disease in infants; papular glove disease in older children

CMV: cytomegalovirus; DNA: deoxyribonucleic acid; EBV: Epstein–Barr virus; HAV–HGV: hepatitis virus A–G; RNA: ribonucleic acid.

Hepatotropic viruses

Hepatitis A virus

Hepatitis A virus (HAV) is a single-stranded ribonucleic acid (RNA) virus classified as a picornovirus. It is transmitted via the fecal–oral route and there is no evidence of maternal to neonate transmission. Transmission via blood transfusion, if it occurs, is exceedingly rare. The distribution of the virus is worldwide although the incidence of HAV disease is higher in less developed areas and has been decreasing in the United States. About 30% of the population of the United States shows evidence of past infection. The incubation period is 15–50 days.

The infection itself is often asymptomatic, but can be associated with clinically significant disease and rarely is implicated in acute liver failure. Symptoms include nausea, vomiting, and anorexia. Sometimes the symptoms are more flu-like with pharyngitis, cough, runny nose, headache, and myalgias. Fever can occur but is not always present. Physical findings may include jaundice, weakness, pruritis, and tender, slightly enlarged liver and spleen. Chronology of the course of HAV infection is shown in Figure **37.1**. A vaccine is available.

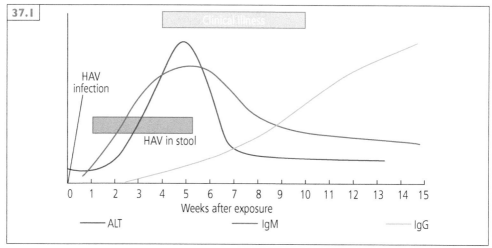

37.1 Time course of hepatitis A virus (HAV) infection. ALT: alanine aminotransferase; Ig: immunoglobulin.

Hepatitis B virus

Hepatitis B virus (HBV) is a deoxyribonucleic acid (DNA) virus of the Hepadnaviridiae family. Since widespread HBV vaccination, the screening of blood products, and the effective prevention of vertical transmission, the incidence of HBV infection is decreasing dramatically. It remains a serious problem in developing areas of the world. The transmission of HBV requires blood contact, thus the four modes of transmission are: 1) via blood, 2) sexual contact; 3) tissue penetration; and 4) mother to neonate. Fecal–oral transmission has never been observed. The incubation period varies from 15 to 180 days and viremia lasts from weeks to years. Most acute infections are self-limited; only 1–5% of adults who become infected progress to chronic hepatitis. However, 90% of neonates and 50% of children develop chronic infections.

Effective prevention in the form of vaccination is available, and infection can be prevented even in infants born to mothers with known active HBV disease, by administration of hepatitis B immune globulin followed by vaccination. Chronic infection is associated with cirrhosis, liver failure, and hepatic cell carcinoma. Histologic changes consist of inflammatory changes with Kupffer cell mobilization and hepatocellular swelling (**37.2**). Individuals who contract

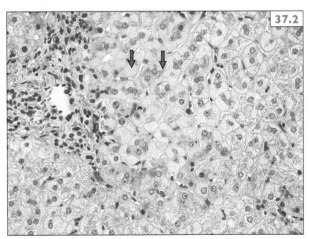

37.2 Ground glass appearance in hepatitis B virus infection (arrows). (Courtesy of Abdur Khan, MD; Women and Children's Hospital of Buffalo.)

HBV at birth have a 30% chance of dying from a liver related cause. Diagrams of the course of an acute infection and a chronic infection are shown in Figures **37.3** and **37.4**, respectively.

The diagnosis and categorizing of HBV is based on serology. The following antigens and antibodies are used: hepatitis B surface antigen (HBsAg), antibody to HBsAg (Anti-HBs), hepatitis B e antigen (HBeAg), antibody to HBeAg (Anti-HBe), antibody to hepatitis B core antigen (Anti-HBc) (the core antigen is not detected in blood), and immunoglobulin (Ig) M antibody to HBcAg (IgM anti-HBc) (*Table 37.3*).

The treatment of HBV infection is interferon or pegylated interferon, a nucleoside or nucleotide analog or combinations of these medications. Who should be treated and under what circumstances and for how long is very controversial. Pediatricians are most likely to face this issue when caring for children of recent immigrants from the developing world and children adopted from developing areas. Typically, these children have vertically acquired disease that responds very poorly to interferon treatment. Because of this poor response, in the past it was recommended not to treat vertically acquired disease. However, with the advent of more effective antiviral drugs such as nucleoside reverse transcriptase inhibitors, and the recognition that vertically acquired disease is not as benign as previously thought, the debate about treatment has reopened. This debate and precise treatment options are beyond the scope of the chapter.

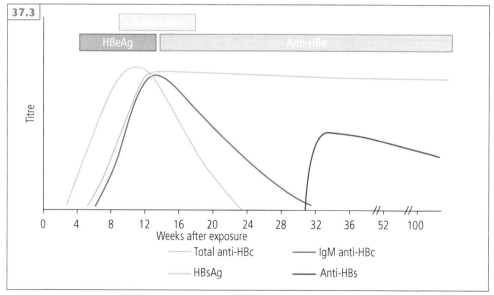

37.3 Time course of acute hepatitis B virus infection. HBeAg: hepatitis B e antigen; Anti-HBe: antibody to HBeAg; HBsAg: hepatitis B surface antigen; Anti-HBs: antibody to HBsAg; Anti-HBc: antibody to hepatitis B core antigen; IgM: immunoglobulin M.

Table 37.3 Hepatitis B virus (HBV) markers

Test	Antigen/antibody	Interpretation
HBsAg	Hepatitis B surface antigen	Detection of acute or chronic infection Used in HBV vaccine development Transient identification of serum HBsAg can be seen after a recent vaccination
Anti-HBs	Antibody to HBsAg	Identifies who has resolved infection with HBV Positive in immune, vaccinated individuals
HBeAg	Hepatitis B e antigen	Detects HBV infection with increased risk of transmitting HBV
Anti-HBe	Antibody to HBeAg	Detects HBV infection with decreased risk of transmitting HBV
Anti-HBc	Antibody to HBV core antigen	Detects acute, resolved, or chronic HBV infection Not present after immunization
IgM anti-HBc	IgM antibody to HBV core antigen	Identifies acute or recent HBV infections
HBV DNA by PCR	Amplified HBV DNA	Detects virus in blood or liver tissue Indicates ongoing infection

DNA: deoxyribonucleic acid; Ig: immunoglobulin; PCR: polymerase chain reaction.

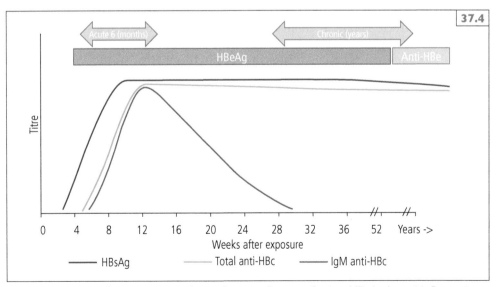

37.4 Time course of progression to chronic hepatitis B virus infection. HBeAg: hepatitis B e antigen; Anti-HBe: antibody to HBeAg; HBsAg: hepatitis B surface antigen; Anti-HBc: antibody to hepatitis B core antigen; IgM: immunoglobulin M.

37.5 Lymphoid aggregate in the portal tract in hepatitis C virus infection (arrow). (Courtesy of Abdur Khan, MD; Women and Children's Hospital of Buffalo.)

Hepatitis C virus

Hepatitis C virus (HCV) is a RNA virus of the Flaviviridae family. A number of genotypes and serotypes exist that have important implications regarding treatment and response to treatment. To date the development of an effective vaccine has been elusive. Like HBV, HCV transmission requires blood contact, so at-risk groups are much the same as for HBV: 1) via blood; 2) sexual contact; 3) tissue penetration; and 4) mother to neonate. Unlike HBV, chronic disease is the rule. Self-limited hepatitis occurs in 15–45% of adults. Also unlike HBV, vertical transmission is not common, occurring in less than 10% of at-risk pregnancies. The pediatrician is likely to encounter HCV in the intravenous drug abusing teenager and occasionally in the child with vertically acquired disease.

The two types of diagnostic tests for HCV are: 1) anti-HCV antibodies of the IgG variety. The third generation assays are 97% sensitive and 99% specific. There is no IgM-based test available. Maternally acquired antibodies can last in the infant up to 18 months, so the antibody-based tests for determining perinatally acquired disease are not reliable before 18 months of age. 2) RNA can be detected in the blood using a polymerase chain reaction (PCR)-based technique and can be followed for response to therapy. These tests can be used as early as 1 month of age. Since viremia is not always present more than one negative test is needed to declare a patient virus free. Liver pathology will demonstrate generalized necroinflammatory and fibrotic changes, along with lymphoid aggregates in portal areas and sinusoids (**37.5**). Variability in alananine aminotransferase can be seen through a typical course of HCV disease (**37.6**).

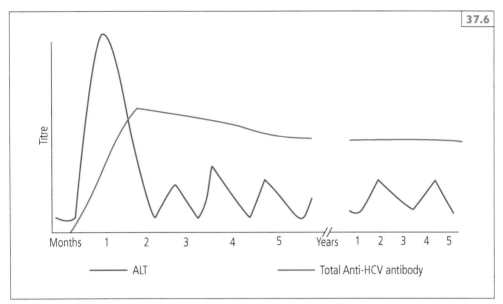

37.6 Time course of hepatitis C virus (HCV) infection. ALT: alanine aminotransferase.

Treatment for hepatitis C is evolving quickly. In adults, treatment with pegylated interferon and ribavirin results in a 50% sustained viral response (SVR) in genotype 1 diseases and an 80% SVR in genotypes 2 and 3. The sparse data for children suggest a similar response rate. In adults, the addition of protease inhibitors such as telaprevir or boceprevir (triple therapy), has improved response rates and decreased treatment times; however, no triple therapy regimen is approved for pediatrics and there are no current studies available in children.

Since treatment is available and because HCV is the most common reason for liver transplant in the United States, appropriately managing these patients is crucial. No standards for monitoring children with HCV have been established. Yearly evaluation of liver function, viral load, and tumor marker determination (alpha-fetoprotein) as well as yearly abdominal ultrasounds are prudent.

Hepatitis D virus

Hepatitis D virus (HDV) infection causes disease only in individuals with acute or chronic hepatitis B. It is a small positive sense RNA virus that codes for a single protein. This protein is coated by HBsAg. Unlike HBV, HDV infects only the hepatocytes and no extrahepatic invasion has been documented. HDV can be acquired at the time of initial HBV infection or can occur later after chronic hepatitis B has been established. IgM and IgG immunologic tests for HDV are available. PCR-based tests are for research only. Clinically, the effect of HDV appears to be to accelerate and worsen the course of HBV. HDV is cytotoxic to hepatocytes; however, the exact mode of action is unknown.

Treatment is pegylated interferon as for HBV. Limited information is available regarding the addition of antivirals such as lamivudine. Post-transplant individuals with HBV/HDV infection have a lower incidence of recurrence than do transplant recipients with HBV alone. The course of HDV infection is shown in Figure **37.7**.

Hepatitis E virus

Hepatitis E virus (HEV) is an RNA virus that presently has a family of its own, hepatitis E-like viruses. It is water borne and fecal–oral transmission is the rule. Pigs are known carriers. It is both endemic and epidemic with a worldwide distribution.

Although rare in the United States, it is extremely common among young adults in developing areas of the world, and recently a number of imported cases have been reported. There have been documented cases of maternal to neonate transmission. For the most part it is a short, self-limited disease characterized by jaundice, malaise, anorexia, fever, abdominal pain, and arthralgias. Asymptomatic infections occur as do severe, fulminant infections. Mortality as high as 10% is reported in pregnant women. Anti-IgG and anti-IgM HEV tests are commercially available but are not United States Food and Drug Administration approved. Detection of fecal RNA is diagnostic but these assays are

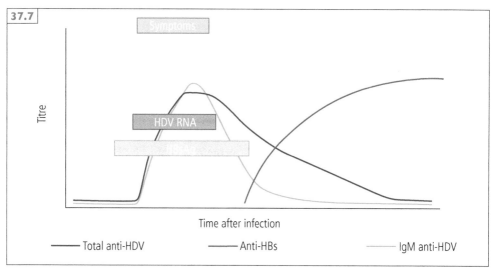

37.7 Time course of hepatitis D virus (HDV) infection. HBsAg: hepatitis B surface antigen; Anti-HBs: antibody to HBsAg; IgM: immunoglobulin M; RNA: ribonucleic acid.

only available on a research basis (through the Centers for Disease Control and Prevention). An effective vaccine has been developed and tested, but is not available. The time course of HEV infection is shown in Figure **37.8**.

Hepatitis G virus

Hepatitis G virus (HGV or GBV) is known to infect humans but has not been definitively shown to cause disease. It is a single-stranded RNA virus of the Flaviviridiae family, closely related to HCV. Risk factors include being an intravenous drug abuser, human immunodeficiency virus (HIV) positive, and having multiple sexual partners. Testing is on a research basis only.

Nonhepatotropic viruses that may cause hepatitis

In immunocompromised individuals and neonates relatively few nonhepatotropic viruses are known to cause hepatitis. In patients throughout the pediatric age range, EBV infection commonly includes an element of hepatitis.

Epstein–Barr virus

EBV is a gamma herpes virus and is most commonly associated with infectious mononucleosis in infants and children. EBV is a double-stranded DNA virus also known as human herpes virus-4 (HHV-4). It has an

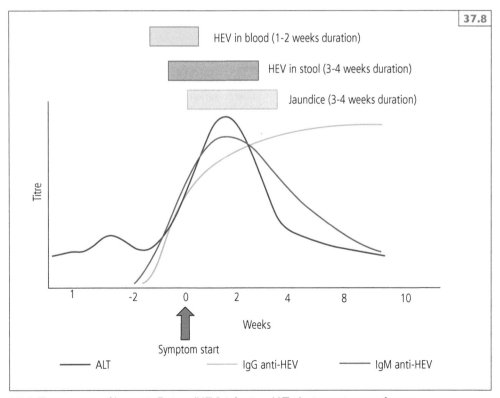

37.8 Time course of hepatitis E virus (HEV) infection. ALT: alanine aminotransferase; IgM: immunoglobulin M.

affinity for lymphocytes, especially B-cells, and thus is associated with a wide range of affected organs. Even in simple, self-limited disease, there is almost always a degree of hepatic involvement. Occasionally, the hepatitis becomes the predominant feature of the disease.

EBV has been implicated in acute liver failure. There is no evidence that treatment of EBV hepatitis is effective. A short course of steroids can shrink lymphoid tissue and relieve symptoms from obstructive tonsils and may improve EBV-associated hematophagocytic lymphohistiocytic syndrome. Steroids have not been shown to change the course of EBV hepatitis. Antiviral treatment does not improve or shorten the course of EBV hepatitis. Because of EBV's propensity for infecting lymphocytes, it is associated with a host of complex syndromes in immunocompromised individuals such as those with HIV and transplant recipients.

There are numerous tests available for the diagnosis of EBV disease and none are specific for liver disease. The heterophile test relies on the presence of antibodies (primarily IgM) to the viral capsid antigen (VCA). False-negative results are common in children under 4 years of age. IgM and IgG antibodies to VCA can be determined independently and both will be positive in acute disease. Antibodies to Epstein–Barr nuclear antigen (EBNA) are not detected for several weeks to several months after primary infection. DNA and RNA PCR tests do not necessarily indicate an acute infection and are most useful when followed over time in an immunocompromised patient (*Table 37.4*).

Table 37.4 Epstein–Barr virus (EBV) diagnostic tests

Test	Antibody/antigen	Interpretation
VCA-IgM	IgM antibody to VCA	Positive in early primary infection False negative under 4 years of age
VCA-IgG	IgG antibody to VCA	Positive in early primary infection; remains positive for years False negative under 4 years of age
Heterophil	Combination of IgM and IgG antibodies to VCA, mostly IgM	Positive in early primary infection; remains positive for years False negative under 4 years of age
Anti-EBNA	Antibody to EBNA	Becomes positive weeks to months after primary infection Positive anti-EBNA excludes active primary disease
EBV DNA by PCR	Amplified EBV DNA	Detects EBV DNA in blood or tissue Does not indicate acute infection Most useful in following immunocompromised patients

DNA: deoxyribonucleic acid; EBNA: Epstein–Barr nuclear antigen; Ig: immunoglobulin; PCR: polymerase chain reaction; VCA: viral capsid antigen.

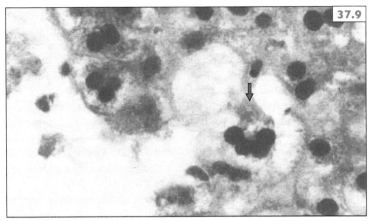

37.9 Cytomegalovirus hepatitis with giant cell transformation (arrow). (Courtesy of John Pohl, MD; Primary Children's Hospital, University of Utah.)

Cytomegalovirus

Cytomegalovirus (CMV) is a DNA virus of the herpes virus group. In older, healthy children it causes a mononucleosis-like illness. Often the initial infection is asymptomatic. Hepatic involvement is encountered in neonates and in immunocompromised individuals. Transmission of the virus can occur transplacentally, during delivery, via saliva, or from breast-milk. It can be introduced through blood or blood products. An antenatally-acquired infection can be asymptomatic, but it also can be associated with congenital anomalies: low birth weight, microcephaly, cerebral calcifications, chorioretinitis, deafness, and retardation. The liver manifestations include conjugated hyperbilirubinemia and hepatosplenomegaly. Definitive diagnosis of CMV as a cause of hepatitis is problematic because of the ubiquity of the virus, the frequency of asymptomatic infections, and possible concomitant infection with other organisms.

A strongly positive, CMV-specific IgM early in life is highly suggestive of CMV-related disease. In older children a fourfold increase in CMV specific antibodies in paired sera samples can be used as a presumptive diagnosis. Finding the virus in the liver of an infant with hepatitis strongly favors CMV as the causative agent (**37.9**).

Treatment is with intravenous gancyclovir or foscarnet. CMV immunoglobulin is also administered intravenously. Long-term follow-up of neonatal hepatitis due to CMV has demonstrated portal hypertension without cirrhosis. Liver transplantation has been needed in infants with liver failure. Children with severe infection and neurologic sequelae have a poor prognosis.

Rubella (German measles)

Rubella was a common, usually self-limited childhood infection prior to the widespread use of vaccination. Today rubella is rare in the United States with only 15 cases reported in 2003. It is seen in under-immunized individuals or in immigrants from areas where vaccination is not practiced. Its major significance was and is as the cause of congenital rubella syndrome (CRS).

If acquired antenatally, rubella is associated with devastating congenital anomalies: ophthalmologic, cardiac, auditory, and neurologic. Rubella is an RNA virus of the Togaviridae family. Transmission is usually via droplet contact from nasopharyngeal secretions. Transplacental transmission is common if the mother contracts the disease during pregnancy. Babies with CRS can shed virus for up to 1 year, thus creating a risk to contacts.

CRS is confirmed by rubella-specific IgM antibodies. PCR and liver tissue confirms rubella as a cause of hepatitis. While mild cases of CRS are reported, crippling congenital anomalies are the rule. Liver involvement is common in CRS. Hepatomegaly is almost always present but is rarely (never) the only manifestation of CRS. It is not unusual for splenomegaly, direct hyperbilirubinemia, cholestasis, and liver enzyme elevation to be present with CRS hepatitis. Liver tissue shows periportal fibrosis and extramedullary hematopoiesis.

Treatment is supportive. Infants with CRS usually recover from hepatitis, but their prognosis remains poor due to other manifestations of CRS.

Herpes simplex virus 1 and 2

Herpes simplex virus 1 and 2 (HSV-1, HSV-2), known collectively as herpes simplex, are two distinct, but similar, double-stranded DNA viruses. In adolescents and adults HSV-1 is primarily associated with gingivostomatitis while HSV-2 causes genital herpes. However, increasingly there is cross-over and either clinical entity is associated with either viral type. Neonatal herpes can be either HSV-1 or HSV-2. There are three distinct presentations of neonatal herpes: 1) disease involving skin, eyes and mouth; 2) central nervous system (CNS) disease with or without skin manifestations; and 3) disseminated, multi-organ disease, prominently liver and lung but frequently also involving CNS. Neonatal herpes can be contracted antenatally, perinatally, and postnatally. The neonate's chances of becoming infected ranges from 60% if the mother has a primary infection to only 2% if the mother has a reactivated infection; however, it is difficult to distinguish a primary infection from a reactivated one. Neonates may not show evidence of disease for 4–8 days after birth. Rapid diagnosis is important because without treatment, the outcome is universally fatal. However, treatment with acyclovir has improved the outlook considerably. Liver transplant may be necessary in neonates with severe liver involvement. Virus can be isolated from skin lesions. PCR has become the test of choice to identify HSV.

Parvovirus B19

Parvovirus B19 is the causative agent for Fifth disease (erythema infectiosum) in young children and 'glove and socks' syndrome in adolescents and adults. In children under 5 years of age and individuals of any age with immune compromise, parvovirus B19 has been reported to cause a range of liver manifestations from acute hepatitis to fulminant liver failure, and to chronic hepatitis with persistent infection. Parvovirus B19 is a single-stranded DNA virus that replicates mainly in human red blood cell precursors, but other sites of replication have been proposed. The virus can be transmitted vertically from mother to fetus, via respiratory tract secretions and via percutaneous exposure to blood. Although patients with parvovirus B19 hepatitis can be quite ill, complete recovery is the usual course, and the need for liver transplantation is rare.

Other hepatitis-associated viruses

A number of viruses have occasionally been associated with hepatitis especially neonatal liver disease. These include: coxsackieviruses, echoviruses, and enteroviruses. HHV-6, the causative agent of exanthema subitum (Sixth disease), has been reported to be the cause of acute and chronic hepatitis in an infant who eventually died. There are several case reports of paramyxovirus hepatitis. Hepatitis in HIV is common, but whether the hepatitis is due to the HIV virus itself or the result of secondary opportunistic infection is debated.

Conclusion

There have been huge gains in our knowledge of the process of hepatitis caused by viruses. Progress in prevention has also been made through public health efforts and vaccinations. Treatments are available for many types of viral hepatitis and medical science is on the threshold of introducing more and better treatments. Drugs developed to treat HIV have been discovered to be effective against viruses that cause hepatitis.

CHAPTER 38

Gallbladder Disease

Mark Davenport

DEFINITION AND EPIDEMIOLOGY

The gallbladder is an off-shoot of the extrahepatic biliary tree with a fundus, body and pouch (of Hartmann) connecting via a cystic duct to the common hepatic duct and therefore forming the common bile duct. Its normal physiologic function is to store and concentrate bile. The dynamic process of discharge is under neurohumoral control (e.g. cholecystokinin) and triggered by luminal presence of lipid within the duodenum. Gallbladder mucosa is actively able to absorb water, chloride and bicarbonate. Thus during its gallbladder phase, bile changes so that sodium concentration almost doubles, bile salt concentration triples, cholesterol increases by fourfold, and bilirubin levels increases about 10-fold. Many of these salts therefore enter a supersaturated state forming the basis for crystallization and stone formation, the usual source of complications and gallbladder pathology.

The incidence of biliary stones in the overall pediatric age-group is unknown. Specific groups may be predisposed. For example, about 20% of children with sickle cell anemia have ultrasound-detectable stones entering adolescence. Other groups at risk for stones include obese children and those receiving oral contraceptives.

CLINICAL PRESENTATION

Stones are often asymptomatic. Stones may cause symptoms by mechanical obstruction somewhere in the biliary tree or at its outlet at the ampulla; or as a predisposition to actual infection and inflammation. Biliary pain is usually felt in the right-upper quadrant, may radiate to the back, is related to fat-laden foodstuffs, and therefore postprandial pain lasts minutes to hours (biliary colic).

Transit of stones into the common bile duct may cause obstruction and surgical jaundice, or if blocking the pancreatic duct at the ampulla, acute pancreatitis.

Acute cholecystitis may have a bacterial overlay, although chemical-induced inflammation is likely. The right upper quadrant pain and any systemic symptoms are much more pronounced with localized guarding and peritonitis. Sometimes, acute cholecystitis leads to an obstruction at the neck of the gallbladder and failure of drainage with gallbladder distension and pus formation, or an empyema.

ETIOLOGY AND PATHOPHYSIOLOGY

The two principal components of gallstones in children are bilirubinate and cholesterol and they have a distinct natural history and origin.

Pigment stones

These are formed from calcium bilirubinate within the gallbladder and are an inevitable consequence of hypersecretion of conjugated bilirubin from the hepatocyte into the biliary canaliculus. This conjugated water-soluble bilirubin is the end-product of the process of red cell degradation and recycling of hemoglobin which begins in the spleen and the reticuloendothelial lymphatic system. In hereditary conditions of red cell deformity, such as sickle cell anemia, spherocytosis, and thalassemia, there is increased red cell turnover and therefore increased throughput of hepatic bilirubin, leading to supersatured bile in the gallbladder and the increased potential for stone formation. Clinically, the stones are invariably black, friable, and multiple (**38.1**).

Cholesterol stones

Cholesterol is secreted into the biliary canaliculus by the transporter proteins ABCG5 and G8. As a highly insoluble product, cholesterol is kept in solution by the formation of micelles with bile salts and phospholipid. Again, with increasing solute concentration in the gallbladder this process may be tipped into crystalization and cholesterol stone formation. This sequence is much more multilayered than is the case for pigment stones, and the interplay of underlying factors is complex. Obesity, a family history of gallbladder disease, and the female gender predispose to stone formation in the pediatric age-group as for adults. Most patients become symptomatic during adolescence.

Cholesterol stones are usually solitary or, if more than one, often faceted (**38.2**). They are harder and on section, multiple layering can be appreciated.

DIFFERENTIAL DIAGNOSIS

- Acute right upper quadrant pain:
  - Retrocecal appendicitis.
  - Acute pancreatitis.
- Chronic right upper quadrant pain:
  - Duodenal ulceration.
  - Choledochal malformation.
  - Biliary dyskinesia – a poorly characterized condition consistent with a nonfunctional gallbladder.

DIAGNOSIS

Liver biochemistry may be entirely normal. Bile duct obstruction leads to rising conjugated bilirubin, γ-glutamyl traspeptidase, and alkaline phosphatase enzyme levels. A raised C-reactive protein and leukocytosis would be expected in any acute inflammatory process. Stones should be visible on ultrasound, usually displaying an acoustic 'shadow' (**38.3**). This technique should also be able to measure any degree of biliary tract dilatation suggestive of obstruction, and thickness of the gallbladder wall suggestive of chronicity. Further imaging of the biliary system may be indicated, particularly if there is a history of jaundice or pancreatitis. Magnetic resonance cholangiopancreatography is noninvasive, and in most individuals it is able to delineate the extrahepatic and intrahepatic ducts (**38.4**). Radioisotope studies may be able to show whether a gallbladder is functional or not and again detect degrees of obstruction. The underlying cause of stones should be investigated to determine if there is a hemolysis etiology. Cholesterol stones might be suspected if the subject is female, overweight, and with a positive family history of gallbladder disease, although the fasting plasma cholesterol is still usually normal.

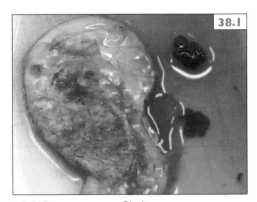

38.1 Pigment stones. Cholecystectomy specimen from 10-year-old boy with sickle cell anemia.

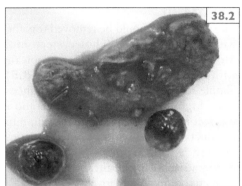

38.2 Cholesterol stones. Cholecystectomy specimen from 15-year-old girl with multiple, idiopathic gallstones. The superficial deep green/black color is caused by oxidation and bile staining.

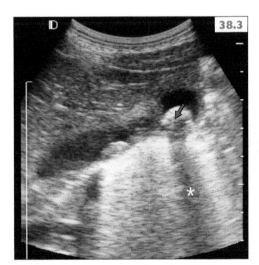

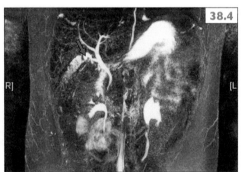

38.4 MRI (T2-weighted) of the biliary system showing a normal extrahepatic biliary tree together with a gallbladder filled with gallstones, pictured here as filling defects (arrow).

38.3 Ultrasound examination of gallbladder showing intraluminal gallstones (arrow) and an obvious acoustic shadow (star).

TREATMENT

Most gallstones should be removed together with the gallbladder (cholecystectomy). Mostly this is performed laparoscopically with a minimal stay in hospital (**38.5**). Simple removal of stones during childhood has a high incidence of recurrence and is not recommended. Stones in the common bile duct should be removed, and the easiest method is from below using endoscopic retrograde cholangiopancreatography and sphincterotomy. Alternatively, actual surgical exploration of the duct from above should be rarely needed, but is possible. Typically the duct itself should be dilated sufficiently to allow drainage.

The treatment of asymptomatic gallstones during childhood is controversial. There is a chance of spontaneous resolution in gallstones dating from infancy where the underlying cause has been removed (e.g. parenteral nutrition). Children with chronic underlying hemolysis (e.g. sickle cell disease) and stones are probably candidates for prophylactic cholecystectomy.

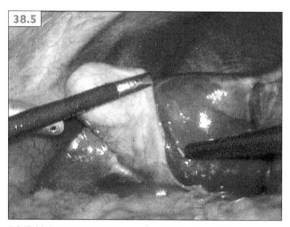

38.5 Video capture image of mobilization of the gallbladder during laparoscopic cholecystectomy.

Hepatotoxins

Daniel Leung, Sanjiv Harpavat

Introduction

The liver metabolizes and secretes a remarkable number of ingested compounds. To accomplish this, hepatocytes process foreign substrates in three steps (**39.1**):

- Step 1: Activation. Cytochrome P450 mono-oxygenases insert an oxygen residue into the compound, rendering the compound more water-soluble but also more toxic.
- Step 2: Detoxification. Enzymes attach another residue to the step 1 metabolite, making it even more water-soluble and neutralizing its toxicity.
- Step 3: Excretion. The water-soluble product is extruded into the cannalicular space and secreted with bile.

Unfortunately, the liver cannot metabolize all compounds safely. Drug-induced liver injury (DILI) occurs when ingested substances induce liver damage. DILI is less common in pediatric populations than adult populations for a number of reasons:

- Fewer children take medications.
- Children are less likely to abuse alcohol or smoke cigarettes (two factors that alter drug metabolism).
- Children are seldom prescribed medications commonly associated with DILI, such as antiarrhythmics.
- Children may metabolize drugs differently, conferring some degree of protection.

However, DILI is a recognized pediatric problem, with acute liver failure complicating as many as one of every six pediatric deaths caused by adverse drug reactions in some surveys.

DILI is most often caused by Step 1 metabolite accumulation, following one of three patterns. Drugs with 'intrinsic hepatotoxicity' cause predictable liver damage when consumed in large amounts. While drugs with this property are rare, acetaminophen (paracetamol) is a well-studied example. In large amounts, acetaminophen is converted to the toxic intermediate N-acetyl-

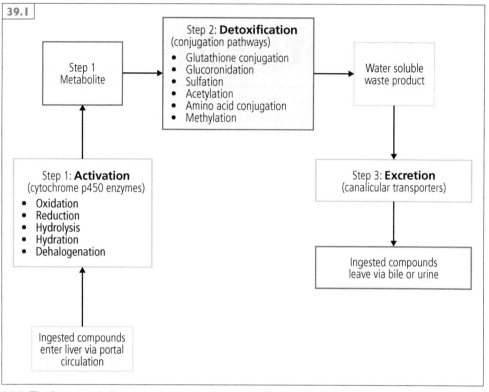

39.1

Step 2: Detoxification
(conjugation pathways)
- Glutathione conjugation
- Glucoronidation
- Sulfation
- Acetylation
- Amino acid conjugation
- Methylation

Step 1
Metabolite

Water soluble
waste product

Step 1: Activation
(cytochrome p450 enzymes)
- Oxidation
- Reduction
- Hydrolysis
- Hydration
- Dehalogenation

Step 3: Excretion
(canalicular transporters)

Ingested compounds
leave via bile or urine

Ingested compounds
enter liver via portal
circulation

39.1 The liver metabolizes compounds via three well-characterized steps.

p-benzoquinoneimine (NAPQI) by cytochrome P450 mono-oxygenases. Normally, Step 2 enzymes would neutralize NAPQI with glutathione; however, excessive NAPQI depletes glutathione reserves and leaves free NAPQI to damage hepatocytes (**39.2**). Acetaminophen toxicity is treated with N-acetylcysteine, which promotes more glutathione production.

More commonly, DILI is less predictable and idiosyncratic. Drugs with the second pattern, 'contingent hepatotoxicity', only cause liver damage in particular individuals at certain times. Their toxicity is probably related to the great variation in Step 1 and Step 2 enzymes. Among individuals, the enzymes can vary in nucleotide sequence, subtly changing the way they recognize substrates or the speed with which they catalyze their reaction. For example, the Step 2 enzyme thiopurine methyltransferase differs between individuals, accounting for the different rates that children with inflammatory bowel disease or liver disease metabolize 6-mercaptopurine (6-MP) (**39.3**). Step 1 and Step 2 enzyme levels also

39.3 (Opposite) Thiopurine methyltransferase (TPMT) promotes production of the hepatotoxin 6-methylmercaptopurine (6-MMP) over the production of the immunosuppressant 6-thioguanine (6-TG). HPRT: hypoxanthine phosphoribosyl transferase; XO: xanthine oxidase; 6-MP: 6-mercaptopurine.

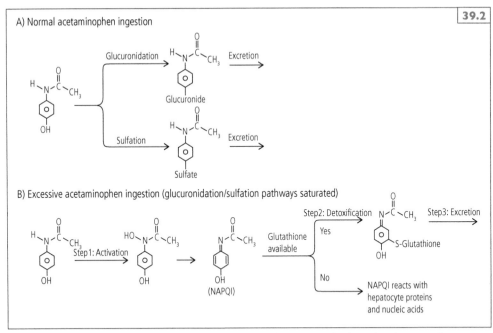

39.2 Acetaminophen hepatotoxicity results when Step 2 enzymes deplete glutathione and can no longer detoxify intermediate substrates. NAPQI: N-acetyl-p-benzoquinoneimine.

vary across developmental time. For example, the Step 1 enzyme CYP1A2 that metabolizes caffeine is expressed at low levels in newborns and high levels in prepubertal adolescents. Hence, caffeine is metabolized slowly in newborns and quickly in adolescents.

Drugs with the third pattern, 'immuno-allergic toxicity', cause liver damage that resembles an autoimmune or allergic insult. These drugs may cause a rise in serum immunoglobulin (Ig) G, anti-antinuclear antibody (ANA) antibodies, and even anti-liver-kidney microsomal (LKM) antibodies as seen in Type 2 autoimmune hepatitis. These drugs can also induce eosinophil-mediated liver damage. In both cases, the Step 1 metabolite is thought to bind to hepatocyte proteins, create neoantigens, and in certain individuals stimulate an immune response. It is unclear why this process may occur suddenly even in individuals with a long and previously uneventful history of taking a medication.

Clinically, all three patterns overlap in the symptoms they produce. When Step 1 metabolites damage hepatocytes, children present with a hepatitis picture of nausea, vomiting, anorexia, and elevated transaminases. When Step 1 metabolites injure cholangiocytes, cholestatic symptoms of pruritis and jaundice occur. Step 1 metabolites can also injure any of the other liver cells, including endothelial cells creating a vaso-occlusive disorder picture. Often, DILI affects multiple cells in the liver and creates a mixed hepatic–cholestatic clinical picture that can occur acutely, subacutely, or chronically. If not addressed, DILI can lead to liver fibrosis, cirrhosis, and ultimately liver failure.

Histologically, hepatotoxins may injure the liver differentially. The hepatic acinus is the functional unit of the liver and is oriented around the afferent vascular system. The acinus consists of an irregular shaped, roughly ellipsoidal mass of hepatocytes aligned around the hepatic arterioles and portal venules just as they anastomose into sinusoids. The acinus

can be divided into zones that correspond to the distance from the arterial blood supply (**39.4**). Hepatocytes closest to the arterioles (zone 1) are the best oxygenated, while those farthest from the arterioles have the poorest supply of oxygen (zone 3). This arrangement also means that cells in the center of the acinus (zone 1) are the first to be exposed to blood-borne toxins absorbed into portal blood from the small intestine. Zonal patterns of injury may or may not be specific to the toxin.

Specific compounds

Some of the most common pediatric causes of DILI, which must be considered in a child who presents with liver abnormalities, are outlined below (in alphabetical order).

Acetaminophen
Excessive acetaminophen ingestion is common, accounting for as many as 30,000 reports yearly to the United States National Poison Data System. Ingestion occurs in two forms: 1) an acute overdose, often by adolescents trying to harm themselves; and 2) chronic overdose, by caregivers giving excessive amounts over a series of days. Chronic overdose is particularly difficult to diagnose, because therapeutic doses (75 mg/kg/day) are only slightly less than doses considered toxic (greater than 90 mg/kg/day). However, children may be slightly protected, because they have a larger capacity to sulfonate acetaminophen before it is converted to NAPQI by Step 1 enzymes. Furthermore, children have more glutathione to bind NAPQI when it is made.

Clinically, patients usually present with subtle symptoms including nausea, vomiting, or malaise. Over the course of a few days, liver-specific symptoms ensue, including right upper quadrant pain and elevated transaminases. In severe cases, liver failure with coagulopathy and encephalopathy occurs. Liver pathology reveals zone 3 hepatocellular injury, reflecting the higher concentration of P450 mono-oxygenases in perivenular hepatocytes. Treatment focuses on delivering N-acetylcysteine as a substrate for glutathione production. Treating early within the first 8–10 hours is the most hepatoprotective.

Amoxicillin/clavulanate

Amoxicillin/clavulanate toxicity is the most common antibiotic cause of DILI worldwide. It presents with a cholestatic picture when taken chronically, suggesting cholangiocyte or cholangiocyte–hepatocyte damage. Liver biopsy also reveals eosinophils, suggesting an immunoallergic process, and in more advanced cases ductopenia also known as 'vanishing bile duct syndrome'. Clavulanate appears to be essential for DILI to occur, because amoxicillin alone will not trigger DILI even in patients shown to be sensitive to amoxicillin/clavulanate. However, it is not known whether clavulanate alone causes DILI. Acute liver failure has been reported but is rare. Treatment consists of stopping the medication.

Antifungals

Whereas griseofulvin has been associated with elevated serum aminotransferases in some cases, ketoconazole is the most common antifungal medication causing DILI. Patients can develop symptoms weeks after starting

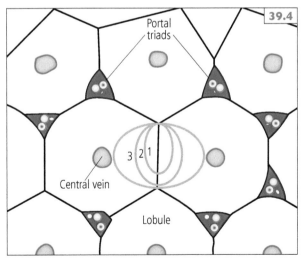

39.4 Hepatocytes belong to different zones in the liver lobule, with zone I hepatocytes closest to the portal tract and zone 3 hepatocytes closest to the central veins.

the medication, and often have hepatocellular necrosis or mixed hepatocellular–cholangiocyte injury on biopsy. Because the hepatocellular injury is found in zone 3, one explanation is that ketoconazole causes contingent hepatoxicity when a Step 1 metabolite abnormally accumulates due to individual variations in Step 2 clearance. Treatment consists of stopping the drug. However, in severe fungal infections with mild increases in transaminases, some clinicians elect to continue the medication and monitor laboratory values carefully.

Erythromycin

Erythromycin and other commonly used macrolide antibiotics can cause DILI. Clinically, patients can have jaundice as well as abdominal pain, elevated serum transaminases, and hepatosplenomegaly. Liver failure and death have been reported. Pathologically, liver biopsies show prominent cholestasis, zone 3 hepatocellular damage, and eosinophils. This pattern suggests immunoallergic toxicity, arising when Step 1 metabolites bind hepatocellular components and induce an immune response. Treatment consists of stopping the macrolide promptly. An isolated report documented success with steroid treatment for clarithromycin (along with nimesulide)-associated hepatotoxicity.

Estrogens/oral contraceptive pills

Oral contraceptive pills (OCPs), particularly those high in estrogen, have been associated with chronic changes in the liver. OCPs are associated with vascular changes, such as hepatic vein thrombosis and peliosis hepatis (cystic dilation of the sinusoids). Furthermore, chronic OCP use correlates with the presence of hepatic adenomas. Because hepatic adenomas can progress to hepatocellular carcinoma, one concern is whether OCPs also induce hepatocellular carcinoma. However, causal data establishing this relationship are lacking. Stopping high estrogen OCPs results in regression of adenomas. Furthermore, OCPs are now made with less estrogen to avoid the risk of hepatic adenoma altogether.

Herbal medications/dietary supplements

Many herbal medications have been shown to cause DILI, though the diagnosis is difficult because herbal use is often not elicited in the history. Up to 10% of DILI cases may be due to herbal medications. Commonly available herbal products include comfrey, bush teas, germander, chaparral, mistletoe, kava kava, jin bu huan, ma-huang, and syosaiko-to. Comfrey, bush teas, and other plant pyrrolizidine alkaloids damage hepatic vein endothelial cells, leading to sinusoidal dysfunction and veno-occlusive disorder.

Isoniazid

Isoniazid (INH) toxicity comes in two forms: 1) mild INH toxicity; and 2) INH hepatitis. Both forms are thought to result in a toxic Step 1 metabolite, and may be aggravated in the presence of rifampin (which induces Step 1 enzyme expression) and malnutrition (which depletes glutathione stores). Mild INH toxicity presents as asymptomatic serum aminotransferase elevation in as many as 20% of individuals, and does not necessarily require drug cessation. INH hepatitis is much rarer, with incidences estimated at 0.1–7.1%. INH hepatitis resembles viral hepatitis with submassive hepatocyte necrosis that may or may not have a zonal pattern. INH hepatitis is life threatening and requires immediate cessation of the drug.

Methotrexate

Methotrexate used to treat inflammatory bowel disease and rheumatologic disorders has been associated with DILI. While the mechanism of damage is unknown, methotrexate given daily (versus weekly) seems to be associated with more liver damage. Multiple histologic changes ensue, including steatosis, stellate cell hypertrophy, and fibrosis. At one point, liver biopsy was standard to track methotrexate-induced liver changes. Now, however, serum liver function tests are followed to detect liver damage, and liver biopsy may or may not be warranted depending on the clinical situation.

6-Mercaptopurine

6-MP and azathioprine can cause mild increases in serum transaminases, though rare cases of severe progressive jaundice have also been reported. 6-MP is metabolized via three pathways (**39.3**). Xanthine oxidase (XO) converts 6-MP to 6-thiouric acid, which has no toxicity. Hypoxanthine phosphoribosyl transferase (HPRT) metabolizes 6-MP to 6-thioguanine (6-TG) nucleotides, the active ingredient involved in immunosuppression. Thiopurine methyltransferase (TPMT) metabolizes 6-MP to 6-methylmercaptopurine (6-MMP), a compound that leads to transaminase elevation. Transaminase levels return to normal once 6-MP doses are reduced. TPMT activity can be checked before starting 6-MP therapy, because low TPMT activity results in higher levels of 6-TG (at the expense of 6-MMP) and potentially dangerous amounts of immunosuppression.

Valproic acid

Similar to INH, valproic acid (VPA) liver toxicity presents in two ways: 1) a mild, asymptomatic increase in transaminases that can be treated with dose reduction; and 2) a severe, progressive form of hepatitis that often is lethal. VPA hepatitis occurs in the first 6 months of starting treatment and is not preceded by serum aminotransferase elevations. Children younger than 2 years, on multiple anticonvulsants, and with other medical problems are most vulnerable. VPA hepatitis presents with nausea, vomiting, and malaise, followed by a coagulopathy and then jaundice. On histology, hepatocellular necrosis and microvesicular fat is present.

VPA is a branched fatty acid, normally metabolized via beta-oxidation in the mitochondria. In the setting of mitochondrial dysfunction, caused by viral illness or inherited defects for example, VPA accumulates. VPA is then metabolized by P450 mono-oxygenases into the substrate 4-EN-VPA. 4-EN-VPA is a potent hepatotoxin in animal models and human cells, and may explain the liver damage seen in VPA hepatitis. Furthermore, both VPA and 4-EN-VPA inhibit further mitochondrial beta-oxidation of lipids, thereby promoting microvesicular steatosis while also shunting more VPA towards 4-EN-VPA production. This feed forward cycle could account for the continuous nature of VPA hepatitis even after VPA has been stopped. Carnitine, a co-factor promoting beta-oxidation, has been tested with some success as an antidote to VPA hepatoxicity.

Metabolic Disorders I

Karen Francolla

- **Wilson disease**
- **Alpha-1 antitrypsin deficiency**

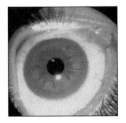
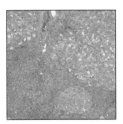
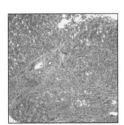
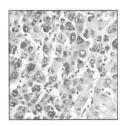

Wilson disease

DEFINITION

Wilson disease (WD), also known as hepato-lenticular degeneration, was first described by American neurologist, Kinnear Wilson, in 1912. He described 'progressive lenticular degeneration': a rare, familial, lethal disease characterized by softening of the lenticular nuclei and chronic liver disease leading to cirrhosis. Since that time, the pathophysiology of WD has been established. WD is a human copper storage disease, resulting in the accumulation of copper primarily in the liver, but also in a number of other organs such as the brain, eyes, and kidneys (**40.1**).

WD is transmitted by autosomal recessive inheritance. It is caused by a mutation in the *ATP7B* gene. The *ATPB7* gene normally codes for a metal-transporting P-type adenosine triphosphatase (ATPase), mainly expressed on hepatocytes. In health, this ATPase functions in the transmembrane transport of copper within hepatocytes. In WD, the absent or reduced function of this ATPase results in the decreased hepatocellular excretion of copper into bile and leads instead to copper accumulation in the liver, and subsequent hepatic injury. Over time, copper may be released into the bloodstream and deposited in secondary organs, such as the brain, cornea, and kidneys. Clinical disease therefore may range over a variable spectrum including abnormal liver function tests to fulminant hepatic failure and cirrhosis, to seizures, psychosis, and other neurologic manifestations.

CLINICAL PRESENTATION

WD can have a wide variety of clinical presentations, making its diagnosis challenging. From a hepatic perspective, signs and symptoms may include asymptomatic elevation of aminotransferases, asymptomatic hepatomegaly, isolated splenomegaly, acute hepatitis, fatty liver, portal hypertension with possible associated gastrointestinal (GI) bleeding, cirrhosis, and/or fulminant hepatic failure. From a neurologic or psychiatric perspective, signs and symptoms may include changes in behavior, decompensation in handwriting or school work, movement disorders, rigid dystonia, dysarthria, drooling, seizures, migraine

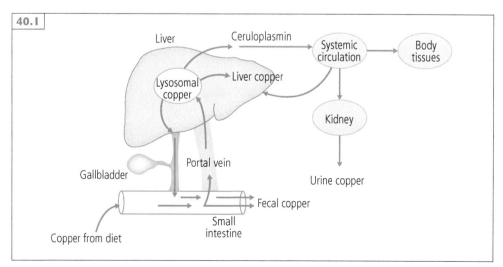

40.1 Schematic diagram of copper storage and excretion. (Adapted from Emerick KM. Wilson's disease. In: Bishop W (ed). *Pediatric Practice Gastroenterology*. McGraw-Hill, New York, 2011.)

headaches, anxiety, depression, insomnia, personality changes, and/or psychosis. Other manifestations may include menstrual irregularities (e.g. amenorrhea, infertility), Coombs-negative hemolytic anemia, aminoaciduria, and nephrolithiasis.

The most common presentation is that of liver disease in the 10–20-year-old patient. This presentation is followed by neurologic and psychiatric symptoms in the 20–40-year-old patient. Less commonly, WD may be diagnosed in the evaluation of hemolytic anemia. However, it can present at almost any age, again making its diagnosis challenging. Clinical symptoms of liver involvement in WD typically do not occur prior to 3–5 years of life. Hepatic presentations of WD include acute hepatitis, fulminant hepatic failure, chronic active hepatitis, and cirrhosis. WD may present solely as elevated aminotransferases in an otherwise asymptomatic patient. Patients less than 20 years old tend to present with liver dysfunction whereas older patients typically present with psychiatric and neurologic manifestations. Neurologic manifestations may initially be subtle behavioral changes such as a decline in school performance, tremors, or slurred speech; if WD remains untreated, neurologic manifestations may progress to dysarthria and dystonia. Copper deposition in the kidneys may lead to nephrocalcinosis, hematuria, or aminoaciduria. Cardiac manifestations may include cardiomyopathy and arrhythmias. Arthritis and arthalgias may also occur.

Copper silently accumulates in the liver in the early pediatric years. After the liver's ability to store copper is surpassed, circulating free copper levels rise and copper begins to accumulate in other systemic organs including the kidneys, corneas, and central nervous system. This change in the distribution of copper in systemic organs accounts for the various clinical presentations of WD.

The ocular manifestations of WD, Kayser–Fleischer (KF) rings and sunflower cataracts, are among the most widely recognized extrahepatic signs of WD. The KF ring is a

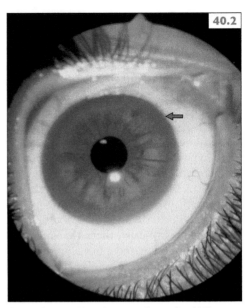

40.2

40.2 Kayser–Fleischer ring (arrow) in Wilson disease.

green/brown colored ring at the corneal edge caused by copper accumulation. Light reflecting off the copper granules deposited there gives rise to the ring's appearance. KF rings do not affect visual acuity and are best diagnosed via slit-lamp examination by an ophthalmologist (**40.2**). Isolated KF rings are not pathognomonic for WD and can be found in other cholestatic liver diseases. KF rings are present in only approximately 50% of patients with primarily liver disease at the time of their diagnosis of WD. They are nearly invariably present in patients with neurologic symptoms, but still may be absent in a small minority of cases. In children, KF rings are typically absent. Like KF rings, sunflower cataracts do not interfere with vision and are diagnosed by slit-lamp examination. Sunflower cataracts represent copper granules deposited in the anterior and posterior lens capsule. Both ophthalmologic manifestations can resolve with chelation therapy.

EPIDEMIOLOGY

WD has an estimated incidence of 1–4 per 100,000 live births worldwide. The heterozygous carrier state is approximately 1 in 90–100 people. WD may present with hepatic, hematologic, neurologic, or psychiatric symptoms. WD presents as liver disease more commonly in children and younger adults than older adults. Its most typical presentation is that of hepatic or hematologic symptoms in the second decade of life. Neurologic and psychiatric presentations are more common in the third and fourth decades. Symptoms may be nonspecific. Typically, there are similarities in the age of onset and clinical presentation of affected members in families. However, it is likely that environmental factors also have an effect on the manner in which the disease is expressed, as occasionally affected family members may have marked differences in biochemical findings and organ involvement at presentation. All patients with WD have some degree of liver involvement, although this may be well compensated and asymptomatic. A high degree of clinical suspicion is therefore necessary in achieving an efficient diagnosis, and thereby minimizing advancement of neurologic or hepatic manifestations.

DIFFERENTIAL DIAGNOSIS

In pediatrics, the initial presentation of WD is typically hepatic in origin. This allows for a more restricted differential diagnosis in pediatrics than is true in adult medicine. Clinical presentation usually falls into one of four main patterns: asymptomatic transaminits, chronic hepatitis, fulminant liver failure, or cirrhosis. The main differential diagnosis for WD in pediatrics is summarized in *Table 40.1*.

DIAGNOSIS

No single diagnostic test in isolation is considered to be a perfect gold standard in the diagnosis of WD. Diagnostic evaluations should begin with evaluation of a serum hepatic panel containing aspartate aminotransferase (AST), alanine aminotransferase (ALT), gamma-glutamyl transferase (GGT), alkaline phosphatase,

---

Table 40.1 Differential diagnosis of Wilson disease in pediatric patients

Clinical presentation	Asymptomatic transaminitis	Chronic hepatitis	Fulminant liver failure
	Viral infections	Hepatitis B, C	Drug/medication toxicity
	Drug/medication toxicity	Nonalcoholic steatohepatitis	Viral hepatitis, non-A–G
	Nonalcoholic steatohepatitis	Autoimmune hepatitis	Autoimmune hepatitis
	Hypothyroidism	Alpha-1-antitrypsin deficiency	Ischemia
	Autoimmune hepatitis	Primary sclerosing cholangitis	Budd–Chiari syndrome
	Celiac disease	Cystic fibrosis	
	Alpha-1-antitrypsin deficiency	Systemic lupus erythmatosus	
	Primary sclerosing cholangitis		
	Muscle disease		

total and direct bilirubin, albumin, prothrombin time with international normalized ratio (INR), and total protein. The aminotransferases, AST and ALT, typically tend to be elevated into the moderate range (100–500 IU/l). The AST value is often greater than that of the ALT. Other laboratory findings consistent, but not diagnostic for WD, include a markedly elevated bilirubin, a low alkaline phosphatase, and a normal total protein. Serum copper levels, serum ceruloplasmin, and urine copper levels are useful in investigating WD as a cause of liver disease. Serum copper measurements are typically low (values often less than 20 µg/dl [3 µmol/l]). However, copper levels can vary depending on the disease activity.

Serum ceruloplasmin values are typically low in WD, although they may be normal. Ceruloplasmin is an acute phase reactant; therefore, any disease that results in hepatic inflammation can cause elevation of ceruloplasmin. Additionally, disorders that reduce liver synthetic function can also reduce the ceruloplasmin. Serum ceruloplasmin testing in isolation has a sensitivity of approximately 80% and specificity of 94% using the standard laboratory value of less than 20 mg/dl (200 mg/l).

Measurement of 24-hour urine copper is also useful in the diagnosis of WD. WD patients typically excrete greater than 40 µg of copper in the 24-hour collection. Urinary copper results >40–100 µg require further work-up. Penicillamine challenge may be helpful when WD is suspected and the 24-hour urine copper is measured. This test involves administration of 500 mg of D-penicillamine at the initiation and at the 12 hour mark into the 24-hour urine collection. A positive result is obtained when >1600 µg of urine copper is excreted in a 24-hour period. Elevated urine copper results can be seen in disorders other than WD, such as chronic liver disease or other diseases leading to fulminant hepatic failure. Therefore, patients with these results require further evaluation with liver biopsy.

Liver biopsy is helpful in supporting a diagnosis of WD (**40.3, 40.4**). In severe liver failure, the risks of liver biopsy may outweigh its benefits. Hepatic biopsy findings in WD

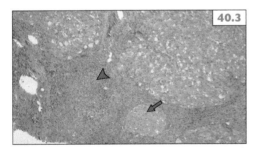

40.3 Liver histology of a child with Wilson disease with portal inflammatory changes (arrowhead) and fibrosis (arrow). (Courtesy of Rafal Kozielski, MD; Women & Children's Hospital of Buffalo.)

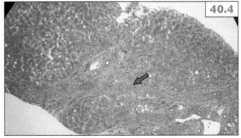

40.4 Liver histology of a child with Wilson disease with extensive fibrosis (arrow) highlighted with trichrome stain. (Courtesy of Rafal Kozielski, MD, Women & Children's Hospital of Buffalo.)

show steatosis. Hepatic copper quantification is the most important test performed in conjunction with biopsy. The specimen must be collected in a copper-free container. Hepatic copper levels typically are greater than 250 µg/g dry weight of liver. However, it is important to highlight that elevated hepatic copper levels are not unique to WD and are seen in the setting of other chronic diseases such as biliary atresia.

The diagnosis of WD is complicated by the fact that no single individual test is diagnostically perfect. Thus, the correct diagnosis of WD is made via the combination of good clinical judgment and well-selected diagnostic testing. A 24-hour urine copper collection and liver biopsy with hepatic tissue copper measurement should be performed in all suspected cases of WD.

PATHOPHYSIOLOGY

Copper is an essential metal which acts as a cofactor for many proteins. In normal human copper metabolism, the dietary intake of copper exceeds physiologic needs and is therefore excreted (**40.1**). The typical Western diet provides 3–4 times the estimated adult physiologic copper requirement. Copper is absorbed in the stomach and proximal small intestine relatively efficiently; therefore, to avoid copper toxicity, the amount of copper absorbed and stored in the body must be finely regulated. The main system for achieving such regulation is the hepatic excretion of copper into bile. Up to 80% of absorbed copper is actually excreted in bile to maintain this homeostasis.

In WD, mutations in the *ATP7B* gene cause impaired biliary copper excretion and defective incorporation of copper into ceruloplasmin. This in turn leads to the progressive accumulation of copper in the liver, subsequently followed by the deposition of copper in other organs. Copper deposition in the liver begins during the first few years of life. At the end of the first or second decade of life, the ability of the liver to store this copper burden is exceeded; free copper is then released into the circulation and penetrates other tissues. Hepatic copper measurements may actually decrease during this time while nonhepatic organ stores, such as those in the brain, eye, and kidney, may increase.

TREATMENT

WD is fatal without treatment. Treatment modalities for WD include diet modification, chelation, zinc, antioxidants, tetrathiomolybdate, and liver transplantation. Choice of specific therapy is dependent upon clinical presentation.

Dietary modification with restriction of consumed copper is nearly universally recommended for WD patients for at least their first year of therapy. Sources of copper in the western diet include nuts, chocolate, mushrooms, shellfish, liver, and other organ meats. Attention must also be paid to environmental sources of copper, such as well water and water delivered via copper pipes into the home.

Copper chelation is the mainstay of treatment. Copper chelation therapy was introduced in the 1950s. Currently, D-penicillamine and trientine are the typical chelation medications utilized in treating WD. Laboratory monitoring and dosing of D-penicillamine and trientine are the same. In children, dosing of these medications is approximately 20 mg/kg/day divided two to three times daily. Pyridoxine (25 mg/day) should be co-administered with both D-penicillamine and trientine. Severe adverse reactions can occur and have been reported to occur at a frequency of approximately 30% of patients treated with D-penicillamine and 5% of patients treated with trientine. These reactions may include hypersensitivity reactions, thrombocytopenia, neutropenia, proteinuria, and autoimmune diseases. Efficacy of treatment is determined by following 24-hour urine copper measurements that is followed every 3 months for the first 2 years and then annually. Drug toxicity needs to be followed closely with a complete blood count, hepatic panel, creatinine, and urinalysis serially. Lifetime adherence to the patient's prescribed medical regimen is essential.

For asymptomatic patients, zinc therapy is often recommended. Zinc therapy works by inhibiting copper uptake from the GI tract and promoting copper excretion. Dosing of zinc varies by patient age. Its main side-effect is gastritis; this occurs in about 10% of patients. Success of therapy is again guided by results of 24-hour copper measurements.

In hepatic failure, liver transplantation is the most appropriate therapy. Plasmapheresis or kidney dialysis may be used as temporizing measures to bridge to transplant. These patients require timely referral to and care by a pediatric liver transplant center.

Screening for WD in asymptomatic relatives should begin at 3 years of age. This screen should include a history and physical examination, hepatic function panel, prothrombin time and INR, slit lamp examination by a pediatric ophthalmologist, 24-hour urine copper, and consideration of genetic testing. The genetic defect in WD has been localized to the *ATP7B* gene on chromosome 13. Screening is made difficult be the large size of this gene and more than 200 unique mutations. For prenatal diagnosis and family members, linkage analysis can be helpful when the proband's mutations are known.

Alpha-1 antitrypsin deficiency

DEFINITION

Alpha-1 antitrypsin (A1AT) deficiency is an autosomal co-dominant disease that causes both liver and lung disease. A1AT deficiency is the most common etiology of neonatal liver disease resulting from a genetic cause. A1AT deficiency is associated with chronic liver disease in 10–15% of affected children. The A1AT protein is the main serum inhibitor of proteolytic enzymes. Injury to the liver occurs as a result of the intracellular accumulation of mutant A1AT protein within hepatocytes. In the lung, tissue damage, ultimately leading to emphysema, occurs secondary to an absence of functional A1AT protein; this absence allows for excessive neutrophil elastase activity which in turn damages the lung tissue.

CLINICAL PRESENTATION

The hepatic manifestation of A1AT deficiency typically occurs in the neonatal period. It is manifest by persistent jaundice and alteration of liver enzymes. Conjugated bilirubin and aminotransferase levels are commonly mildly to moderately elevated. Alkaline phosphatase and GGT measurements may also be elevated. The liver may be enlarged on physical examination. Clinically, the infant may be small for gestational age. Other less common presentations include GI bleeding, bruising, or bleeding from the umbilical stump. Liver injury may advance to cirrhosis, although the time to cirrhosis is variable.

Approximately 10% of infants will manifest liver dysfunction, ascites, and hepatosplenomegaly. Severe fulminant liver failure may also occur in infancy, though infrequently. Liver dysfunction may also present in late childhood or the teenage years. In these cases, the patient may present with abdominal distention resulting from either ascites or hepatosplenomegaly, GI bleeding from esophageal variceal hemorrhage, or isolated splenomegaly. In the adult patient, A1AT deficiency should be considered as the possible etiology of chronic hepatitis, portal hypertension, cirrhosis, or hepatocellular carcinoma. Emphysema resulting from A1AT deficiency is generally reserved for the adult patient who is typically male and a tobacco smoker.

EPIDEMIOLOGY

A1AT deficiency is one of the world's most common genetically inherited diseases. The normal A1AT protein is the M type (protease inhibitor M, or PiMM). The two most common mutant alleles encode protease inhibitor S or Z (PiS or PiZ). Other much more rare alleles have been associated with mutant proteins resulting in liver disease. Classic A1AT deficiency occurs in patients homozygous for the mutant protease inhibitor Z; these patients are designated as PiZZ. Liver disease is also known to occur in PiSZ heterozygotes. The PiZ allele frequency is approximately 14.5 per 1000 people in the United States, and the PiZZ genotype is estimated to occur at a frequency of 1 in approximately 2000-4000 births in this population. The PiZ allele tends to be more common in people of northern European descent, and appears with lower frequency in African Americans, Latinos, and Asians. Approximately 10–15% of PiZZ individuals will manifest evidence of liver disease within the first years of life.

DIFFERENTIAL DIAGNOSIS

The differential diagnosis of A1AT deficiency is dependent upon the age of presentation. In neonates, it classically presents as a direct hyperbilirubinemia with jaundice. Biliary atresia may have a similar presentation and requires exclusion, as do other types of extrahepatic obstruction, inborn errors of metabolism, such as tyrosinemia and galactosemia, and congenital infections. In the older pediatric patient, the differential diagnosis must be broadened to include other infectious and metabolic causes, as well as autoimmune causes, anatomic defects, and toxic effects of medication and alcohol.

DIAGNOSIS

The diagnosis of A1AT deficiency is made via protease inhibitor typing. This is accomplished via electrophoresis which is used to separate the various forms of A1AT present in serum. Measurement of the total serum A1AT level may also be helpful before phenotyping results are available; the majority of PiZZ patients have low serum A1AT levels, defined as approximately 10–15% of the normal value. However, it is important to note that A1AT is an acute phase reactant, so levels may be artificially elevated. This makes the serum A1AT measurement unreliable at times. Deoxyribonucleic acid (DNA) testing for the most common A1AT mutations is also commercially available. On liver biopsy, A1AT disease is suggested by the presence of periodic acid-Schiff-positive, diastase-resistant globules in the endoplasmic reticulum of hepatocytes (**40.5**). Other histologic features include bile ductular injury, paucity of bile ducts, portal fibrosis, inflammatory infiltrates, and/or cirrhosis. These histologic findings are not specific for deficiency and, alone, are insufficient for a diagnosis of A1AT deficiency.

PATHOPHYSIOLOGY

The A1AT protein is a member of the serpin family of serine protease inhibitors. It is a 52 kD protein synthesized by the liver whose main function after release into the circulation is the inhibition of neutrophil proteases. The gene encoding this protein is located on the long arm of chromosome 14. In the PiZZ individual, the loss of protease inhibition allows the actions of destructive enzymes, such as elastase, to be unopposed in the lung; this results in tissue damage and progressive emphysema. Lung involvement typically becomes symptomatic after age 30 years with its peak in the 4th and 5th decades; its onset is hastened by smoking. Conversely, in the liver, the mechanism of hepatocyte injury is secondary to a gain of function in the mutant protein. This gain of function results from a mutation that substitutes lysine for glutamate at position 342 of the protein. The abnormally folded protein is secondarily retained in the endoplasmic reticulum; it has a higher propensity to form polymers than the wild type protein. Accumulation of this mutant protein in the endoplasmic reticulum may be one mechanism for hepatocyte injury; another proposed mechanism includes defective autophagy, the cellular mechanism for clearance of the accumulated proteins.

TREATMENT

Avoidance of tobacco smoking is critical for reducing lung damage in association with A1AT deficiency. Unfortunately, at this time, no medical therapy has been demonstrated to be effective in treating hepatic manifestations of A1AT deficiency. Therapies being investigated for the treatment of A1AT deficiency include cyclosporine A to avoid mitochondrial damage, chemical chaperones to prevent abnormal misfolding of protein, and modifiers of glycosylation to improve secretion of A1AT. Orthotopic liver transplantation is curative for liver disease manifestations of A1AT, but only halts further progression of emphysema. Liver transplant is reserved for patients with severe complications of liver involvement including portal hypertension and cirrhosis. Disease progression may be slow, and liver transplantation may be avoided for many years.

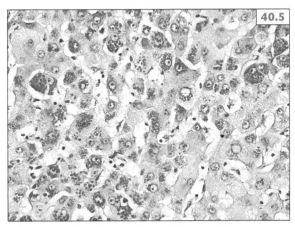

40.5 Liver biopsy from patient with α-1-antitrypsin deficiency stained with periodic acid-Schiff (PAS). The hepatocytes are mildly swollen with numerous PAS-positive globules. (Courtesy of Gloria Young, MD, Hackensack University Medical Center.)

CHAPTER 41

Metabolic Disorders II

Achiya Amir, Vicky Ng

- **Galactosemia**
- **Hereditary tyrosinemia type 1**
- **Hereditary fructose intolerance**

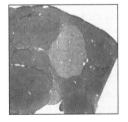
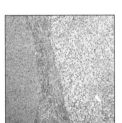
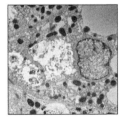

Galactosemia

DEFINITION AND EPIDEMIOLOGY

Galactosemia is a disorder of galactose metabolism that can result in life-threatening complications including feeding problems, failure to thrive, hepatocellular damage, bleeding, and sepsis in untreated infants. Galactose metabolism is important for energy production, glycogen stores, and galactosylation of glycolipids and glycoproteins. This chapter will focus on classic galactosemia (OMIM 230400), a potentially lethal inherited disorder caused by the deficiency of galactose-1-phosphate-uridyltransferase (GALT). Despite adequate treatment with a lactose/galactose restricted diet, children with galactosemia remain at increased risk for developmental delays, speech problems, and abnormalities of motor function.

Galactosemia affects about 1 in every 30,000–60,000 babies.

CLINICAL PRESENTATION

Presentation is dependent on galactose exposure. Disease onset is typically acute and occurs in the early neonatal period as infants are fed lactose-containing breast milk or cow-milk formulas. The main organs affected by galactosemia are the liver, brain, kidneys (Fanconi syndrome), gonads, and the optical lenses. Presenting symptoms are usually nonspecific and range from feeding difficulties to sepsis, acute liver failure, or metabolic crisis. Over time, symptoms may be alleviated as the alternative metabolic pathways of galactose gain more functionality and endogenous galactose production decreases; hence galactose intolerance decreases.

Findings in symptomatic neonates with classic galactosemia include:

- Gastrointestinal (GI) – vomiting, diarrhea.
- Liver – neonatal liver failure, jaundice, ascites, hepatomegaly, splenomegaly, elevated liver enzymes, hyperbilirubinemia, hypoglycemia.
- Hematology – easy bruising, coagulopathy.
- Central nervous system – lethargy, hypotonia, convulsions, coma.
- Behavioral changes – irritability, feeding difficulties.
- Renal tubulopathy – metabolic acidosis, glucosuria, phosphaturia, aminoaciduria.
- Constitutional – Gram-negative sepsis, failure to thrive.
- Other findings – cataract, pseudotumor cerebri.

DIAGNOSIS

The diagnosis of galactosemia is established by measurement of erythrocyte GALT enzyme activity and galactose-1-phosphate (gal-1-P) concentration, and GALT molecular genetic testing. Clinically, galactosemia should be suspected in patients with any combination of the above described constellation of symptoms. Suspected galactosemia should be diagnosed or ruled out quickly and diligently as the disorder may be life-threatening, given that initial treatment is simple and most effective the earlier the diagnosis is made. Testing urine for reducing substances is a screening test to detect various substances in the urine that chemically react with an indicator metallic dye called cupric sulfate. The most common reducing substances examined include glucose or galactose. However, false-negative results may occur if an infant has been fasting or is already on a galactose-free diet. False-positive results may occur in patients with liver disease. Hence, diagnosis should always be confirmed with quantitative measurement of erythrocyte concentration of gal-1-P and erythrocyte GALT enzyme activity. It is important to note that erythrocyte GALT enzyme activity may be falsely elevated by a recent red blood cell (RBC) transfusion (false-negative).

Another option is using urinary sugars gas chromatographic analysis to reveal elevated urinary galactose and galactitol. Galactitol will always be present in patients' urine, in spite of a galactose-free diet and RBC transfusions.

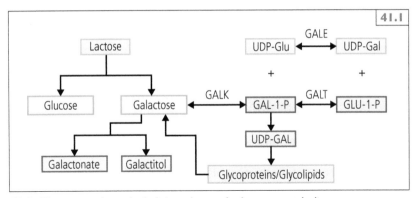

41.1 Diagram to show the Leloir pathway of galactose metabolism.
Gal-1-P: galactose-1-phosphate; GALE: galactose epimerase; GALK; galactokinase;
GALT: galactose-1-phosphate uridyltransferase; Glu-1-P: glucose-1-phosphate;
UDP: uridine diphosphate.

Galactosemia can be detected in virtually 100% of affected infants in countries that include testing for galactosemia in their newborn screening programs. Newborn screening utilizes a small amount of blood obtained from a heel prick to assay GALT enzyme activity and to quantify total RBC gal-1-P and galactose concentrations. The newborn with questionable results on newborn screening should continue to be treated with soy-based formula pending definitive results of confirmatory testing.

Galactosemia is inherited in an autosomal recessive fashion; the gene encoding the GALT enzyme is located on chromosome 9p13. To date at least 223 disease-causing mutations have been identified, ranging from mild enzymatic deficiency to nondetectable enzyme activity. The most common mutations are the severe p.Q188R among Caucasians and the relatively mild p.S125L among African-Americans. Genetic testing is also available for prenatal diagnosis in affected families with a known mutation. A clear genotype–phenotype association has been established. Molecular testing for specific GALT mutations is the most sensitive and specific laboratory test.

PATHOPHYSIOLOGY

Galactose is a monosaccharide, predominantly derived from hydrolysis of lactose or 'milk sugar', the main type of sugar found in milk and dairy products. The Leloir Pathway of galactose metabolism is depicted in Figure **41.1**. In addition to formation of glucose-1-phosphate, the main end-product galactose may be phosphorylated for further integration into glycoproteins or glycolipids, (up to 5% of the GALT metabolic capacity), reduced to galactitol, or oxidized to galactonate.

Infants with classic galactosemia have no GALT activity and are unable to oxidize galactose to carbon dioxide. In the absence of GALT activity, gal-1-P, galactose, and galactitol accumulate in a retrograde fashion and may be detected. With the one exception of galactitol accumulation etiologic for new cataract formation, the exact pathogenic mechanisms of galactosemia are less well understood. However, research suggests that the main factors are probably the toxic effects of accumulated gal-1-P and galactitol on the brain, liver, and kidneys. Endogenous galactose production, metabolite depletion, and abnormal glycosylation of glycoproteins and glycolipids may account in part towards the long-term complications. Indeed, existing evidence suggests that damage may begin *in utero*.

TREATMENT

Treatment of galactosemia is based on elimination of dietary galactose. For initial treatment as soon as galactosemia is suspected, galactose should be immediately removed from the diet (i.e. changing feeds to a soy-milk-based formula). Restriction of all lactose-containing foods (dairy products, tomato sauces) including lactose-containing medications (tablets, capsules, sweetened elixirs) should occur, with the goal of reversal of acute symptoms and biochemical manifestations. Once galactose is removed from the diet, improvement in symptoms, renal and hepatic functions, and cataract is to be expected shortly after. Supporting measures should be aimed at treating symptoms such as sepsis, coagulopathy, jaundice, and electrolyte imbalances.

For long-term treatment, a lactose-free diet is the rule. Most authorities nowadays endorse a relatively 'liberal' lactose-free diet only, and approve fruits, vegetables, legumes, bread, and mature hardened cheeses with negligible galactose levels. As most children have metabolic bone disease, calcium supplements are usually also required.

A promising future direction is use of galactokinase (GALK) inhibitors that will induce a GALK deficiency-like disease which carries a more benign course. Other future directions are aimed at stimulating residual GALT activity (e.g. folic acid, progesterone), replacement of depleted metabolites (inositol), gene therapy, and hepatocyte transplantation.

PROGNOSIS

A lactose-free diet will prevent and reverse metabolic crises or liver failure. Cataracts typically do not develop after the neonatal period. However, regardless of newborn screening, early diagnosis, and institution of a strict galactose-restricted diet, long-term complications continue to affect most patients. These include hypergonadotrophic hypogonadism, decreased bone density, developmental delay, and motor abnormalities including ataxia, mental retardation, and speech and language defects including verbal dyspraxia. These complications evolve independently of the time that dietary restriction was begun. Early detection and intervention of these complications are key elements in the long-term follow-up of these patients.

Hereditary tyrosinemia type 1

DEFINITION AND EPIDEMIOLOGY

Tyrosinemia is a genetic disorder characterized by elevated levels of the amino acid tyrosine, a building block of proteins. Tyrosinemia is caused by the deficiency of one of the enzymes required for the multistep process that breaks down tyrosine. There are several different types of tyrosinemia, each with distinctive symptoms and caused by the deficiency of a different enzyme. This chapter will focus on hereditary tyrosinemia type 1 (HT1, OMIM 276700), the most severe form. Synonyms of HT1 include fumarylacetoacetate hydrolase (FAH) deficiency and hepatorenal tyrosinemia. HT1 is characterized by liver failure, renal tubular dysfunction associated with growth failure and rickets, neurologic crises, and risk of hepatocellular carcinoma.

The estimated global incidence of HT1 is approximately 1 in 100,000 births, but the geographical variation is wide and this number is probably lower in most countries. HT1 is more prevalent in Scandinavia (1:60,000 live births), and Quebec, Canada (1:846–1:16,000).

CLINICAL PRESENTATION

Children with HT1 may present with a number of different symptoms. The clinical presentation of HT1 can be divided into two forms.

The onset of the acute form occurs during the first few months of the child's life with severe liver involvement. Acute liver failure is often notable for a marked coagulopathy not corrected by vitamin K supplementation and, paradoxically, only modestly elevated serum liver transaminase and often only slightly elevated serum bilirubin. Progression to the known complications of end-stage liver failure includes ascites, jaundice, and GI bleeding. Untreated affected infants may die from liver failure within weeks or months of first symptoms.

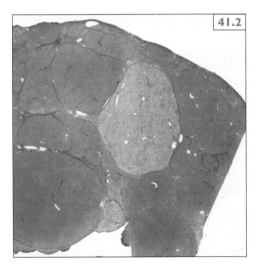

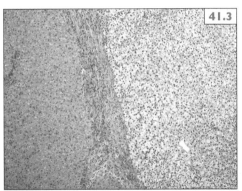

41.2, 41.3 Hereditary tyrosinemia. Macroscopic (**41.2**) and microscopic (**41.3**) views of a hepatic nodule in a patient with hereditary tyrosinemia type 1. (Courtesy of Dr. Glenn Taylor; The Hospital for Sick Children, Toronto, Canada.)

The onset of the chronic form is gradual and the symptoms are often less severe. Renal tubular involvement (involving a Fanconi-like renal syndrome with generalized aminoaciduria, phosphate loss, and renal tubular acidosis) is often the major manifestation, although other symptoms include failure to thrive, hepatomegaly, liver dysfunction (**41.2, 41.3**), bone abnormalities caused by rickets due to the continued renal loss of phosphate, and a typical 'boiled cabbage' odor.

Tyrosinemia should be suspected in any infant or child with evidence of hepatocellular necrosis, cirrhosis, or coagulopathy for which the cause is not evident.

Untreated children may have repeated neurologic crises similar to those seen in older children with acute intermittent prophyria. These crises include abdominal, pain, changes in mental status, painful paresthesias, autonomic signs (hypertension and tachycardia), and progressive paralysis up to respiratory failure requiring mechanical ventilation. Other clinical manifestations include: hepatocellular carcinoma, pancreatic Langerhans islets hypertrophy, diabetes mellitus, hypertrophic cardiomyopathy, and deposition of corneal crystals.

DIFFERENTIAL DIAGNOSIS

Hypertyrosinemia in a pediatric patient is a nonspecific finding, and can be associated with all forms of liver failure as well as with a diverse group of conditions involving the pathway of tyrosine catabolism:
- Hepatocellular dysfunction due to acute or chronic liver disease.
- Transient tyrosinemia of the newborn.
- Hereditary genetic enzymatic deficiencies:
  - HT1– fumarylacetoacetate (FAA) deficiency.
  - HT2 – Tyrosine aminotransferase deficiency.
  - HT3 – 4-hydroxyphenylpyruvate dioxygenase (HPD) deficiency.
- Scurvy.
- Hyperthyroidism.

DIAGNOSIS

Tyrosinemia type I is characterized by the following biochemical findings:
- Increased succinlyacetone excretion in the urine of a child with liver failure or severe renal disease is pathognomonic of tyrosinemia type 1. Many laboratories require that measurement of succinylacetone be specifically requested when ordering urine organic acids.
- Elevated urinary concentrations of tyrosine metabolites (p-hydroxyphenylpyruvate, p-hydroxyphenyllactate, and p-hydroxyphenylacetate) detected on urinary organic acids testing.
- Increased urinary excretion of the compound delta-aminolevulinic acid (δ-ALA) secondary to inhibition of the enzyme δ-ALA dehydratase by succinylacetone in liver and circulating RBCs.
- Elevated plasma concentration of tyrosine, methionine, and phenylalanine on plasma amino acid analysis; however, elevated plasma tyrosine concentration can also be a nonspecific indicator of liver damage or immaturity.
- Very low or undetectable FAH enzyme activity as measured in cultured skin fibroblasts or hepatocytes. Specific reference ranges vary among laboratories.

Supportive findings include prolonged prothrombin time and markedly elevated serum concentration of alpha-fetoprotein (average 160,000 ng/ml; normal: <1000 ng/ml for infants 1–3 months of age).

The inheritance pattern of HT1 is autosomal recessive. HT1 is caused by mutations in a gene encoding the FAH enzyme located on chromosome 15q23. Molecular genetic testing by targeted mutation analysis for the four common FAH mutations and sequence analysis of the entire coding region are clinically available and can detect mutations in more than 95% of affected individuals.

Prenatal diagnosis may be considered in affected families by measuring the concentration of succinylacetone in amniotic fluid, FAH enzyme level in amniotic fluid cells, or by genetic testing.

PATHOPHYSIOLOGY

Tyrosine is a nonessential amino acid, derived from the degradation of phenylalanine. The complete tyrosine degradation pathway is expressed in only two cell types – hepatocytes and renal proximal tubules. FAH deficiency causes up-stream accumulation of FAA in the liver and kidneys (**41.4**). FAA accumulation results in apoptotic cell death and profound disregulation of gene expression in the involved cells. The kidney injury is mediated by FAA accumulation as in the liver, but also through succinylacetone accumulation which induces renal Fanconi syndrome independently.

The elevated tyrosine levels found in HT1 are not a direct effect of the FAH deficiency, but rather due to reduced activities of the upstream tyrosine aminotransferase (TAT) and 4-HPD enzymes, secondary to the genes expression disturbances. Tyrosine per se is not toxic to the liver or kidney; however, at high concentrations it may cause corneal ulcerations, dermatologic hyperkeratosis, and possible neurodevelopmental delay. Tyrosine itself, therefore, is mostly of diagnostic and monitoring interest.

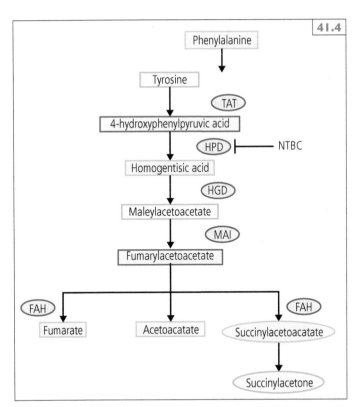

41.4 Hereditary tyrosinemia type I metabolic pathway. FAH: fumarylacetoacetate hydrolase; HGD: homogentisic acid lipoxygenase; HPD: hydroxyphenylpyruvate dioxygenase; MAI: maleylacetoacetate isomerase; NTBC; 2-[2-nitro-4-fluoromethylbenzoyl]-1,3-cyclohexanedione; TAT; tyrosine aminotransferase.

Another secondary biochemical alteration is the inhibitory effect of accumulated succinyl-acetone on heme synthesis, which leads to intermittent porphyria-like symptoms.

TREATMENT

NTBC (2-[2-nitro-4-trifluoromethyl-benzoyl]-1,3-cyclohexanedione) was approved by the United States Food and Drug Administration in April 2002 for the treatment of HT1. NTBC reduces the metabolic flow of tyrosine degradation as it inhibits HPD (the second step in the tyrosine degradation pathway) thus preventing the accumulation of FAA and its conversion to succinylacetone (**41.4**). NTBC should be prescribed (1 mg/kg/day) with the support of a metabolic specialist as soon as the diagnosis of HT1 is confirmed. Rare side-effects of NTBC have included transient low platelet and neutrophil counts, and photophobia, although significant side-effects have not been reported.

Dietary management should be started immediately upon diagnosis, with a nutritionally complete diet with controlled intake of phenylalanine and tyrosine. Medical formulas are available to supplement low-protein diets. Restriction diet alone does not prevent progression of the disease.

Close monitoring is required for prevention of secondary complications including metabolic control, development of corneal ulcerations, and hepatocellular carcinoma, and for long-term neurologic development.

Surveillance in collaboration with a metabolic specialist is paramount to ensure resolution of primary manifestations and as prevention of secondary complications. Monitoring may include periodical liver evaluation, renal studies, skeletal evaluation, HT1 markers, as well as periodic ophthalmologic examinations, liver imaging, and neurologic assessments.

Recent clinical experience indicates that liver transplantation should now be reserved for those children with severe liver failure at clinical presentation who fail to respond to NTBC treatment, or patients who have documented evidence of malignant changes in hepatic tissue. Future approaches are hepatocyte transplantation and gene therapy directed at the liver.

PROGNOSIS

If untreated, HT1 typically is a devastating disease with early death. With NTBC treatment, the long-term prognosis is good; patients regain normal liver and kidney function, and may continue this treatment for years. Monitoring for complications is essential, particularly for hepatocellular carcinoma development; annual α-fetoprotein measurement and imaging (computed tomography or magnetic resonance imaging) are recommended.

Genetic counseling should be offered to affected families including evaluation of relatives at risk and prenatal testing in future pregnancies.

Hereditary fructose intolerance

DEFINITION AND EPIDEMIOLOGY

Hereditary fructose intolerance (HFI, OMIM 22960) is an inborn error of fructose metabolism caused by a deficiency of the enzyme aldolase B. The key identifying feature of HFI is the appearance of symptoms with the introduction of fructose (or any of its common precursors, sucrose and sorbitol) to the diet. Symptoms can widely range from mild abdominal discomfort to severe liver and renal impairment; cases of sudden death have been reported. Treatment of HFI is based around strict avoidance of fructose in the diet.

The incidence of hereditary fructose intolerance is estimated to be 1:20,000–1:30,000 individuals each year worldwide.

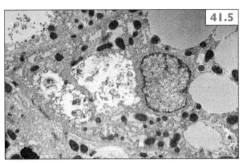

41.5 Electron microscopy of liver biopsy from a patient with hereditary fructose intolerance. Note the cellular damage portrayed as 'fructose holes', the fat lobules in the size of the nucleus, and general cellular swelling. (Courtesy of Dr. Michael Stormon; The Children's Hospital at Westmead, Sydney, Australia.)

CLINICAL PRESENTATION

Patients affected by HFI are healthy and completely asymptomatic, provided they do not ingest foods containing fructose or any of its common precursors, sucrose and sorbitol. Newborns fed breast milk do not manifest symptoms, as breast milk contains lactose (comprised of glucose and galactose). Clinical symptoms such as vomiting, nausea, restlessness, pallor, sweating, trembling and lethargy can occur at the time of weaning when fructose and sucrose are added to the diet in the form of baby foods (vegetables, fruits, fruit juice and sweetened foods). The severity of symptoms depends on age at exposure and fructose load. Prolonged fructose ingestion in infants leads ultimately to liver and/or renal failure and death. Patients may develop a strong distaste for sweet food, as confirmed by a detailed dietary history from older patients; indeed, most older patients do not have a history of dental caries.

Symptoms associated with HFI may be categorized as resulting from acute and chronic exposure to fructose. The early symptoms of HFI may involve multiple systems and might include nausea, vomiting, tremor, dizziness, lethargy, and coma. Tissue toxicity results in hepatomegaly, hepatic failure, and renal dysfunction, and may present as failure to thrive with accompanying feeding difficulties, chronic vomiting and/or diarrhea, jaundice, and evidence of chronic liver disease (**41.5**).

Physical examination may confirm signs of liver disease including scleral icterus, jaundice, hepatomegaly, and splenomegaly.

Laboratory abnormalities are consistent with the deleterious effects of aldolase B deficiency with downstream effects of fructose-1-phosphate accumulation and microenvironmental phosphate depletion and include:
- Hypoglycemia.
- Hypophosphatemia.
- Hypokalemia.
- Hypermagnesemia.
- Hyperuricemia.
- Lactic acidosis.
- High pyruvate.
- Findings consistent with liver failure: coagulopathy, hyperbilirubinemia, elevated transaminases, hyperammonemia.
- Findings consistent with proximal renal tubular dysfunction (Fanconi syndrome).

DIAGNOSIS

A detailed nutritional history correlating onset of symptoms with intake of fructose-containing foods is often a key component in the diagnostic process. Most often, young infants with HFI present for work-up with vomiting, hepatomegaly, poor feeding, and failure to thrive. Older infants and children usually present with similar symptoms or occasionally for evaluation of anomalous behavior or a storage disorder. The significant abnormal laboratory findings include hypoglycemia, fructosuria, and aminoaciduria. Suspicion is fostered by the presence of reducing substances in urine. Upon suspicion of a potential diagnosis of HFI, all food and pharmaceutical sources of fructose, sucrose, and sorbitol should be eliminated from the diet; resolution of symptoms (typically observed within days to weeks) is further supportive of the diagnosis. Nonetheless, HFI requires confirmatory investigations:

- Direct measure of aldolase B activity – definitive diagnosis can be made by enzyme assay of liver tissue.
- Past diagnostic tests, rarely performed nowadays, include a fructose tolerance test and magnetic resonance spectroscopy, demonstrating metabolic changes following a fructose load.
- Genetic studies – HFI is an autosomal recessive disorder. The affected gene encoding the aldolase B enzyme is located on chromosome 9q22.3. Carriage rate has been reported to be at least 1.3% in the UK. To date, 45 different mutations have been identified to be disease causing in ~90% of patients. The mutation A149P predominates and is present in 57% of patients. Molecular biology being an easy, inexpensive and noninvasive mode of diagnosis has circumvented the utilization of former diagnostic modalities, now reserved for inconclusive studies or cases with new mutations. Testing for the three most common mutations will cover ~75% of patients.

PATHOPHYSIOLOGY

Fructose is a fruit sugar that naturally occurs in the body. Man-made fructose is used as a sweetener in many foods, including baby foods and drinks. After ingestion, fructose is degraded and phosphorylated to fructose-1-phosphate and then spliced by aldolase B (expressed in liver, kidneys, and small intestine) into dihydroxyacetone phosphate and D-glyceraldehyde. A deficiency of adolase B results in an accumulation of fructose-1-phosphate and trapping of phosphate. The downstream effects of aldolase B deficiency are the inhibition of glucose production and reduced generation of adenosine triphosphate. Figure 41.6 highlights the key deleterious effects of aldolase B deficiency.

TREATMENT AND PROGNOSIS

Treatment of the acute symptoms involves correction of metabolic derangements, hypoglycemia and coagulopathy. Long-term management is accomplished by complete and permanent removal and avoidance of foods that contain fructose and sucrose. Sorbitol must also be eliminated due to its conversion to fructose in the human body. Fructose is replaced in the diet by glucose, maltose, or other sugars. Attention must be given to food additives and medications which often contain sucrose or sorbitol within pill coatings and medication suspensions. Health institutions must be attentive to the use of fructose or sorbitol IV solutions in afflicted patients, as numerous cases of subsequent acute, potentially fatal, hepato-renal failures have been described. Patients may be advised to wear a medical alerting bracelet, and emergency treatment of an acute hypoglycemia should include glucose and milk-based IV/oral preparations.

Strict dietary elimination of fructose/sucrose/sorbitol will result in an immediate clinical improvement, reversal of organ dysfunction including hepatic pathologic changes, and help achieve neurocognitive potential and catch-up growth. Nevertheless, these dietary restrictions are difficult to follow, and experienced dietician assistance is usually required. A strict exclusion diet will result in normal life expectancy.

Genetic counseling should be offered to affected families including evaluation of relatives at risk and prenatal testing in future pregnancies.

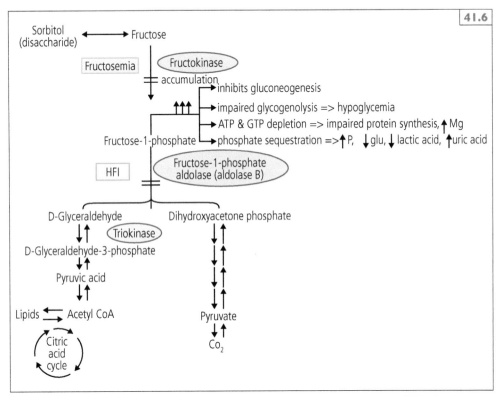

41.6 Hereditary fructose intolerance (HFI) metabolic pathway and pathogenesis. ATP: adenosine triphosphate; GTP: guanosine triphosphate.

CHAPTER 42

Metabolic Disorders III

Laurie A. Tsilianidis, David A. Weinstein, Roberto Zori

- Glycogen storage disease
- Niemann–Pick disease

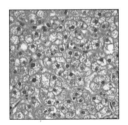
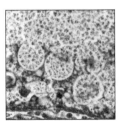
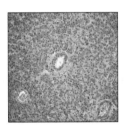
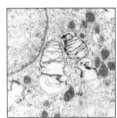

Glycogen storage disease

DEFINITION AND EPIDEMIOLOGY

Glycogen storage disease (GSD) is a heterogeneous group of genetic disorders characterized by defective glycogen utilization or synthesis. There are 13 distinct types of GSD affecting liver, muscle, and other tissues. This chapter will describe those types of GSD that involve the liver as shown in *Table 42.1*.

The overall incidence of GSD is estimated to be 1 in 100,000 births. Mild forms of GSD are likely under diagnosed.

GSD II (Pompe disease) is due to an acid maltase deficiency and mainly causes myopathy, in particular of cardiac muscle, with minimal liver involvement.

CLINICAL PRESENTATION

Classic features of hepatic GSD include fasting hypoglycemia, hepatomegaly (except GSD 0) and poor growth in children who are undertreated. Transient hypoglycemia in the neonatal period and difficulty weaning from overnight feeds is common.

ETIOLOGY AND PATHOPHYSIOLOGY
Glycogen synthase deficiency (GSD Type 0)

Mutations in the hepatic glycogen synthase gene (*GYS2* on 12p12.2) cause decreased hepatic glycogen synthesis. Hepatomegaly is not a feature of this disease, but it is classified as a form of GSD due to lack of access to glycogen during periods of fasting. Patients with GSD 0 have fasting ketotic hypoglycemia, and hyperglycemia and hyperlactatemia occur postprandially. Most children are cognitively and developmentally normal. Short stature and osteopenia are common, but other long-term complications have not been reported.

Table 42.1 Deficient enzyme and typical features of glycogen storage diseases (GSDs) that involve the liver

Type	Deficiency	Features
GSD 0	Glycogen synthase	No hepatomegaly; ketotic hypoglycemia; postprandial hyperlactatemia
GSD I	Glucose-6-phosphatase	Hepatomegaly; most severe hypoglycemia; elevated lactate, uric acid, and triglycerides; no response to glucagon
GSD III	Debranching enzyme	Firm hepatomegaly; AST/ALT often >1000 I/U; may have elevated CK
GSD IV	Branching enzyme	Hepatomegaly; amylopectin accumulation in liver and heart; cirrhosis may develop in infancy
GSD VI/IX	Phosphorylase/phosphorylase kinase	Hepatomegaly with fasting ketosis
GSD XI	GLUT-2 transpoter	Hepatomegaly; ketotic hypoglycemia; postprandial hyperlactatemia; chronic glucosuria and diarrhea

ALT; alanine aminotransferase; AST: aspartate aminotransferase; CK: creatine kinase.

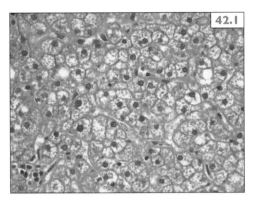

42.1 Glycogen storage disease. Hepatocytes with abundant clear cytoplasm with pyknotic nuclei.

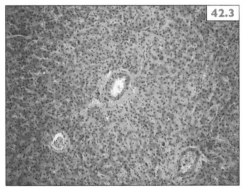

42.2 Electron micrograph of hepatocyte with glycogen accumulation.

Glucose-6-phosphatase deficiency (GSD Type I)

GSD I (Von Gierke disease) results from deficient activity of glucose-6-phosphatase, the enzyme complex that catalyzes the final common step in glycogenolysis and gluconeogenesis. Fasting results in hypoglycemia and increased production of lactate, uric acid, and triglycerides. Massive hepatomegaly results from glycogen and fat accumulation in the liver (**42.1, 42.2**). The subtype GSD Ib is caused by a defect in the transporter (*G6PT1* gene on 11q23) that moves glucose-6-phosphate across the endoplasmic reticular membrane where hydrolysis by glucose-6-phosphatase occurs. Clinical manifestations are similar to GSD Ia (caused by mutations in the *G6PC* gene on 17q21), but patients additionally develop neutropenia and inflammatory bowel disease that phenotypically mimics Crohn disease. Hepatic adenomas, renal insufficiency, and poor growth are known complications, but the risk of complications is dramatically reduced in the setting of optimal metabolic control (**42.3**).

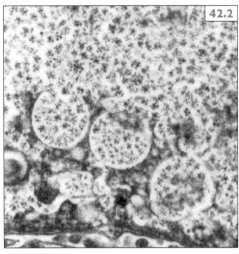

42.3 Hepatic adenoma with characteristic solitary artery without other portal structures.

Glycogen debranching enzyme deficiency (GSD Type III)

GSD III (Cori disease or Forbes disease) is caused by mutations in the *AGL* gene on 1p21 resulting in deficient activity of glycogen debranching enzyme. Debranching enzyme has two separate catalytic sites that remove branched outer chains from glycogen. Defects in this enzyme result in the accumulation of structurally abnormal glycogen, called limit dextrin. GSD IIIa affects both liver and muscle and accounts for 85% of patients with GSD III; type IIIb affects only the liver. During infancy and childhood, hepatomegaly and hypoglycemia can be severe. In adolescence and adulthood, the hypoglycemia tends to become milder and a progressive myopathy becomes the predominant feature. A hypertrophic cardiomyopathy can occur, and marked elevations in hepatic transaminases and creatine kinase concentrations are seen prior to commencement of treatment.

Glycogen branching enzyme deficiency (GSD Type IV)

GSD IV (Andersen disease) is caused by a deficiency of the glycogen branching enzyme encoded by the *GBE1* gene (3p14). Lack of this enzyme leads to structurally abnormal glycogen accumulation (amylopectin). GSD IV is a clinically heterogeneous disorder that affects liver and/or muscle. GSD IV can present as fetal akinesia deformation sequence with arthrogryposis, hydrops, polyhydramnios, and pulmonary hypoplasia. Most children present in the first year of life with hepatomegaly, and rapid progression to cirrhosis is common.

Phosphorylase deficiency (GSD Type VI)

GSD VI (Hers disease) is caused by mutations in the *PYGL* gene located at 14q21-22. Although glycogen phosphorylase is the rate-limiting step in glycogenolysis, this is a mild disorder that presents with ketotic hypoglycemia or hepatomegaly.

Phosphorylase kinase deficiency (GSD Type IX)

GSD IX results from deficiency of phosphorylase kinase, an enzyme made up of four subunits α, β, γ, and δ. The α-subunit is encoded by the *PHKA* gene at Xp22.2-p22.1. Inheritance is X-linked, and mutations in this subunit account for 75–80% of cases of GSD IX. The β-subunit is encoded by the *PHKB* gene located on chromosome 16q12-q13. The γ-subunit, which contains the catalytic site of the enzyme, is encoded by the *PHKG* gene on chromosome 16p11-p12. While most children with GSD IX have a mild phenotype similar to GSD VI, severe variants associated with very elevated hepatic transaminases, cirrhosis, and metabolic instability can occur. Treatment improves growth, normalizes laboratory abnormalities, and appears to decrease the risk of cirrhosis.

Fanconi–Bickel syndrome (GSD Type XI)

Fanconi–Bickel syndrome (FBS) is a rare disorder caused by mutations in the *GLUT-2* gene located at 3q16-q26.3. GLUT-2 is a facilitative glucose transporter located in hepatocytes, pancreatic β-cells, enterocytes, and proximal renal tubular cells. Deficiency of GLUT-2 leads to fasting ketotic hypoglycemia alternating with postprandial hyperglycemia in a pattern that can be confused with GSD 0. However, chronic glucosuria, diarrhea, and hepatomegaly are classic features of FBS and are not typical of GSD 0.

DIFFERENTIAL DIAGNOSIS

- Hyperinsulinism.
- Adrenal insufficiency.
- Growth hormone deficiency.
- Early diabetes mellitus.
- Disorders of gluconeogenesis.
- Hereditary fructose intolerance.
- Disorders of amino acid metabolism.
- Congenital disorders of glycosylation.
- Respiratory chain defects.
- Disorders of fatty acid oxidation.
- Ketone utilization defects.

DIAGNOSIS

Definitive diagnosis of GSD previously required a liver biopsy and assay of enzyme activity, but now all types can be diagnosed noninvasively. When a particular type of GSD is suspected based on characteristic clinical and biochemical abnormalities, mutation analysis is recommended to confirm the diagnosis.

TREATMENT

The goal of treatment of all types of GSD is to maintain normal blood glucose levels and minimize the metabolic derangements associated with hypoglycemia. Uncooked cornstarch can be used as a slowly digested dietary source of glucose; the dose and frequency are individualized based on GSD type and patient age. In all types of GSD, complex carbohydrates are preferred over simple sugars to prevent excess glycogen storage. In GSD I, galactose, sucrose, and fructose are nonutilizable sugars that cannot be converted to glucose, and are restricted. The gluconeogenic pathway is intact in all hepatic forms of GSD except type I, and a high protein diet (at least 3 g/kg) can be used to provide substrate.

PROGNOSIS

The prognosis for all types of GSD except GSD IV is excellent with appropriate treatment. Long-term complications, once believed to be universal with the more severe forms of GSD, can be avoided with good metabolic control and near normalization of laboratory tests. Liver transplantation should be viewed as a treatment of last resort for all types of GSD except GSD IV. Liver transplantation has been associated with progression of renal disease in GSD Ia and cardiac disease in GSD III.

Niemann–Pick disease

DEFINITION, ETIOLOGY, AND EPIDEMIOLOGY

Niemann–Pick types A, B, and C are lysosomal diseases grouped together historically because of similar clinical presentations. Lysosomal diseases are the result of defects of lysosomal enzymes leading to an excess of incompletely catabolized substances within lysosomes. Types A and B are sphingolipidoses caused by deficiencies of acid sphinogomyelinase, leading primarily to an excess of sphingolipids (**42.4, 42.5**) Niemann Pick type C is a lipid storage disorder characterized primary by storage of other lipid compounds.

Niemann–Pick types A and B are autosomal recessive conditions caused by mutations in the acid sphingomyelinase (ASM) gene *SMPD1*. Type A refers to the severe phenotype while Type B describes the milder form thought to have residual enzyme activity. Both types are panethnic but Type A has a higher incidence amongst Ashkenazi Jews. Worldwide population frequency is estimated to be 0.5–1 in 100,000.

Niemann–Pick type C disease (NPC) is a neurovascular, autosomal recessive, lysosomal lipid storage disorder of impaired intracellular transport of endocytosed cholesterol associated with impaired intracellular lipid trafficking, leading to accumulation of cholesterol and glycosphingolipids in the brain, liver, spleen, and lung. Incidence is estimated to be at least 1 in 120,000. It is caused by gene mutations in *NPC1* in 95% of cases and *NPC2* in 4%. Cases found without a mutation are thought to be due to a third unknown gene.

CLINICAL PRESENTATION

In Neimann–Pick types A and B, the extreme excess of sphinoglipids accumulates in affected organs, predominantly the central nervous system (CNS), liver, spleen, and lung. This accumulation leads to hypertrophy and progressive loss of function. Sphingolipids are present in all systems but

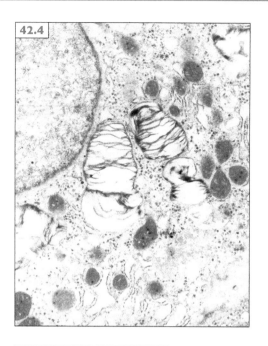

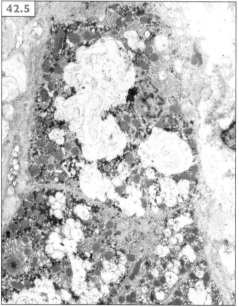

42.4, 42.5 Electron micrograph images demonstrating hepatocytes with intra- and extralysosomal sphingolipid accumulation in a 6-month-old infant with Niemann–Pick type A presenting with hepatosplenomegaly and hypotonia.

are of special significance to the central and peripheral nervous system. In type A the newborn period is unremarkable except for occasional prolonged jaundiced. Within the first few months the child develops hepatosplenomegaly sometimes with lymphadenopathy. Bone marrow studies are frequently performed and commonly reveal the typical Niemann–Pick lipid full foam cells of macrophage/monocyte origin. Bone marrow suppression is common. Neurologic degeneration follows soon, usually by 3–6 months, frequently heralded by feeding difficulties and constipation secondary to decreased tone and weakness. Aspiration pneumonia secondary to reflux is suspected in the first year of life, but infiltration is usually the basis of lung disease. Growth is also affected and developmental regression becomes pronounced in the second half of the infant's first year of life. By the second year the child becomes emaciated and spastic, and death is common by the third year.

The clinical signs of Niemann–Pick type B are more variable and have a milder phenotype. Hepatospenomegaly is noticed in infancy or childhood and progression is slow with survival to adulthood. Interstitial lung disease may become prominent in adolescence. Neurological disease is not a major feature. The cherry red spot indicative of storage within retinal cells is seen in about half of type A affected individuals while it is rarely seen in type B.

NPC has a very heterogeneous clinical presentation with wide variation in age of onset, progression, and symptomatology. Presentation can occur at any time between the perinatal period and adulthood. Onset of neurologic disease predicts prognosis, leading to a classification into early infantile, late infantile, juvenile, and adolescent/adult onset. A perinatal form with severe systemic disease also exists.

The neonatal period for NPC is generally normal or characterized by transient neonatal jaundice. Systemic findings usually predate the neurologic symptoms. Behavioral complaints usually appear first and neurologic regression can slowly progress over decades. Seizures, ataxia, cataplexy, dystonia, dementia, or psychiatric manifestations may develop as the disease progresses. Findings especially suggestive of NPC are prolonged neonatal cholestasis, splenomegaly, cataplexy, and vertical supranuclear gaze palsy. Drooling/dysphagia and hepatomegaly may bring the child to the attention of a pediatric gastroenterologist. Patients frequently die in the second or third decade although mild cases can survive past 60 years of age.

DIAGNOSIS

Niemann–Pick types A and B are diagnosed by deficient ASM activity in peripheral leukocytes or in cultured fibroblasts. Type C disease may also have moderately decreased activity. Because of disease variability in NPC, a clinical tool, the NP-C suspicion index, has been developed and validated to aid in the detection of NPC (www.npc-si.com). NPC should be in the differential diagnosis of patients with severe neonatal jaundice, isolated splenomegaly, and any suspicion of a neurodegenerative condition. Diagnosis requires a fibroblast culture and molecular genetic testing of *NPC1* and *NPC2* genes.

Other storage conditions with hepatosplenomegaly and neurologic deterioration, such as Gaucher disease, may be confused with Niemann–Pick but these other storage disorders have normal levels of ASM activity. Confirmation by molecular diagnosis is also available.

TREATMENT

Treatment for types A and B is symptomatic and curative therapies being used or considered include bone marrow transplant, enzyme replacement gene therapy, and small molecule therapies. NPC treatment is also tailored to symptoms and miglustat is a promising systemic therapy.

CHAPTER 43

Hepatic Tumors

Rohit Gupta, Laura S. Finn, Karen F. Murray

- **Introduction**

BENIGN TUMORS

- **Infantile hepatic hemangioma**
- **Mesenchymal hamartoma**
- **Focal nodular hyperplasia**
- **Hepatocellular adenoma**
- **Nodular regenerative hyperplasia**

MALIGNANT TUMORS

- **Hepatoblastoma**
- **Hepatocellular carcinoma**
- **Fibrolamellar carcinoma**
- **Embryonal (undifferentiated) sarcoma of liver**
- **Epithelioid hemangioendothelioma**
- **Angiosarcoma**
- **Hepatobiliary rhabdomyosarcoma**

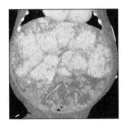
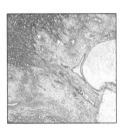
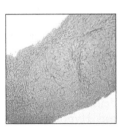
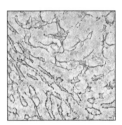

Introduction

Hepatic tumors most commonly present as a palpable abdominal mass. Primary hepatic neoplasms represent a small percentage of solid tumors in children. The majority of liver masses are malignant.

Serum alpha-fetoprotein (AFP) is not elevated in all malignant liver tumors; radiologic and pathologic assessment is vital for making the diagnosis.

BENIGN TUMORS

Infantile hepatic hemangioma

DEFINITION

Infantile hepatic hemangioma (IHH), formerly infantile hemangioendothelioma, is the most common benign hepatic tumor of infancy. Lesions are typically focal, multi-focal or diffuse, the latter two having a slight female predominance without any racial predilection. Hemangiomas can either be clinically silent or have serious clinical complications. The term hemangioendothelioma should be avoided to prevent confusion with epithelioid hemangioendothelioma, an adult liver tumor with malignant potential, and the pediatric soft tissue kaposiform hemangioendothelioma.

CLINICAL PRESENTATION

Most IHH are diagnosed before the first year of life manifesting as an asymptomatic abdominal mass. Life-threatening complications include high output congestive heart failure (CHF) resulting from arteriovenous shunting of blood along with Kasabach–Merritt syndrome of coagulopathy due to platelet sequestration. Hypothyroidism, detected in patients with diffuse hemangiomas and in a subset with multi-focal lesions, is a result of increased activity of type 3 iodothyronine deiodinase produced directly from the tumor. Hypothyrodism

in addition to the arteriovenous shunting can exacerbate the cardiac dysfunction. The majority of patients with multi-focal liver tumors have hemangiomas at other sites including skin, trachea, chest, adrenal glands, and the dura mater.

DIAGNOSIS AND PATHOPHYSIOLOGY

Biopsies are rarely indicated to differentiate IHH from other hepatic lesions, and due to the increased risk of bleeding, a biopsy of these masses is usually avoided.

Plain abdominal radiograph might show evidence of hepatomegaly and occasionally fine hepatic calcifications. Features suggestive of a high flow lesion on chest radiograph include cardiomegaly and pulmonary edema if the child is in CHF. Hepatic artery and vein enlargement along with tapering of the abdominal aorta below the origin of celiac axis are features suggestive of high flow across the hemangioma. Ultrasound plays a critical role both in initial detection and localization and in follow-up of IHH. Lesions are either hypoechoic or of variable echogenicity relative to normal hepatic parenchyma on ultrasound. Doppler flow analysis can provide information regarding arteriovenous shunting. Multi-phase computed tomography (CT) with arterial, portal, or venous and delayed phases helps characterize the lesions further; however, magnetic resonance imaging (MRI) is the preferred modality of imaging as it allows for confident diagnosis. Multi-focal lesions (**43.1**) that are small show homogenous signal intensity while the presence of central hemorrhage, necrosis, and fibrosis results in heterogenous signal intensity. Angiography is usually reserved for patients in whom embolization therapy is anticipated.

Classification

Differentiation of IHH from various other hepatic lesions is primarily based on clinical and radiologic features. Hepatoblastoma can be distinguished by imaging features of intense centripetal enhancement and elevated AFP levels. A mesenchymal hamartoma is a hypovascular, multi-cystic, and multi-loculated mass with characteristic enhancement of the septa and solid portions of the tumor. Metastatic neuroblastomas and angiosarcomas can be differentiated on the basis of imaging features as well as elevated urinary catecholamines typical of a neuroblastoma.

Focal

- Glucose transporter-1 (GLUT-1) negative; clinically asymptomatic, often seen on prenatal imaging.
- High flow shunting can cause CHF along with anemia and thrombocytopenia.
- T2-weighted MRI: hyperintense, heterogeneous enhancement due to areas of central necrosis, thrombosis, or hemorrhage.
- Undergoes regression by 12–14 months of age.
- Considered to be a rapidly involuting congenital hemangioma (RICH).

Multi-focal

- GLUT-1 positive; clinically asymptomatic and often has associated extrahepatic lesions.
- Patients can develop CHF.
- On T2-weighted MRI: hyperintense, homogenous enhancement, aortic tapering below the origin of celiac axis suggesting arteriovenous shunting.
- Usually has a proliferative phase that is followed by involution.

Diffuse

- GLUT-1 positive.
- Clinically presents as massive hepatomegaly.
- Abdominal compartment syndrome and hypothyroidism can be present.
- On imaging: near total hepatic parenchymal replacement (**43.2**).
- Clinically diffuse IHH follows a complicated course.

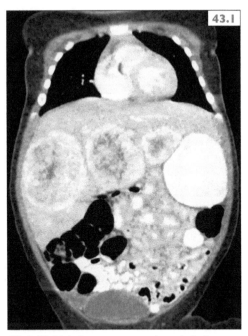

43.1 Multiple heterogeneous hepatic lesions with thick peripheral rim of enhancement consistent with multi-focal hemangioma on CT abdomen.

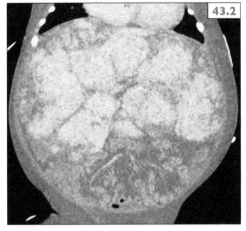

43.2 Contrast enhanced CT scan showing a markedly enlarged liver with innumerable arterially enhancing areas that are present diffusely throughout the liver in diffuse infantile hepatic hemangioma.

Histologically, IHH are composed of closely packed small capillary-sized vessels lined by variably plump endothelial cells and adjacent pericytes. Endothelium in multi-focal and diffuse lesions is typically GLUT-1 positive while focal lesions are negative, consistent with a RICH.

TREATMENT

Aggressive management of CHF results in improved survival as most deaths in patients with IHH are related to CHF. Thyroid hormone supplementation has a positive impact in the improvement of cardiac dysfunction. Multi-focal and diffuse hemangiomas that have potential for a complicated clinical course can be treated with corticosteroids, propranolol, interferon α-2a or vincristine if necessary. Embolization can be assessed in the context of the patient's clinical status, and in most severe cases, liver transplantation is the definitive treatment.

Mesenchymal hamartoma

DEFINITION AND EPIDEMIOLOGY

In mesenchymal hamartoma (MH) most lesions are identified by the age of 5 years as a painless abdominal mass; there is a slight male predominance.

CLINICAL PRESENTATION

Cystic lesions can sometimes present with rapid abdominal distension secondary to fluid accumulation. Serum AFP levels are typically not elevated, but occasionally a mild elevation above the age-adjusted reference range can be seen.

DIFFERENTIAL DIAGNOSIS

For predominantly solid lesions, hepatoblastoma should be considered as they also present in young children. Significant elevation of AFP levels along with a solid appearance and calcifications would favor hepatoblastoma over MH; however, overlapping features may warrant histopathologic review for diagnostic confirmation. Solitary IHH with degenerative changes and embryonal sarcoma of the liver (ESL) are distinguished by characteristic imaging features for hemangioma and the older age of presentation for ESL. Predominantly cystic lesions must be differentiated from simple cysts, hydatid disease, hepatic abscess, choledochal cyst, enteric duplication cyst, and pedunculated mesenteric lymphangioma.

DIAGNOSIS AND PATHOPHYSIOLOGY

Imaging features are dependent upon the cellular components of the lesion. Most tumors are predominantly cystic with either thin or thick septa or predominantly solid with a few small cysts. On ultrasound the cystic portions are anechoic with thin or thick echogenic septa, while solid portions appear echogenic. CT and MRI studies can provide better characterization of solid versus cystic structures within the tumor (**43.3**).

43.3 CT abdomen showing numerous hypodense cysts with heterogeneously enhancing solid components in mesenchymal hamartoma.

43.4 A low-power view demonstrates typical heterogeneity of mesenchymal hamartoma with epithelial (hepatocyte-rich) region, left, adjacent to myxoid region that becomes cystic, as seen in the lower right of the image.

43.5 At higher power, atypical ductular structures lie within fibromyxoid stroma; cyst degeneration occupies the space at right in mesenchymal hamartoma.

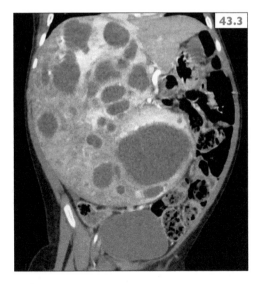

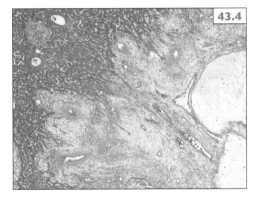

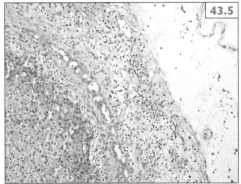

The multiple hypotheses proposed for the pathogenesis of MH include developmental malformation (ductal plate), vascular and toxic insult, or a neoplastic proliferation that is disorganized and limited. MH is typically seen as a large solitary mass with clear margins that contains cysts of varying sizes. The histopathologic appearance is diverse as various epithelial or mesenchymal elements may predominate (**43.4**). The epithelium includes irregular bile ducts and ductules and typically peripherally placed cords of bland hepatocytes (**43.5**). Loose fibromyxomatous stroma dissects the lesion and often contains thin-walled vascular channels. A link between MH and ESL, an aggressive malignant liver neoplasm, has been suggested based on rare reports of a shared chromosomal translocation (19q13.4) and ESL arising within a MH.

TREATMENT

MHs have the potential for rapid growth and questionably for malignant transformation and hence complete surgical excision is the preferred and definitive treatment.

Focal nodular hyperplasia

DEFINITION AND EPIDEMIOLOGY

Focal nodular hyperplasia (FNH) is a benign tumor resulting from the proliferation of hepatocytes, Kupffer cells, and vascular and biliary elements. FNH is usually seen in adult women but infrequently can occur in children and adolescents. A central stellate scar (coalescence of fibrous septa) is a characteristic feature of FNH, although is not present in all cases. The diagnosis of FNH is often made incidentally in children between the ages of 2 and 5 years and usually in females.

CLINICAL PRESENTATION

FNH is an asymptomatic liver tumor. Large mass lesions can be associated with abdominal pain. AFP levels are not elevated in FNH.

FNH most likely represents a hyperplastic response to a vascular abnormality. An increased prevalence has been seen in children who have received chemotherapy or radiation therapy for solid malignancies, probably due to resulting vascular injury.

DIFFERENTIAL DIAGNOSIS

The homogenous appearance of FNH on imaging can be differentiated from hepatoblastomas and hepatocellular carcinomas, which are more heterogeneous due to hemorrhage, necrosis, and calcification; AFP levels in FNH are also normal. ^{99m}Tc sulfur colloid scan can help differentiate FNH from hepatic adenoma. A needle biopsy of FNH must be distinguished for hyperplastic regenerative nodules of cirrhosis.

DIAGNOSIS AND PATHOPHYSIOLOGY

Multi-phase CT scan including the arterial, portal venous, and delayed phases is the test of choice for making the diagnosis of FNH. During the early arterial phase FNH appears as a contrast-enhanced homogenous lesion that becomes isodense to hepatic parenchyma on delayed phase.

The tumors are typically single well-circumscribed, unencapsulated, lobular masses that are paler than the surrounding normal liver. A central fibrous scar is invariably present from which fibrous septa radiate to separate the lesion into smaller nodules (**43.6, 43.7**). Microscopically hyperplastic hepatocytes lack an acinar arrangement and are interrupted by variably inflamed fibrous septa; numerous ductules are present at the interface between hepatocytes and septa but do not communicate with the biliary tree. Numerous vessels, particularly arteries with subintimal fibrosis, course through the septa and central scar (**43.8, 43.9**).

TREATMENT

FNH is a slow-growing tumor with no known malignant potential. Rare complications, such as hemorrhage or rupture, are managed conservatively. Surgical resection or possibly ablative therapy or embolization can be performed in symptomatic cases.

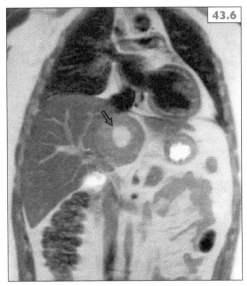

43.6 MRI abdomen showing a mildly hyperintense liver mass in the caudate lobe with central T2-hyperintense scar (arrow) in focal nodular hyperplasia.

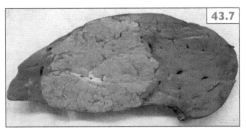

43.7 Focal nodular hyperplasia The pale well-circumscribed cerebriform cut surface bulges from the adjacent normal liver parenchyma; note the slightly eccentric scarred region in which vascular profiles are apparent.

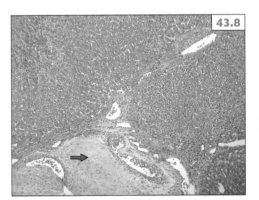

43.8 Focal nodular hyperplasia; a low-power view shows a 'central scar' with aberrant ectatic vascular spaces and fibrous septa that radiate into the adjacent hepatocytes (arrow).

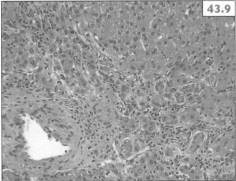

43.9 Focal nodular hyperplasia: numerous ductular profiles haphazardly interdigitate with hepatocytes, adjacent to an irregular thick walled vessel.

Hepatocellular adenoma

DEFINITION AND EPIDEMIOLOGY

Hepatocellular adenoma (HA) is strongly related to the use of hormonal birth control in women of childbearing age. In pediatrics, most patients are females over the age of 10 years who have a history of oral contraceptive use. HA is also associated with glycogen storage disease (I and III), galactosemia, and familial diabetes mellitus.

CLINICAL PRESENTATION

Patients usually present with abdominal pain or mass and the primary clinical concern is the possibility of intratumoral hemorrhage with rupture, resulting in intraperitoneal hemorrhage and hypovolemic shock. There usually is no elevation of AFP in HA.

DIFFERENTIAL DIAGNOSIS

Arterial phase hyperattenuating lesions include FNH, hepatocellular carcinoma, and fibrolamellar carcinoma in addition to HA. A central stellate scar helps differentiate FNH from HA. Findings of cirrhosis, portal hypertension, and metastasis usually accompany hepatocellular carcinoma. Fibrolamellar carcinoma commonly has calcifications and an eccentric scar.

DIAGNOSIS AND PATHOPHYSIOLOGY

Pathologic composition determines radiologic appearance. HAs are usually hyperechoic lesions on ultrasound secondary to increased lipid content or hemorrhage; however, in the setting of glycogen storage diseases or fatty infiltration of the liver, adenomas can appear hypoechoic. Hepatic arterial phase enhancement with contrast can be seen on CT, in addition to features consistent with lipid or hemorrhage.

HA may be difficult to distinguish from a well-differentiated hepatocellular carcinoma on a needle biopsy. Most tumors (80%) are solitary and multiple lesions are often associated with anabolic androgen therapy or glycogen storage disease. HA are tan or variegated due to hemorrhage or necrosis. HA are smooth, well-circumscribed, and fleshy varying in size anywhere from 1 to 30 cm, but typically measure 5–15 cm. HA are composed of sheets of hepatocytes that lack an acinar arrangement and often have cytoplasmic glycogen or lipid. They contain scattered thin-walled vessels and Kupffer cells are inconspicuous (**43.10**).

TREATMENT

Spontaneous regression has been seen after discontinuing oral contraceptives or after instituting dietary therapy for glycogen storage disease. Increasing size and prolonged duration of contraceptive therapy increase the risk of hemorrhage and are valid indications for surgical resection. Sporadic cases of hepatocellular carcinoma arising from HA have been reported.

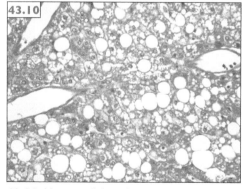

43.10 Hepatocellular adenoma. Many hepatocytes contain variably sized cytoplasmic lipid droplets that enlarge the cells leading to compression of sinusoids. Multiple thin-walled vessels are distributed randomly within the lesion.

Nodular regenerative hyperplasia

DEFINITION AND CLINICAL PRESENTATION

Nodular regenerative hyperplasia (NRH) is a rare benign transformation of hepatic parenchyma into small regenerative nodules without any fibrosis. NRH is an incidental finding in most cases and most patients with NRH are asymptomatic with laboratory evaluation of liver function yielding normal results.

DIFFERENTIAL DIAGNOSIS

When nodules are large, differentiation from FNH or HA sometimes requires liver biopsy. NRH does not demonstrate arterial phase enhancement on imaging and thus can usually be distinguished from other hepatic tumors.

DIAGNOSIS AND PATHOPHYSIOLOGY

The imaging appearance varies depending on the size of the nodules, and smaller nodules might remain undetected. Since the nodules are composed of normal hepatocytes, even larger nodules might not be appreciated. Findings associated with portal hypertension including splenomegaly, gastroesophageal varices, and ascites can be seen.

The atrophic liver is diffusely studded with small tan nodules that are typically less than 1 cm in diameter. Small nodules may be challenging to appreciate on a needle biopsy but are recognized by their usual periportal location and compression of intervening parenchyma, which is highlighted with reticulin staining. The nodules are composed of hyperplastic, otherwise normal appearing, hepatocytes that often acquire cytoplasmic glycogen or lipid as the nodule enlarges; they have less lipofuscin or other pigment (i.e. hemosiderin) than the internodular hepatocytes. The surrounding parenchyma often shows acinar atrophy without any fibrosis (**43.11–43.13**).

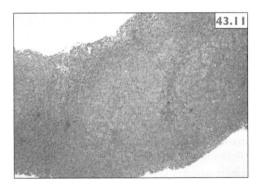

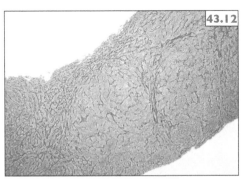

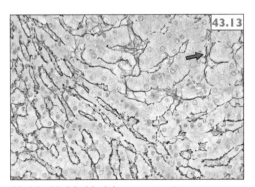

43.11–43.13 Nodular regenerative hyperplasia. **43.11**: Only slight tinctorial differences on an H&E stain hints at the distorted lobular architecture. Fibrosis is not evident; **43.12** reticulin stain of the same field dramatically demonstrates the hyperplastic hepatocellular nodules that compress intervening parenchyma; **43.13** higher magnification illustrates the thick hepatocellular plates of a nodule (arrow) and the nearly perpendicular orientation of its sinusoids compared to the adjacent atrophic parenchyma.

Etiopathogenesis of NRH is not entirely understood, although animal models suggest a possible decrease in blood flow causing acinar atrophy and compensatory hyperplasia in the adjacent acini where blood supply is preserved. Associated endothelial injury can be due to underlying autoimmune, inflammatory, or neoplastic disease or secondary toxic effects of immunosuppressive therapy. Endothelial injury subsequently results in obliteration of small venules and thus leads to portal hypertension.

TREATMENT

There is no specific treatment for NRH. Malignant transformation to hepatocellular carcinoma can occur rarely. Portosystemic shunting might be required in patients who suffer clinical complication secondary to portal hypertension.

MALIGNANT TUMORS

Hepatoblastoma

DEFINITION AND EPIDEMIOLOGY

Hepatoblastoma (HB) is the most common primary hepatic tumor in preadolescent children. The majority of the cases are identified by the age of 5 years and there is a slight male predominance. The increasing incidence of HB is most likely related to increased survival of premature patients; low birth weight infants are at increased risk of developing HB. Multiple syndromes associated with HB include: familial adenomatous polyposis, Beckwith–Wiedemann syndrome, Li–Fraumeni syndrome, trisomy 18, and type 1A glycogen storage disease.

CLINICAL PRESENTATION

HB presents as an abdominal mass with associated weight loss, anorexia, and abdominal pain. About 90% of patients have elevated serum AFP levels and these levels generally correlate with disease extent. Metastatic disease may involve the lungs most commonly, but also the brain, bones, lymph nodes, and eyes. A high index of suspicion in the appropriate clinical setting is crucial towards making the diagnosis.

DIFFERENTIAL DIAGNOSIS

Other tumors to be considered in young children include IHH and MH. Being a vascular tumor, IHHs are hyperintense compared to adjacent liver parenchyma on contrast enhanced images and do not cause an elevation in AFP. MH, a predominantly cystic benign lesion, is usually associated with a normal AFP level.

DIAGNOSIS AND PATHOPHYSIOLOGY

Ultrasound typically demonstrates a hyperechoic, solid, intrahepatic mass. CT scan typically shows a well-circumscribed slightly hypoattenuating mass compared to adjacent normal liver parenchyma. A more homogenous appearance on CT is associated with epithelial HB whereas mixed tumors are predominantly heterogeneous. CT and MRI are also helpful in delineating the segmental involvement and the proximity of the tumor to the portal vein which helps determine resectability. Use of contrast, especially with MR-angiography, helps to define its vascular supply, again to assist in surgical planning.

HB is typically a single mass in the right lobe of the liver that is variegated tan to light brown to green on cut surface, with frequent areas of hemorrhage and necrosis. Microscopically, HBs are subdivided into either the epithelial (56%) or the epithelial/ mesenchymal (44%) types. The epithelial type is further subdivided into fetal (31%), embryonal (19%), macrotrabecular (3%), and small-cell undifferentiated (3%) subtypes. Fetal HB comprises cords of hepatoid cells while embryonal tumors have smaller cells with higher nuclear:cytoplasmic ratios, and the small-cell tumors resemble other 'small round blue cell' tumors of childhood. Most tumors contain a mixture of fetal and embryonal cells. The most common mesenchymal elements are cartilage and osteoid in mixed HBs (**43.14**).

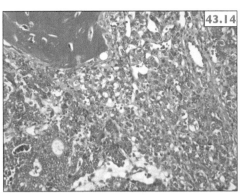

43.14 Hepatoblastoma. The mixed (epithelial/ mesenchymal) hepatoblastoma contains both fetal (right) and embryonal (left) epithelial components, the former bearing a close resemblance to normal hepatocytes. A segment of bone projects into the upper left portion of the field.

TREATMENT

Surgical resection is the mainstay of treatment and resectability of the tumor determines the prognosis. The use of neoadjuvant chemotherapy can frequently allow resection of initially unresectable tumors leading to improved prognosis and survival. The need for liver transplantation should be determined on a case-by-case basis. Pulmonary metastasis is not an absolute contraindication to liver transplantation as these lesions are sensitive to chemotherapy. Contraindications to resection include extensive bilateral liver involvement, vascular invasion of major hepatic veins and inferior vena cava, multi-focal disease, and distant metastasis.

PROGNOSIS

Outcome largely depends on staging at presentation in addition to several other factors, detailed below, that bear prognostic importance. Failure to decrease serum AFP levels by two logs with initial therapy suggests a poor prognosis. Pure fetal histology is associated with a better prognosis, while undifferentiated histology carries a poorer prognosis. The presence of mesenchymal elements is associated with an improved prognosis. Preoperative PRETEXT staging system utilizes the number of liver segments involved to help stage the disease.

Hepatocellular carcinoma

DEFINITION AND EPIDEMIOLOGY

Hepatocellular carcinoma (HCC) is the second most common primary liver tumor in the pediatric population, with a male predominance. The incidence of HCC parallels the prevalence of hepatitis B and C viral infection rates in the population. Other risk factors include inborn errors of metabolism (tyrosinemia, urea cycle defects), biliary atresia, biliary cystic diseases, chronic cholestasis, glycogen storage diseases, alpha-1 antitrypsin deficiency, and Wilson disease.

CLINICAL PRESENTATION

HCC is a tumor of older children with the median age at diagnosis of 12 years. HCC has been reported in children less than 5 years of age. Clinical presentation includes an incidental finding of a mass that accompanies other symptoms such as abdominal pain, anorexia, and weight loss. Pre-emptive monitoring of patients with risk factors mentioned above aids in timely diagnosis and intervention. Screening with serum AFP and abdominal ultrasound can help detect tumors prior to their clinical manifestation. A thorough evaluation is warranted whenever there is a deviation or a sudden change in clinical status in patients with known HCC.

DIFFERENTIAL DIAGNOSIS

Differentiation from hypervascular tumors of the liver such as HA, FNH, HCC, metastases, and fibrolamellar carcinoma is based on imaging characteristics and clinicopathologic correlation.

DIAGNOSIS AND PATHOPHYSIOLOGY

Smaller lesions can be hypo-, iso- or hyperechoic to the liver parenchyma on ultrasound, while bigger lesions tend to be heterogeneous. Vascular invasion can be analyzed with Doppler evaluation. Multiphase CT scan shows an early arterial phase enhancement as the main blood supply is via the hepatic artery. On MRI, HCC is hyperintense on T2-weighted images. Larger tumors will have a mosaic pattern secondary to the presence of intratumoral hemorrhage, necrosis, fat, or calcifications.

HCC can be solitary, multinodular, or rarely a diffuse infiltrative tumor. Histologically, tumors are comprised of intermediate to large, polygonal cells with central nuclei and a moderate amount of eosinophilic or clear cytoplasm that are separated by bile canaliculi; they may be so well-differentiated as to resemble normal liver. They typically grow as thick trabeculae that are separated by sinusoid-like spaces (**43.15**) but can occasionally have a pseudoglandular architecture. Necrosis and hemorrhage as well as vascular invasion are commonly seen.

TREATMENT

Complete surgical resection of the tumor confers the best chance for survival; however, HCC is often unresectable at presentation in the pediatric population. Systemic chemotherapy is not very effective. Liver transplantation for HCC is still controversial; however, recent reports suggest improved survival postorthotopic liver transplantation when following restricted inclusion guidelines.

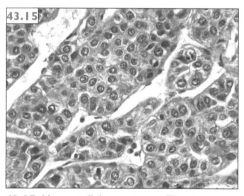

43.15 Hepatocellular carcinoma. The tumor cells resemble small hepatocytes and grow as thick cords, mimicking cell plates of normal liver. The trabeculae are surrounded by endothelial cells and separated by vascular spaces.

Fibrolamellar carcinoma

DEFINITION AND EPIDEMIOLOGY
Fibrolamellar carcinoma (FLC) is a variant of HCC seen in adolescent and young adults who lack any evidence of underlying liver disease.

CLINICAL PRESENTATION
As with standard HCC, the typical presentation includes an abdominal mass or pain, along with constitutional symptoms of weight loss, anorexia, and malaise. Less commonly, jaundice, gynecomastia, or venous thrombosis have been reported as presenting symptoms. Unlike HCC, serum AFP levels are not elevated.

DIFFERENTIAL DIAGNOSIS
FNH, HA, HCC, and metastases in the similar age group have to be differentiated from FLC. Imaging and histologic features help make that distinction.

DIAGNOSIS AND PATHOPHYSIOLOGY
A solitary circumscribed mass with heterogenous appearance on ultrasound can be seen. CT scan is the preferred modality of imaging and provides better definition and aids in visualization of the central scar that commonly is calcified. Nonenhancement on arterial phase of the central scar helps differentiate FLC from other lesions.

On gross examination, FLC is a well-circumscribed firm mass with characteristic radiating fibrous septa that resemble FNH. Microscopically neoplastic cells are large and polygonal with abundant granular eosinophilic cytoplasm that often contains hyaline or 'ground-glass'-like inclusions. Nuclei are large hyperchromatic and vesicular with prominent nucleoli. The name is derived from the distinct feature of fibrous stroma and thick hyalinized collagen that surrounds individual or groups of cells (**43.16**).

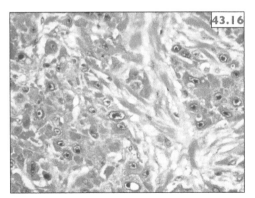

43.16 Fibrolamellar carcinoma. Large tumor cells have abundant granular cytoplasm and vesicular nuclei with prominent nucleoli. Strands of dense hyalinized collagen interdigitate between the cells.

TREATMENT AND PROGNOSIS
Surgical resection is the mainstay of treatment along with adjunctive chemotherapy. Chemoembolization and liver transplantation can also be utilized based on tumor characteristics. The best prognosis is achieved by complete tumor resection with negative surgical margins. Other indicators of better prognosis include younger age at presentation, absence of lymph node involvement, and vascular invasion.

Embryonal (undifferentiated) sarcoma of liver

DEFINITION AND EPIDEMIOLOGY
Embryonal (undifferentiated) sarcoma of liver (ESL) is a rare but highly malignant hepatic neoplasm of mesenchymal origin seen in young children. Most cases are identified in children less than 10 years of age. There is no sex predilection.

CLINICAL PRESENTATION
There are no specific clinical features. Abdominal mass with accompanying abdominal pain is seen in the majority of patients, but rarely, it can present acutely with complications of tumor rupture. Serum AFP levels are not elevated.

DIFFERENTIAL DIAGNOSIS
Differentiation from cystic appearing lesions, such as MH, hydatid cyst, abscess, or cystic degeneration within HB or HCC, can be done based on age at presentation, travel history, and serum AFP levels.

DIAGNOSIS AND PATHOPHYSIOLOGY
The solid tumor is either iso- or hyperechoic relative to normal liver parenchyma on ultrasound. A cyst-like appearance can be seen on CT and MRI which is in contrast to ultrasound and the gross pathologic appearance of ESL. MRI is the preferred modality for imaging and helps determine resectability with regards to vascular or biliary tree involvement. The tumors are usually >10 cm and up to 30 cm in size and predominantly solid on the periphery, whereas the center has cystic gelatinous spaces, hemorrhage and necrosis. It is well demarcated and often demonstrates a fibrous pseudocapsule.

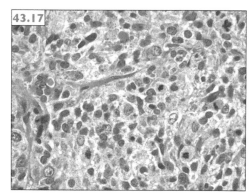

43.17 Embryonal sarcoma. The moderately cellular tumor comprises hyperchromatic ovoid undifferentiated cells and has numerous mitotic figures. Eosinophilic globules (left) lie within the cytoplasm of a pleomorphic tumor cell.

Microscopically, the tumor cells are spindled, oval or stellate with hyperchromatic and often very pleomorphic nuclei and frequent mitoses (**43.17**). They are arranged loosely or compactly within fibrous or typically mucopolysaccharide-rich stroma. Multiple intra- or extracellular periodic acid Schiff-positive eosinophilic globules of varying size are characteristically present and entrapped dilated bile ducts can be seen at the periphery.

TREATMENT
Previously considered to carry a poor prognosis, the mean 12-month survival of ESL has significantly improved. Complete surgical resection is the mainstay of treatment. Neoadjuvant chemotherapy renders unresectable tumors amenable to surgical excision. Liver transplantation for unresectable tumors can also be considered.

Epithelioid hemangioendothelioma

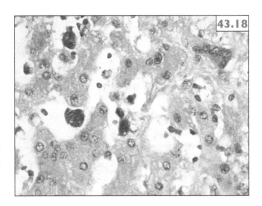

DEFINITION AND EPIDEMIOLOGY
Epithelioid hemangioendothelioma (EHE) is a rare slow-growing vascular tumor of the liver that primarily affects adult patients, with only rare cases reported in late childhood (12–14 years of age). EHE is considered a low-grade malignant neoplasm in contrast to the more aggressive angiosarcoma.

CLINICAL PRESENTATION
Nonspecific symptoms include right upper quadrant pain, and weight loss. There is a slight female predominance. The serum AFP is generally not elevated.

DIFFERENTIAL DIAGNOSIS
EHE can be differentiated from angiosarcoma as it follows a prolonged course while angiosarcoma is rapidly progressive. Findings consistent with the primary tumor on history and physical examination in combination with laboratory markers helps to differentiate EHE from metastatic lesions.

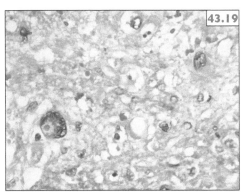

43.18, 43.19 Epithelioid hemangioendothelioma. **43.18:** Hyperchromatic atypical epithelioid cells infiltrate hepatic sinusoids and destroy hepatic plates; **43.19:** a sclerotic area of tumor contains only a few atypical and multinucleated tumor cells that lack obvious vascular features.

DIAGNOSIS AND PATHOPHYSIOLOGY
Single to multiple nodules are seen peripherally located with adjacent capsular retraction. EHE nodules are predominantly hypoattenuating compared to normal liver parenchyma on noncontrast CT. A target-like appearance of EHE on MRI is not infrequent and is due to reduced signal secondary to central hemorrhage, coagulative necrosis, and calcification which contrasts to the higher signal intensity at the periphery due to edematous connective tissue and viable tumor tissue.

These tumors are often multifocal involving both lobes of the liver. Peripheral masses close to the capsule cause subcapsular retraction secondary to a fibrotic reaction. Lesions are firm, white to tan in color, and range from a few millimeters to 14 cm. Histologically, EHE is composed of dendritic and epithelioid cells that show vascular differentiation. Epithelioid cells have nuclear atypia and contain abundant eosinophilic cytoplasm. Some have a signet-ring appearance, where a cytoplasmic vacuole represents an intracellular vascular lumen. Immunohistochemistry is usually necessary to demonstrate endothelial differentiation where EHE is positive for factor VIII (von Willebrand factor), CD34, and/or CD31. The tumor often grows along pre-existing sinusoids and hepatic or portal vein branches allowing persistence of acinar landmarks despite extensive invasion (**43.18**). As the tumor evolves, its fibromyxoid stroma becomes progressively sclerotic (**43.19**).

TREATMENT

EHE is not readily amenable to chemo-therapy and thus surgical resection and liver transplantation are the mainstay of treatment. The presence of multiple lesions diffusely throughout the liver parenchyma makes surgical excision challenging. Even in the face of metastatic disease, the prognosis is considered better than other hepatic malig-nancies. Infiltration of the Glisson's capsule, mitoses, or nuclear atypia bears no prognostic importance; however, high cellularity cor-relates with poor clinical outcome.

Angiosarcoma

Angiosarcoma is a rare rapidly progressive vascular tumor of the liver that carries a poor prognosis. It most commonly affects elderly men and is only rarely reported in children. Abdominal pain, anorexia, and weight loss in combination with hepatomegaly is the most common clinical presentation.

Features seen with IHH, such as anemia, thrombocytopenia, and consumptive coagu-lopathy, are commonly seen in angiosarcoma. Hepatic involvement can be in the form of a single dominant nodule or multiple nodules. Biopsies are rarely done so as to avoid the possible complication of significant bleeding. As in EHE, endothelial markers confirm vascular differentiation. Pediatric angiosarcomas often have a 'kaposiform' component comprising bundles of spindled cells with slit-like vascular spaces.

Imaging with multiphase CT or MRI is key to making the diagnosis. A hypoattenuating lesion is seen on CT in both arterial and venous phases. Delayed persistent enhance-ment with incomplete centripetal filling due to central fibrosis or necrosis can also be seen. Metastatic involvement of the liver can be differentiated from an angiosarcoma based on clinicopathologic and imaging characteristics. Arterial embolization can be utilized in appropriate clinical setting and based on tumor features.

Hepatobiliary rhabdomyosarcoma

Rhabdomyosarcoma (RMS) involving the liver is extremely rare and presents in early childhood (median age at presentation of 3.4 years). RMS originates from the biliary tree and less commonly from the gallbladder, cystic duct, and the ampulla of Vater. It commonly presents with obstructive jaundice, abdominal pain, fever, vomiting, and weight loss. Laboratory evaluation discloses mild transaminitis in association with moderate elevation of serum bilirubin. Ultrasound or CT scan can help delineate the hepatobiliary anatomic features and demonstrate dilatation of the hepatic/bile ducts suggesting obstruction. Biliary tree dedicated MRI is the imaging test of choice. The tumor, often a 'grape-like mass' (sarcoma botryoides) that projects into the duct lumen, comprises round to spindled cells that may have eosinophilic cytoplasm and cross-striations. Immunohistochemically the cells are positive for muscle lineage markers such as desmin, myogenin, and myogenic regulatory protein D. Typically the tumors remain localized and are not entirely amenable to resection and thus, instead of surgery, chemotherapy or radiation therapy is initiated first.

Biliary obstruction either from the RMS or secondary to chemotherapy might necessitate stent placement or even an external biliary drain. Neoadjuvant chemotherapeutic and multidisciplinary strategies have signifi-cantly improved the prognosis of hepato-biliary RMS.

CHAPTER 44

Liver Transplantation

Yuliya Rekhtman

- **Introduction**
- **Transplant methodology**
- **Post-transplant management**

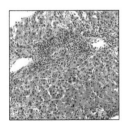
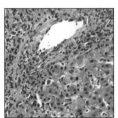
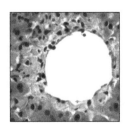
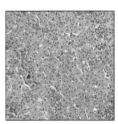

Introduction

Solid organ transplantation is one of the greatest breakthroughs in transplant science over the last 50 years. An improvement in surgical techniques and medical management along with advances in immune suppression has facilitated our advancement in liver transplant medicine. Currently, liver transplantation is performed in over 100 centers around the world. Reports of 1-year survival range from 83% to 93% in the United Kingdom, United States, and Australia.

In 2011, 6341 liver transplants were performed in the United States, making it the second most commonly transplanted organ after the kidney. In 2011, 536 pediatric liver transplants were performed, with 59 from living donors (United Network for Organ Sharing [UNOS] data). Currently, there are approximately 900 children age 18 years and younger on the UNOS waiting list for liver transplant. The most common indications for pediatric liver transplantation are outlined in the *Table 44.1*. Allocation of organs available for transplantation is currently based on the designated adult and pediatric scoring systems. The Model for End-Stage Liver disease (MELD) and Pediatric End-Stage Liver Disease (PELD) scoring systems were designed to prioritize listing by severity of illness rather than waiting time. These scores have been shown to predict the risk of death within 3 months. The PELD scoring system is used in children aged 12 years younger, and is based on a child's age, extent of growth failure, serum bilirubin, international normalized ratio (INR), and serum albumin. For children over 12 years and adults, the MELD scoring is used. MELD only takes into account bilirubin, serum creatinine, and INR.

Despite many accomplishments, liver transplantation still presents many clinical and surgical challenges requiring a multidisciplinary team approach to achieve optimal care of such children.

Table 44.1 Common indications for liver transplantation in children in the United States

Cholestatic liver disease (~54%)	Biliary atresia (42%) Total parenteral nutrition-associated cholestasis Alagille syndrome Progressive sclerosing cholangitis Progressive familial intrahepatic cholestasis Neonatal hepatitis
Fulminant or acute liver failure (~13%)	Drug induced (e.g. acetaminophen, valproic acid) Idiopathic
Metabolic liver disease (~13%)	Primary (e.g. alpha-1-antitrypsin deficiency, tyrosinemia) Secondary (e.g. urea cycle defect, bile acid synthesis defects)
Tumor (~5%)	Hepatoblastoma Hepatocellular carcinoma
Other (~7%)	Caroli disease Nonalcoholic steatohepatitis
Cirrhosis of unknown etiology (~8%)	

INDICATIONS

Indication for transplantation may be either disease-related or function-related. The liver has many functions including protein synthesis essential for homeostasis, metabolism including synthesis of bile acids that are essential for absorption, and detoxification with excretion. Defects in any of these hepatic functions can lead to irreversible liver damage along with defects in other systems and organs. Congenital defects often compromise multiple functions and can lead to excessive retention of bile acids. In children with Alagille syndrome, for example, liver transplantation may be indicated to address severe intractable pruritus secondary to bile acid deposition despite normal hepatic synthetic function. The current scoring system used for organ allocation does not account for quality of life parameters, recurrent infections as seen with defective immunoglobulin synthesis, or mental health changes.

Transplant methodology

TRANSPLANT LIVER ANATOMY

The native liver can be divided into eight surgical segments (**44.1**). Each segment has separate vasculature and innervations allowing relatively straightforward separation.

Orthotopic liver transplantation (previously called 'cadaveric') refers to a procedure in which the failing liver is removed and replaced with a healthy liver from a deceased donor. This is the most common method used for liver transplantation in the United States and most of the western world. A donated liver may be given to one or sometimes two recipients ('split liver' donation). For example, the left lateral segment can be given to an infant while the rest of the adult liver can be transplanted to an adult recipient.

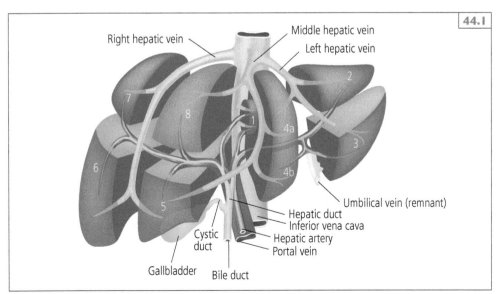

44.1 Functional anatomy of the liver with Couinaud's segments. Segment 1 is the caudate lobe; segment 2, 3, 4a, and 4b make up the left lobe; segments 5, 6, 7, and 8 make up the right lobe.

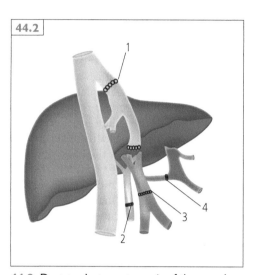

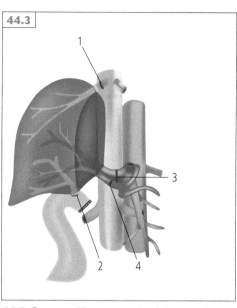

44.2 Duct-to-duct anastomosis of the vessels. 1: Inferior vena cava; 2: bile duct; 3: portal vein; 4: hepatic artery.

44.3 Roux-en-Y anastomosis of the vessels. 1: Inferior vena cava; 2: bile duct to Roux conduit; 3: portal vein; 4: hepatic artery.

Living-related donor transplantation is a procedure in which a healthy living person donates part of their own liver to a related recipient. This procedure is increasingly used in response to the shortage of cadaveric donors. Living-related donation has been particularly useful in children because of the shortage of cadaveric livers of the appropriate small size. A patient could potentially receive a right lobe, left lobe, or left lateral segment depending on the size of the recipient and the donor.

ANASTOMOSIS

In most cases of a whole liver transplantation, several anastomotic connections are made. The hepatic artery, portal vein and inferior vena cava from the recipient are connected to the donor graft vessels. There are also two types of biliary anastomosis used in liver transplantation which include duct-to-duct and Roux-en-Y anastomoses. If the biliary anatomy of a donor and recipient are compatible, a duct-to-duct anastomosis is performed (**44.2**). A Roux-en-Y anastomosis is used when anatomy of the recipient is abnormal, particularly in the patient with a previous Kasai operation for biliary atresia or in a patient receiving a partial liver transplantation (**44.3**). In this procedure the donor liver is drained by anastomosing the biliary system to a segment of the recipient's small intestine.

The type of biliary connection is a critical factor in predicting and addressing postoperative complications in both early and late postoperative periods.

Post-transplant management

Post-transplant management requires a multidisciplinary approach with the main clinical goals of minimizing transplant complications, ensuring patient/graft survival, monitoring and treating side-effects of medications, and providing adequate nutrition to achieve appropriate recovery, growth, and development of the recipient.

IMMUNOSUPPRESSION

Post-transplant immunosuppression management differs between institutions. Nevertheless, early post-transplant immunosuppression generally includes high-dose steroids, with or without an interleukin (IL)-2 receptor antagonist (e.g. basiliximab) and initiation of long-term therapy, typically a calcineurin inhibitor (CNI). Benefits of tacrolimus over traditional CNI cyclosporine include its improved efficacy, reduced toxicity profile, and ease of drug level monitoring. Mycophenolate mofetil (MMF) is often used as an adjunct to therapy in patients who have underlying autoimmune disease or who cannot tolerate CNI. Sirolimus (rapamycin) is often used as a rescue therapy for chronic graft rejection or as adjunct therapy. Physicians should be aware of the side-effects of each drug used in post-transplantation management (*Table 44.2*).

POSTOPERATIVE COMPLICATIONS

Postoperative complications can be classified by their time of onset. Immediate complications include primary graft non-function, acute rejection, hepatic artery thrombosis, biliary leak, and infection. Late complications include portal vein stenosis or thrombosis, biliary obstruction, rejection, and infection. Other complications include *de novo* autoimmune hepatitis or recurrence of primary liver disease (for example, recurrence of hepatitis C infection).

Rejection

In general, organ allograft rejection can be defined as an immunologic reaction to the presence of a foreign tissue and has the potential to cause graft dysfunction and failure. Acute rejection occurs within the first 3 months after transplantation and is characterized by an increase in transaminases, hyperbilirubinemia, and potential coagulopathy along with characteristic

Table 44.2 Side-effects of commonly used immunosuppressive drugs

Steroids	Hypertension, diabetes, osteoporosis, growth delay, cataracts
Cyclosporine	Nephrotoxicity, hypertension, hypercholesterolemia
Tacrolimus	Nephrotoxicity, diabetes, neurotoxicity
Sirolimus	Bone marrow suppression, hyperlipidemia
Mycophenolate mofetil	Bone marrow suppression, colitis, gastrointestinal discomfort

pathologic findings on biopsy. Acute rejection pathologically is defined as inflammation of the allograft, elicited by a genetic disparity between the donor and recipient, which primarily affects interlobular bile ducts and vascular endothelia especially of the portal veins and hepatic venules (**44.4–44.6**). The Banff criteria propose a consensus for a pathologic definition of acute rejection, taking into account histologic features of liver parenchyma and biliary and vascular changes in defining a liver rejection score (*Table 44.3*).

Management of the acute rejection primarily includes a combination of steroid use and increased immune suppression.

Chronic rejection is managed in a similar manner as acute rejection with the goal of preserving the graft. Unfortunately, chronic rejection is harder to reverse and results in escalation of maintenance therapy. Biopsy specimens from chronic rejection patients outline feature of chronic bridging inflammation and fibrosis along with portal area changes (**44.7–44.9**).

Table 44.3 Banff Criteria – Rejection Activity Index

Category	Criteria	Score
Portal inflammation	Mostly lymphocytic inflammation involving, but not noticeably expanding, a minority of the triads	1
	Expansion of most or all of the triads, by a mixed infiltrate containing lymphocytes first, with occasional blasts, neutrophils and eosinophils	2
	Marked expansion of most or all of the triads by a mixed infiltrate containing numerous blasts and eosinophils with inflammatory spillover into the periportal parenchyma	3
Bile duct inflammation damage	A minority of the involved ducts are cuffed and infiltrated by inflammatory cells with only mild reactive changes such as increased nuclear:cytoplasmic ratio of the epithelial cells	1
	Most or all of the ducts infiltrated by inflammatory cells. Prominent degenerative changes in the ducts with nuclear pleomorphism, disordered polarity and cytoplasmic vacuolization of the epithelium	2
	As above for score 2, with most or all of the ducts showing degenerative changes or focal luminal disruption	3
Venous endothelial inflammation	Subendothelial lymphocytic infiltration involving some, but not a majority of the portal and/or hepatic venules	1
	Subendothelial infiltration involving most or all of the portal and/or hepatic venules	2
	As above for score 2, with moderate or severe perivenular inflammation that extends into the perivenular parenchyma and is associated with perivenular hepatocyte necrosis	3

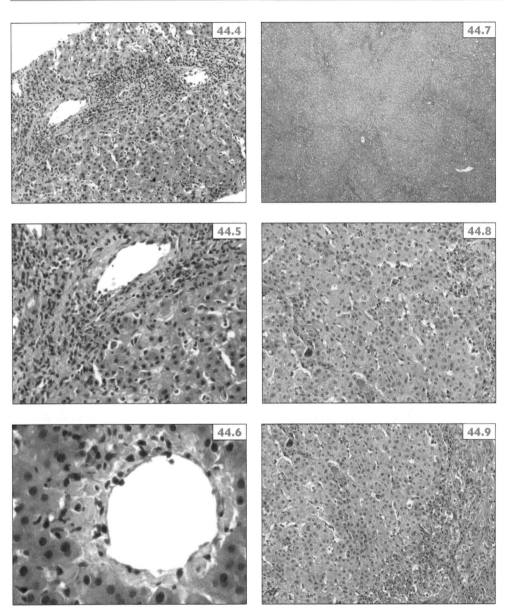

44.4–44.6 Acute rejection. **44.4**: Central venulitis; **44.5**: endotheliitis; **44.6**: triaditis.

44.7–44.9 Chronic rejection. **44.7**: Ductular proliferation and cholestasis; **44.8**: ductopenia and cholestasis; **44.9**: ductular proliferation and cholestasis.

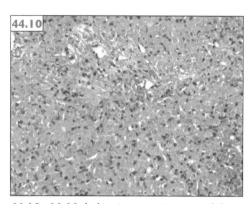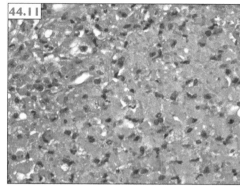

44.10, 44.11 Ischemic necrosis seen with hepatic artery thrombosis.

Hepatic artery thrombosis

Hepatic artery thrombosis (HAT) typically occurs in the immediate postoperative period. It is a surgical emergency and requires urgent intervention. Patients with a history of HAT should have an evaluation for coagulopathy and generally require long-term anticoagulation therapy. Biopsies can show hepatocyte foamy degeneration or necrosis (**44.10**, **44.11**). Diagnosis is often made with radiographic studies.

Biliary stricture

Biliary strictures usually occur at the site of biliary anastomosis and are a consequence of the technical difficulties surrounding surgery on these small structures. Biliary strictures can also be secondary to bile duct ischemia resulting from vascular insufficiency, particularly hepatic artery stenosis or thrombosis. Biliary strictures are fairly common in pediatric liver transplant patients, occurring in up to 35% of patients in some studies. Management depends on the size of the stricture and type of anastomosis. Techniques for diagnosis include endoscopic retrograde cholangiopancreatography (ERCP) for duct-to-duct anastomosis or percutaneous transhepatic cholangiogram (PTC) for Roux-en-Y anastomosis with serial dilatations. Surgical revision is often required.

Portal vein thrombosis

Portal vein thrombosis is typically a late complication of transplantation and is reported in about 10% of pediatric patients, frequently in those patients receiving partial liver transplantation.

Infections

Early post-transplant infections can have a devastating consequence on graft survival and overall patient care. Close monitoring for opportunistic and hospital-acquired infectious organisms with an appropriate therapeutic intervention and management is essential for a favorable outcome (*Table 44.4*). By 6 months after transplantation, 80% of pediatric patients will have achieved stable graft function and will require low intensity immunosuppression. The infection risk at this time period will be more from community-acquired infections rather than from opportunistic organisms. Approximately 5–10% of liver transplant patients will have a chronic viral infection including cytomegalovirus (CMV) and Epstein–Barr virus (EBV). Additionally, 5–10% of patients will have recurrent or chronic rejection necessitating more intensive immunosuppression, thus increasing the risk of opportunistic infections such as *Pneumocystis jiroveci*, opportunistic fungal infections, CMV, or EBV.

Table 44.4 Control of infection in the first 6 months after transplant

Organism	Therapy
Cytomegalovirus	Ganciclovir, acyclovir, cytomegalovirus immune globulin, valganciclovir
Epstein–Barr virus	Ganciclovir, valganciclovir
Candida spp.	Nystatin, fluconazole, ketoconazole
Aspergillus spp.	Caspofungin
Pneumocystis spp.	Sulfamethoxazole/trimethoprim, pentamidine

VACCINATION IN THE POST-TRANSPLANT PERIOD

Current recommendations for vaccination are to restart an immunization schedule within 3–6 months after transplant with inactivated vaccines. Live vaccination has been a topic of the debate with no consensus across the transplant centers. Some authorities consider live vaccinations safe and effective 6 months after transplant with serum antibody measurements for measles, mumps, and rubella obtained in these patients 12 months after transplantation.

POST-TRANSPLANT LYMPHOPROLIFERATIVE DISORDER

Post-transplant lymphoproliferative disorder (PTLD) is a heterogeneous group of lymphoproliferative diseases ranging from benign polyclonal B-cell proliferation, as seen in acute EBV infections (infectious mononucleosis), to a malignant monoclonal lymphomatous lesion. Clinical presentation varies from an infectious mononucleosis-like illness with diffuse lymphadenopathy (60%) to a gastrointestinal syndrome (33%) with diarrhea, blood in the stool, and elevated transaminases. Less common clinical manifestations include isolated or multi-system infiltrative disease involving lymph tissue throughout the body. PTLD occurs in 3–10% of pediatric liver transplant recipients. Risk factors include young age (less than 5 years of age), EBV naïve recipients, and higher levels of immunosuppression.

GROWTH AND DEVELOPMENT

Factors affecting growth after transplant include anorexia, fat malabsorption, increased energy requirements, decreased protein synthesis, relative growth hormone insensitivity, and frequent hospitalizations. In general, 37–47% of catch-up growth occurs after 6 months post-transplantation. Catch-up growth occurs more predictably in younger children. Long-term prednisone use (greater than 2 years of steroid use) is a significant factor associated with growth failure in children. Growth appears not to be related to graft function.

ACKNOWLEDGMENT

Sara Baig for drafting and providing special illustrations and Therese Cermak, MD, for pathology images.

CHAPTER 45

Gastrointestinal Tract Polyps and Polyposis Syndromes

Katharine Eng, Marsha Kay, Robert Wyllie

- **Introduction**
- **Juvenile polyps**

HAMARTOMATOUS POLYPOSIS SYNDROMES

- **Juvenile polyposis syndrome**
- **PTEN hamartoma tumor syndrome**
- **Peutz–Jeghers syndrome**

ADENOMATOUS POLYPOSIS SYNDROMES

- **Familial adenomatous polyposis**
- **Neoplasms of the gastrointestinal tract**
- **Conclusion**

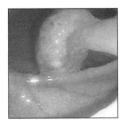
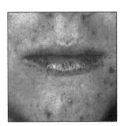
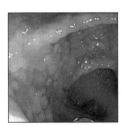
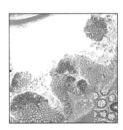

Introduction

Polyps are abnormal growths of tissue that arise from the gastrointestinal (GI) mucosa and project into the GI lumen. GI polyps can be commonly encountered during childhood and are one of the most common causes of rectal bleeding in this age group. The majority of these polyps are benign and located in the colon, with the most frequent being juvenile polyps, usually diagnosed between 2 and 5 years of age. However, with increasing age, juvenile polyps are less likely to be encountered and either adenomatous polyps or polyps associated with underlying genetic abnormalities become more likely. This is particularly true if polyps are present in larger numbers, are located outside the colon, or if there is a positive family history of polyps.

CLINICAL PRESENTATION

The typical presentation of colonic polyps is painless rectal bleeding. Rectal examination may sometimes reveal a palpable polyp. Rarely, there may be symptoms of abdominal pain due to intussusception from a polyp, altered bowel habits, or prolapse of the polyp. Patients with a significant number of polyps may present with iron deficiency anemia, protein-losing enteropathy, and diarrhea. Other children may in comparison be asymptomatic, and the polyp may be discovered as part of a screening protocol for an inheritable polyposis syndrome, work-up of a GI disorder, or other complaints.

Some of the familial polyposis syndromes may also have extraintestinal manifestations. Mucosal pigmentation, particularly of the lips, is one of the most characteristic features of Peutz–Jeghers syndrome (PJS). Pigmentation can occur in other areas as well, such as the buccal mucosa, skin around the eyes, nostrils, hands and feet, and perianal region. Patients with familial adenomatous polyposis (FAP) can have extraintestinal manifestations including subcutaneous cysts, desmoid tumors, dental abnormalities, exostosis, and pigmented ocular lesions. In patients with juvenile polyposis syndrome (JPS), dysmorphic features, such as abnormal facies, macrocephaly, and cleft lip or palate, have been occasionally noted, along with mental retardation. Edema may also be found on physical examination in those patients with infantile JPS secondary to hypoalbuminemia.

DIFFERENTIAL DIAGNOSIS

The differential diagnosis for painless rectal bleeding (the most common presentation of colonic polyps) is broad, varies with age, and includes anal fissure, trauma, allergic colitis, infectious colitis, inflammatory bowel disease, Meckel diverticulum, and congenital vascular anomalies.

DIAGNOSIS

Colonoscopy is the preferred technique for diagnosis and therapy. It has replaced barium contrast imaging as the first-line modality to evaluate rectal bleeding in the setting of suspected polyps. A polypectomy should be attempted at the time of colonoscopy if safe and feasible, and tissue should be sent for histology, which is important to determine future management. The main risks of endoscopic polypectomy are bleeding and perforation. Bleeding following polypectomy may occur in 2–3% of cases, but is usually controllable with additional endoscopic therapy. Colonic perforation following polypectomy is an infrequent complication in the pediatric age group, but can occur, especially with resection of larger polyps or in the poorly prepared colon.

Once a polyp has been identified during endoscopy, a careful family history should be taken regarding family members with bowel cancer, the age of onset of the cancer (and in particular, one should ask if cancer or polyps have occurred in a first- or second-degree relative before 50 years of age), and the site of the cancer. Genetic studies may also be used to help delineate the diagnosis of a polyposis syndrome. It is important to distinguish between an isolated one or two (and up to four) juvenile polyps and those patients with a greater number that would constitute a polyposis syndrome that requires additional evaluation and monitoring.

Laboratory and additional evaluations
A complete blood count and iron studies may reveal an iron deficiency anemia. Imaging studies, such as double-contrast barium enema, may demonstrate polyps, but colonoscopy has higher sensitivity and also provides the benefit of biopsy and removal. Thus, colonoscopy remains the gold standard and barium studies are infrequently performed. Computed tomography (CT) colonography is not yet a mature technology, nor adequately studied in pediatric patients, but is increasing in sensitivity for detection of small polyps. CT colonography has the advantage of being a less invasive technology and has the theoretical advantage of identifying polyps that may be 'hidden' behind mucosal folds that may have been overlooked during colonoscopy. There are, however, disadvantages to this technology including radiation and need for bowel preparation. If polyps are found on CT, colonoscopy with polypectomy is still required, and therefore, colonoscopy with polypectomy is still recommended as a primary intervention in pediatric and adult patients suspected of having colonic polyps.

Histopathologic classification
In children, GI polyps generally fall into two major categories: adenomas and hamartomas. Solitary polyps and the bulk of polyps found in the pediatric age group are most commonly hamartomas, which are predominantly of the juvenile type and likely benign. Solitary adenomas, on the other hand, are rare and may have malignant potential. However, of the familial syndromes occurring in pediatric patients, FAP (adenomatous polyps) is more common than either PJS or JPS (both hamartomatous polyps). Knowing the histologic classification is important in determining the diagnosis and management. Therefore, it is important to retrieve these polyps at the time of polypectomy to send them for histologic evaluation.

Juvenile polyps

CLINICAL PRESENTATION
Juvenile polyps of the large intestine present with painless rectal bleeding or perianal polyp protrusion, usually around a mean age of 4 years. These have a near negligible risk for malignant change and are thought to be benign. They may be single or multiple (but less than five), and are the most frequent type of GI polypoid lesion encountered in pediatric patients. The majority of juvenile polyps are located in the rectosigmoid colon, with the remainder distributed throughout the remainder of the colon; therefore, a full colonoscopy is needed for a complete evaluation. Rectal examination may sometimes reveal a palpable polyp if it is located in the distal rectum.

ETIOLOGY AND PATHOPHYSIOLOGY
The etiology of a juvenile polyp is not known, unless it is associated with a polyposis syndrome.

The gross appearance of juvenile polyps is spherical to slightly lobular in form, with most being pedunculated with long stalks (**45.1**). Microscopically, juvenile polyps have a Swiss cheese appearance with dilated cysts filled with mucin. The lamina propria is noted to have a prominent inflammatory infiltrate that can be haphazardly arranged. Smooth muscle cells are not noted in the stroma, in contrast to the hamartomatous polyps of PJS (**45.2**).

TREATMENT
Although the risk of developing malignancy is negligible, polyps should be removed, even if discovered incidentally, in order to alleviate symptoms and for histologic diagnosis. Management of juvenile polyps will be influenced by the number of polyps (less than five or greater than or equal to five), the absence or presence of upper GI tract juvenile polyps, and the absence or presence of a family history of any polyposis syndromes. It is important to distinguish between the more common juvenile polyp versus a polyposis

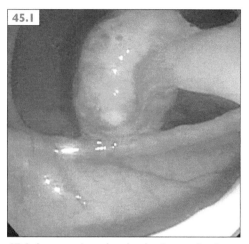

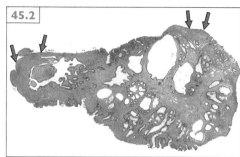

45.2 Low-power view of a juvenile polyp. The polyp is composed of irregular and dilated colonic glands embedded in an inflamed stroma. Juvenile polyps often demonstrate surface erosions, as in this case (arrows). (Courtesy of Thomas Plesec, MD; Anatomic Pathology, the Cleveland Clinic.)

45.1 Large pedunculated polyp in a pediatric patient with juvenile polyposis syndrome.

syndrome. If after a full colonoscopy, less than five polyps are found and there is no relevant family history of multiple juvenile polyps, endoscopic polypectomy is considered to be sufficient and conclusive treatment. Parents should be aware, however, that juvenile polyps may be the first feature of JPS, and that if new symptoms arise, the patient should undergo an additional evaluation including a repeat colonoscopy if indicated.

HAMARTOMATOUS POLYPOSIS SYNDROMES

The hamartomatous polyposis syndromes includes JPS, PTEN harmartoma tumor syndrome (which includes Cowden syndrome [CS] and Bannayan–Riley–Ruvalcaba syndrome [BRRS]) and PJS. These syndromes are a rare group of hereditary autosomal dominant disorders, with variable penetrance.

Juvenile polyposis syndrome

DEFINITION, EPIDEMIOLOGY, AND CLINICAL PRESENTATION

JPS is a rare polyposis syndrome (incidence of ≤1 in 100,000) with multiple hamartomatous polyps and an increased risk of malignancy. The majority of the polyps are found in the colon, although the remainder of the GI tract may be affected. The typical presentation is in the first or second decade of life, and should be considered in patients who present with five or more juvenile polyps in the colon, with juvenile polyps in any other part of the GI tract, or with a juvenile polyp and a relevant family history. JPS has been classified into three different categories: juvenile polyposis of infancy (which can present with diarrhea, rectal prolapse, and protein-losing enteropathy); juvenile polyposis coli (polyp growth occurs only in the colon); and generalized juvenile polyposis (polyps can involve the stomach, small bowel, and colon). Those patients with juvenile polyposis coli and generalized juvenile polyposis can develop 50–200 polyps during their lifetime.

DIAGNOSIS

Many JPS patients may be asymptomatic, although one may see prolapse of a polyp on rectal examination. The typical presentation is similar to the isolated juvenile polyps, such as isolated rectal bleeding. There have also been multiple extraintestinal manifestations that have been reported with JPS, including abnormal facies, macrocephaly, cleft lip or palate, supernumery teeth, and mental retardation. Edema may also be found on physical examination in patients with infantile JPS, likely attributed to hypoalbuminemia. Other extraintestinal manifestations include heart defects, double renal pelvis and ureter, as well as a bifid uterus and vagina. Less frequently, JPS can occur as part of CS or as part of BRRS, with their own unique associated extraintestinal manifestations, which will be discussed later. Due the overlap between JPS, CS, and BRRS, however, the true incidence of extraintestinal manifestations is difficult to determine.

ETIOLOGY AND PATHOPHYSIOLOGY

JPS has an autosomal dominant inheritance pattern with variable penetrance. Approximately 50–60% of cases are familial, while the others occur sporadically. JPS has been associated with germline mutations in three genes (*SMAD4*, *BMPR1A*, and *ENG*), all of which are part of the transforming growth factor-beta signaling pathway. The role of the *PTEN* gene mutation currently remains controversial, and it is thought that this mutation likely represents CS or BRRS patients who have not yet shown the extraintestinal clinical features seen in those patients.

The gross appearance of juvenile polyps is spherical to slightly lobular in form, with most being pedunculated with long stalks. However, in patients with JPS, polyps can also have a multilobulated appearance of a papillary or villiform shape. The histologic appearance of juvenile polyps in JPS is the same as a solitary juvenile polyp.

TREATMENT

JPS is associated with an increased lifetime risk of colorectal carcinoma, thought to arise from dysplastic changes within the hamartomas. The incidence of colorectal cancer has been reported to be up to 20% in one study, with a mean age of 34 years and by 60 years of age, an estimated cumulative risk of 68%. There is no consensus established for optimal screening or surveillance, but generally affected individuals with JPS should undergo surveillance colonoscopy with random biopsies of flat mucosa and polyps every 2 years, or earlier if symptoms arise. Upper GI surveillance through upper endoscopy should also be introduced in the middle teens to mid-20s. In those patients with dysplasia, colon cancer, a high polyp burden with symptoms that can't be adequately resolved endoscopically, at high risk for repetitive endoscopic procedures, or those patients who may be unreliable for attending screening, a colectomy is warranted, although this procedure is performed infrequently in the pediatric age group. Asymptomatic first-degree relatives of patients with JPS should be screened for the disease, as they are at risk for juvenile polyposis and colorectal cancer.

PTEN hamartoma tumor syndrome

PTEN hamartoma tumor syndrome is a term that has been used to encompass CS and BRRS. These disorders are caused by a *PTEN* gene mutation. The polyps within the GI tract resemble juvenile polyps in both gross and histologic appearance; however, patients with CS and BRRS have extraintestinal manifestations that distinguish them from JPS.

Extraintestinal manifestations of CS include mucocutaneous lesions, such as facial trichilemmomas, papillomatous papules, and acral keratoses, as well as other extraintestinal manifestations, such as macrocephaly, and thyroid, endometrial, and breast manifestations, which can include cancer. CS patients are also at risk for other cancers, which include cervical and ovarian cancer, uterine adenocarcinomas, meningiomas, and transitional cell carcinomas of the bladder. Extraintestinal manifestations of BRRS syndrome, on the other hand, include developmental delay, macrocephaly, joint hyperextensibility, pectus excavatum, scoliosis, lipomas, and genital pigmentation.

Unlike CS, there is no formal diagnostic criteria for BRRS due to the scarcity of this syndrome, but this condition should be considered if there is a family history of BRRS or CS and if a patient has one or more associated extraintestinal manifestations.

Peutz–Jeghers syndrome

DEFINITION AND EPIDEMIOLOGY

PJS is a rare GI hamartomatous polyposis syndrome (prevalence of 1 in 50,000 to 1 in 200,000 live births) associated with an increased risk of GI and extraintestinal cancers. This syndrome is characterized by mucocutaneous pigmentation and hamartomatous polyps throughout the GI tract. PJS polyps arise primarily in the small intestine (more commonly in the jejunum than in the ileum or the duodenum), and to a lesser degree in the stomach and colon. These polyps may cause bleeding and anemia, but more concerning is the risk for repetitive small bowel intussusception that can cause intestinal obstruction, vomiting, and pain. Patients with PJS can develop recurrent episodes of small bowel obstruction, intussusception, and bleeding, which can lead to recurrent bowel resections. The average age of onset of symptoms is in early 20s, but this can present in childhood.

DIAGNOSIS

Diagnosis of PJS can be made when one of the following is present:
- Two or more histologically confirmed PJS polyps.
- Any number of PJS polyps along with characteristic mucocutaneous pigmentation.
- Any number of PJS polyps if there is a family history of PJS in close relative.
- Characteristic mucocutaneous pigmentation along with a family history of PJS in a close relative.

Mucosal pigmentation (small, 1–5 mm pigmented macules), particularly of the lips is one of the most characteristic features of PJS (**45.3**). Pigmentation can also occur in other areas, such as the buccal mucosa, skin around the eyes, nostrils, hands and feet, and perianal region. These lesions usually appear in the first year of life, but may fade during puberty and adulthood, which can be a challenge in the diagnosis of older patients with this condition.

ETIOLOGY AND PATHOPHYSIOLOGY

PJS has an autosomal dominant inheritance pattern, with both familial and sporadic transmission. There has been a germline mutation identified, specifically the *STK11/LKB1* gene on chromosome 19p13.3, as the molecular cause in 70% of PJS families and in 50% of sporadic PJS patients. *STK11/LKB1* is a tumor suppressor gene that has an important role in G1 cell cycle arrest, p53-dependent apoptosis, cell polarity, and cellular energy levels.

The typical appearance of a PJS polyp is usually that of a pedunculated polyp with a long stalk. They may be multilobulated and can have a papillary or villiform shape. In comparison to the inflammatory appearance of juvenile polyps, there is hyperplasia of the smooth muscle layer noted on pathology. The hyperplastic smooth muscle is noted to extend out in a tree-like manner toward the epithelial layer (arborization) (**45.4**).

TREATMENT

Patients with PJS can develop recurrent episodes of bowel obstruction, intussusception, and bleeding, which can lead to recurrent bowel resections. In addition, patients with PJS are at higher risk for malignancy, in both the GI tract and in extraintestinal sites, particularly in adulthood. Studies have reported a lifetime risk of cancer anywhere from 37% to 93%, with the most common malignancy being that of colorectal cancer, followed by breast, small bowel, gastric, and pancreatic cancers. There is also an increased lifetime risk of gynecological, lung, and esophageal cancer. Because of the dual risk of complications related to polyps and the risk of malignancy, screening is recommended for any patients at risk for PJS, and if symptomatic, a co-ordinated therapeutic approach is required.

Endoscopic surveillance should include an upper endoscopy and colonoscopy starting at 8 years of age, or earlier if symptomatic. If polyps are noted, endoscopic examinations should be repeated every 2–3 years. Some form of examination of the small bowel is also needed, such as wireless video

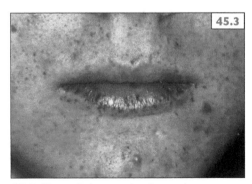

45.3 Mucosal pigmentation in a patient with Peutz–Jeghers syndrome. (Courtesy of Warren Hyer; Paediatric and Adolescent Gastroenterology, St Mark's Hospital.)

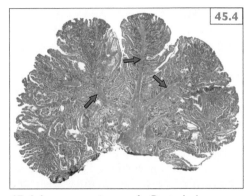

45.4 Low-power image of a Peutz–Jeghers syndrome polyp. The polyp is composed of small bowel mucosa without epithelial dysplasia. These polyps are characterized by broad, arborizing bands of smooth muscle (arrows) that divide the polyp into smaller compartments. (Courtesy of Thomas Plesec; MD; Anatomic Pathology, the Cleveland Clinic.)

capsule endoscopy, magnetic resonance enterography, or barium study. The location and sizes of the polyps will influence their management. It is important to note that endoscopic or surgical resection of polyps does not lower the cancer risk, is not curative or always possible, and it is performed primarily for the complications, or to avoid the complications of PJS polyps.

ADENOMATOUS POLYPOSIS SYNDROMES

Familial adenomatous polyposis

EPIDEMIOLOGY AND CLINICAL PRESENTATION

FAP is the most common of the polyposis syndromes in childhood (occurring in 1 in 10,000 births) and is inherited in an autosomal dominant manner, although spontaneous mutations can occur in about 20–30% of cases. The classic diagnosis of FAP is based on the presence of more than 100 adenomatous colorectal polyps, although patients with attenuated FAP may have fewer polyps. There are other FAP variants as well, including Turcot syndrome (association with brain tumors such as medulloblastoma) and Gardner syndrome (association with extraintestinal manifestations such as desmoid tumors, sebaceous or epidermoid cysts, and osteomas).

Patients with classic FAP may ultimately have hundreds to thousands of adenomatous colonic polyps. These adenomatous polyps begin to appear in childhood or adolescence, and will increase in quantity with age. Patients with FAP may be surprisingly asymptomatic given the large number of polyps, but symptomatic patients may present with bloody or mucousy stools and diarrhea. There may also be extraintestinal manifestations noted, which can include epidermoid cysts, desmoid tumors, fibromas, lipomas, and osteomas (especially of the mandible), which would suggest a variant of FAP (formerly known as Gardner syndrome). While these extraintestinal findings may be benign, it can suggest FAP in at-risk patients. By the fifth decade of life, progression to neoplasia is almost universal in patients with FAP who have not undergone colectomy. Of note, there is also a milder former of FAP, called attenuated FAP, that presents with fewer adenomas (fewer than 100) and has a later presentation as compared to classic FAP.

DIAGNOSIS

On endoscopic examination, numerous adenomatous polyps can be seen which are small, nodular, and typically sessile (**45.5**). These are usually of variable size, distinguishing them from lymphonodular hyperplasia in the colon, which are usually more uniform in size and seen in younger children. On histologic examination, there can be a variety of adenomatous polyps, which can include tubular, tubulovillous, and villous adenomas. The dysplasia noted in all adenomas can be categorized from low to high grade (**45.6**).

ETIOLOGY AND PATHOPHYSIOLOGY

FAP is an autosomal dominant condition in which there is a germline mutation in the adenomatous polyposis coli (*APC*) gene, which is located on chromosome 5q21. In 20–30% of cases, however, the mutation is spontaneous with no familial association. The *APC* gene is thought to be a tumor suppressor gene, and it is thought to play a role in a variety of cellular functions, including differentiation, apoptosis, and proliferation. There are more than 400 mutations of the *APC* gene that have been described in FAP, and the localization of the mutation within the gene can correlate with phenotype and severity of clinical manifestation.

TREATMENT

FAP is an autosomal dominant disorder, and thus many children present to their physician because of a family history of this genetic disorder. In order to determine the appropriate screening, the first step would be determination of which FAP mutation is present in the index case. While there are no formal recommendations for timing of genetic testing in children, in those families with a known mutation, genetic screening of primary relatives should start around age 10 years. In those that test gene positive in a family with a known mutation, it is advised they undergo screening colonoscopy beginning at age of 10–12 years, with repeat endoscopies every 1–2 years, as well as seeing a genetic counselor. Those patients that are gene test negative in a family with an identified *APC* gene mutation have the same colorectal cancer risk as the general population, and they do not need to undergo special screening endoscopy, beyond the standard recommendations for colorectal screening. However, in those families where there is no known mutation found in the index case, genetic testing is not informative, and it is not possible to offer predictive genetic testing to asymptomatic at-risk relatives. These patients will still need to undergo the same regular endoscopic screening as those that test gene positive.

A diagnosis of FAP can be confirmed by finding adenomas on colonoscopy with determination of polyp location and density. This can be helpful, along with the family and psychosocial situation, to help determine the type and timing of surgery. Once a diagnosis of FAP is made, it is advised to undergo a prophylactic proctocolectomy. The only therapy that can eliminate the inevitable risk of colorectal cancer is colectomy. If there is no severe dysplasia present, colectomy is usually performed in the mid to late teens or early 20s. Regular upper endoscopies starting in the early 20s should also be performed, as gastric and duodenal polyps can develop, as well as duodenal ampullary carcinoma, which is the second most common cause of death in FAP patients and is the most common cause in those who have undergone colectomy. Other extracolonic malignancies to screen for include follicular or papillary thyroid cancer, childhood hepatoblastoma, and CNS tumors.

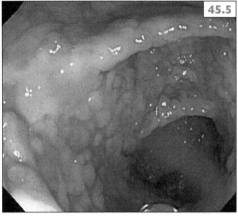

45.5 Multiple small sessile adenomatous polyps of variable size in a pediatric patient with familial adenomatous polyposis.

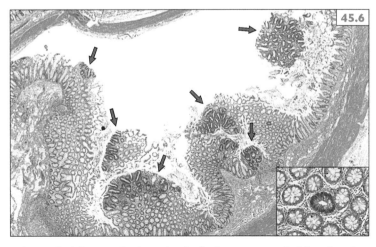

45.6 Low-power photomicrograph of a histologic section from a total colectomy in a patient with familial adenomatous polyposis (FAP). Numerous small tubular adenomas are identified in only one section (arrows), which are characterized by low-grade dysplasia – elongated, 'penciiate' nuclei that are stratified and hyperchromatic. Adenomas begin as dysplastic aberrant crypt foci (inset), and finding more than one of these in a colon is considered virtually pathognomic for FAP. (Courtesy of Thomas Plesec, MD; Anatomic Pathology, the Cleveland Clinic.)

Neoplasms of the gastrointestinal tract

Gastrointestinal neoplasms, either primary or metastatic, are uncommon and often unanticipated in children; however, recognition and prompt diagnosis is important to the care of the pediatric patient. What may appear as an irregular polyp on colonoscopy may actually represent a tumor. Presenting symptoms of GI neoplasms can be nonspecific and variable, and can include abdominal pain, distension, weight loss, vomiting, a palpable mass, and GI bleeding. Neoplasms may be found during surgery for bowel obstruction, intussusception, or perforation, or may be incidentally found during a radiologic study or an endoscopy for work-up for other reasons. For example, Burkitt lymphoma, the most common lymphoma arising from the pediatric GI tract, is most frequently found in the ileocecal region, where it can be a lead point for intussusception or found as an abdominal mass. The most commonly encountered neoplasms of the GI tract in children come from lymphoid and epithelial tissues, with mesenchymal tumors being less frequent. Definitive diagnosis will often require a biopsy for histopathologic examination, and may need cytogenetics and immunotyping. Endoscopic polypectomy of a gastric, small bowel, or colonic tumor may be hazardous and associated with an increased risk of complications, which include perforation and severe bleeding, which may result in exsanguination, as tumors may be eroding through the bowel wall. Therefore, endoscopic biopsy may be a safer initial step if a polypoid lesion suspicious for cancer is encountered upon upper endoscopy or colonoscopy.

Conclusion

Pediatric GI polyps can be commonly encountered during childhood and are often solitary, with the majority of these polyps being benign. However, it is important to gather a detailed family history, particularly when a pediatric patient presents with multiple GI polyps, as this may be a presentation of a polyposis syndrome. Diagnosis of a polyposis syndrome will depend on the location, number, and histologic type of polyps, as well as family history. It is imperative to identify GI polyposis syndromes, as they can be associated with extraintestinal manifestations as well as an increased lifetime risk of cancer. The care of these patients should include a multidisciplinary approach, with involvement of pediatric gastroenterologists, polyposis registries, genetic counseling, endoscopic surveillance, and pediatric and colorectal surgeons. When approaching GI polyps, it is also important to rule out a neoplastic etiology. Knowledge of the various presentations and underlying manifestations of pediatric polyps can help enable appropriate patient care.

CHAPTER 46

Ulcerative Colitis

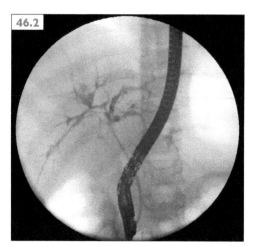

46.2 Primary sclerosing cholangitis: a chronic inflammatory condition of the intra- and extrahepatobiliary collecting system. Endoscopic retrograde cholangiopancreatography shows 'beading' of the intrahepatic bile ducts. (Courtesy of Michael Manfredi, MD; Children's Hospital Boston/Harvard Medical School.)

may develop extraintestinal manifestations including erythema nodosum, oral inflammation, sclerosing cholangitis (**46.2**), autoimmune hepatitis, arthritis, and uveitis. More than 80% of patients with primary sclerosing cholangitis have UC; the disease is progressive and can lead to cirrhosis, liver failure, and need for liver transplantation.

ETIOLOGY
The precise cause of IBD is not known; however, it is thought to be a multi-factorial process due to an aberrant immune response in genetically susceptible individuals and their interaction with a myriad of environmental factors including diet and microbes.

Genetics and the immune system
The proposed role of genetics in IBD has long been an observation of investigators noting strong heritability patterns within families. Twin studies have since shown up to a 19% concordance between monozygotic twins with UC, nearly one-half the rate seen in CD. Genome-wide association studies have shown over 100 susceptibility loci of IBD, of which roughly one-third are shared between UC and CD. Many of the genes implicated in UC control immune functions such as autophagy, microbial recognition, and regulation of both the adaptive and innate immune systems.

Environment
Smoking is a well-documented protective factor in the development of UC, whereas it is a risk factor in CD. Other protective factors include breast feeding and early appendectomy. Known predisposing factors include, nonsteroidal anti-inflammatory drug use, stress, and living in northern climates.

While no specific microbes have been identified as causative agents in IBD, a 'dysbiosis' and reduction in bacterial diversity has been described in the intestinal flora of children with IBD. The role of bacteria in the pathogenesis of IBD is further supported by numerous genetic knock-out animal models of the disease which do not develop colitis in a germ-free environment.

DIFFERENTIAL DIAGNOSIS
The differential diagnosis of UC is quite broad including infections such as *Clostridium difficile*, *Salmonella* and *Shigella* spp., and *Escherichia coli*, inflammatory conditions such as CD, and vasculitis as seen with Henoch–Schönlein purpura and Behçet disease. Other etiologies including allergic colitis, necrotizing enterocolitis, radiation- or chemotherapy-induced colitis, and graft versus host disease should be considered.

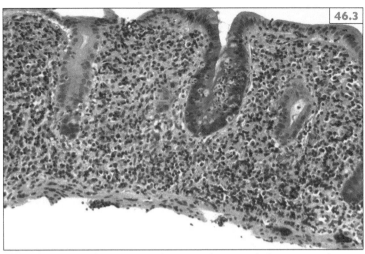

46.3 Superficial inflammatory infiltrate with mucosal ulceration and crypt abscess and regeneration seen in ulcerative colitis. (Courtesy of Jeffery Goldsmith, MD; Children's Hospital Boston/Deaconess Medical Center.)

DIAGNOSIS

When UC is suspected in children, a prompt referral to a pediatric gastroenterologist should be made. Considering typical symptoms may mimic those seen with infectious colitis, stool studies should be performed to rule out *Salmonella* spp., *Shigella* spp., and enterohemorrhagic *E. coli*. Given a nearly 10-fold higher incidence in UC as compared to healthy individuals, evaluation for the presence of a *C. difficile* infection should be investigated. A thorough physical examination and history including family, travel, and recent antibiotic exposure are critical. An initial laboratory evaluation should include a complete blood count, erythrocyte sedimentation rate, C-reactive protein, electrolytes, and albumin which may demonstrate evidence of anemia, chronic and acute inflammation and, at times, hypoalbuminemia and electrolyte disturbances.

Depending upon the severity of symptoms, children may require hospitalization for management of their hydration status, intolerance of oral intake, profound anemia, and the need for expedited evaluation with endoscopic studies and surgical consultation. Bowel rest and empiric antibiotics are often initiated, but have been shown to be of little benefit. Rapid determination of the cause of the colitis is of critical importance and will allow for the initiation of potentially life-saving therapy including medications such as intravenous steroids, potent immunosuppressants, and biologics.

While imaging studies may suggest colonic inflammation or demonstrate hallmarks of UC, such as a 'lead pipe appearance', colonoscopy is the only definitive study that allows for gross visualization and histopathologic confirmation of UC (**46.3**). Classic macroscopic findings of UC include friable, edematous, granular and ulcerated

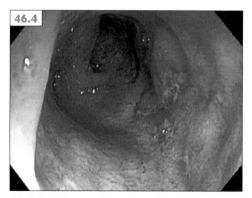

46.4 Friable, granular, and erythematous mucosa seen in continuous distribution in ulcerative colitis.

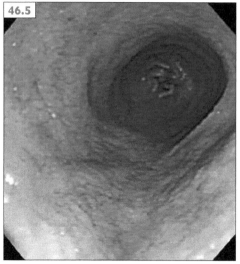

46.5 A featureless colon seen in ulcerative colitis. Note the lack of normal vasculature and haustrae.

mucosa (**46.4**) starting at the anal verge and progressing proximally. There may be a clearly demarcated proximal end-point with a loss of normal vascular pattern and haustrae (**46.5**). In children in particular, atypical findings are fairly common at presentation with rectal sparing occurring in 26% of children and patchy disease in 21%, leading to nearly 10% of cases being labeled as 'indeterminate colitis'.

TREATMENT

Understanding the extent and severity of the disease is critical in determining the most appropriate therapy. A new paradigm in the treatment of IBD is becoming standard where 'mucosal healing' is held as the goal of therapy as opposed to simply controlling symptoms, particularly in the prevention of long-term sequelae such as colorectal cancer. Risk of colorectal cancer is high with an estimated incidence of 18% after 30 years of UC.

Distal and left-sided colitis

Approximately 5% of children present with proctitis and 20% with left-sided disease at diagnosis. For mild to moderate distal disease, therapies such as topical corticosteroids and 5-aminosalicylic acid (5-ASA) can be used for induction of remission. Maintenance therapy can be achieved with oral and topical 5-ASA agents. Given their anti-inflammatory effects, 5-ASA agents are often used as an adjunctive therapy to help prevent the development of colon cancer in any of the UC phenotypes.

For more extensive disease, oral corticosteroids and 5-ASA agents may be necessary for initial induction and maintenance therapy. Disease extension is common and may require more potent immunosuppressants such as azathioprine/mercaptopurine.

Pancolitis

Approximately 75% of children present with pancolonic disease, nearly double that seen in the adult population. For this more severe inflammation and extensive distribution, children will often need to be induced with either oral or intravenous steroids. Thereafter, they may be maintained on immunomodulators, such as mercaptopurine or azathioprine, in combination with 5-ASA agents or as monotherapy.

Severe and fulminant colitis is a medical emergency and may result in the urgent need for a colectomy either prophylactically or in the setting of colonic perforation, hemorrhage, or other complication (**46.6, 46.7**). The favored approach is a laparoscopic total proctocolectomy with creation of a J pouch and ileal pouch anal anastomosis. Hospitalized children will often receive intravenous methylprednisolone as a first-line therapy to help induce a remission. Rescue therapies, such as tacrolimus, cyclosporine, and infliximab, are used in the setting of steroid nonresponse and increasingly as first-line therapies.

PROGNOSIS

The disease course is highly variable, with 70% of children entering a remission within 3 months of presentation. Longitudinal studies suggest prolonged remission in 55%, relapsing, chronic, and intermittent symptoms in 40%, and continuous symptoms in the remaining 5–10% of children. Approximately 20% of children will require colectomy within 5 years of diagnosis with a higher rate in those with more extensive disease. In children with pancolitis, surveillance colonoscopy for colorectal cancer is recommended 8–10 years after diagnosis and every 1–3 years thereafter depending upon findings and duration of disease.

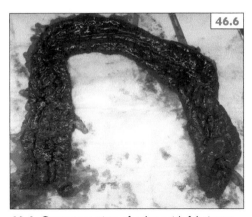

46.6 Gross resection of colon with fulminant pancolitis. Note the ileocecal valve and appendix on the right and the continuous distribution of inflammation from rectum to cecum.

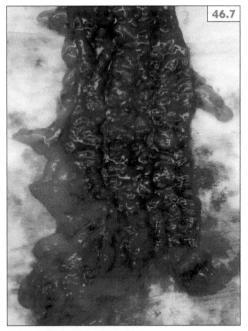

46.7 Mucosa of a colectomy specimen is friable, ulcerated, and hemorrhagic.

CHAPTER 47

Infectious Colitis

Raza A. Patel, Mark Deneau

DEFINITION AND EPIDEMIOLOGY

Infectious diarrhea is a lethal but preventable problem as well as a major economic burden. Most deaths occur in the developing world, where diarrhea is a leading cause of mortality in malnourished pediatric patients. Contaminated water sources are the primary reservoir for pathogenic organisms, making global access to clean drinking water a primary target of public health efforts. In the developed world, infections tend to occur only in travelers or from sporadic food industry outbreaks. Death is rare, and generally occurs only in immunocompromised patients.

This topic encompasses a broad array of infectious organisms (*Tables 47.1, 47.2*) with variable epidemiology, pathogenesis, prognosis, and treatment. A full discussion of each pathogen is beyond the scope of this chapter and summaries of organisms can be found as addendum at the end of the chapter (*Tables 47.3, 47.4*). The focus here will be on general management of the patient with dysentery.

CLINICAL PRESENTATION AND PATHOPHYSIOLOGY

Infectious colitis is distinguished clinically from generalized gastroenteritis by stooling pattern. Inflammation of infected colonic mucosa results in frequent, small volume bowel movements which may be mucoid and bloody. Patients may experience symptoms of dyschezia and tenesmus.

Fever is generally present in infectious colitis. Significant complications are unusual in healthy individuals but can include systemic spread ('typhoid fever' from *Salmonella typhi*), or toxic megacolon and bowel necrosis with viscous perforation.

The clinical picture of small bowel infections from viruses or toxigenic bacteria is classically large volume, watery diarrhea. Complications occur from dehydration and electrolyte imbalance.

Hemolytic uremic syndrome (HUS) is a clinical triad of simultaneous microangiopathic hemolytic anemia, thrombocytopenia, and acute renal injury. Mortality

Table 47.1 Differential diagnosis for infectious enterocolitis

Frequently reported organisms	Other reported/rare organisms
Bacterial	**Bacterial**
Campylobacter spp.	*Actinomyces* spp.
Shigella spp.	*Listeria* spp.
Clostridium difficile	*Aeromonas hydrophila*
Spirochetes	*Mycobacterium* spp.
Escherichia coli	*Chlamydia* spp.
Yersinia spp.	*Treponema pallidum*
Salmonella spp.	*Klebsiella oxytoca*
	Neisseria spp.
Viral	**Parasite**
Adenovirus	*Anisakis simplex*
Herpes simplex	*Enterobius vermicularis*
Cytomegalovirus	*Ascaris lumbricoides*
Protozoal	*Leishmania* spp.
Balantidium coli	Coccidians
Entamoeba histolytica	**Fungal**
Cryptosporidium spp.	*Aspergillus* spp.
Parasite	*Candida* spp.
Schistosoma spp.	Zygomycetes
Trichuris trichiura	*Histoplasma* spp.
Strongyloides spp.	

Table 47.2 Histologic differentiation

Histology

ASLC	Chronic infectious	IBD
Focal cryptitis	Focal active colitis	Focal active colitis
± neutrophilic infiltrate (epithelium and lamina propria)	Neutrophilic infiltrate (epithelium and lamina propria)	Neutrophilic infiltrate (epitheliotropic)
Normal crypt architecture	Parallel tubular crypts	Distortion of crypt architecture
Can see normal crypt architecture/ basal lymphoplasmacytosis	Basal lymphoplasmacytosis	Paneth cell metaplasia
± crypt abscess		
Minimal monocyte infiltration		
Reduced goblet cell mucin		
Edema		

ASLC: acute self limited colitis; IBD: inflammatory bowel disease.

rate can exceed 50%, making HUS a feared complication of infectious colitis. It is an unusual complication of Shiga toxin-producing strains of enterohemorrhagic *Escherichia coli* (EHEC), occurring in <10% of infections. *Shigella* species also cause HUS, primarily in southern Africa, India, and Bangladesh. HUS should be suspected in any child with a diarrheal illness who is experiencing oliguria, hematuria, bruising, or petechiae. Symptoms classically begin 5–10 days after the onset of diarrhea, but can be delayed by several weeks. Antibiotics or antimotility drugs given during a diarrheal illness do not decrease the risk of HUS, do not shorten the duration of a diarrheal illness, and have been identified as a risk factor for HUS in the case of EHEC (O157:H7). Stool culture is not part of the diagnostic criteria. Few children with EHEC develop HUS, and perhaps only one-half of HUS patients have positive stool cultures. This stresses the importance of clinical evaluation and outpatient follow-up rather than unnecessary anxiety or inappropriate reassurance from positive or negative cultures.

Clostridium difficile is a gram-positive bacterium that is nonpathogenic in up to 50% of infants and 5% of adults. Symptoms and complications of pathogenic *C. difficile* are similar to those of other infectious colitides. Outbreaks of *C. difficile* infection occur in both the community and hospital settings, with certain comorbid states (inflammatory bowel disease) and medications (antibiotics, acid suppression) increasing the risk for infection. Diagnosis of *C. difficile* is most commonly done by toxin assay. Treatment regimens include the use of antibiotics (metronidazole, vancomycin, fidaxomicin) and often include use of a probiotic (*Lactobacillus rhamnosus* GG, *Saccharomyces boulardii*) to reduce the risk of refractive or recurrent disease. Novel therapies in chronic/recurrent disease include fecal transplant.

Significant postinfectious and extraintestinal manifestations may occur with some pathogens. *Campylobacter* spp. infections are associated with Guillain–Barré syndrome; *Yersinia* spp. infections are associated with a proliferative glomerulonephritis; and several pathogens cause reactive arthritis and erythema nodosum. Amoeba species can disseminate and cause abscesses anywhere in the body, particularly within the liver.

ETIOLOGY AND EPIDEMIOLOGY
Invasive bacterial and amoebic species are spread from host humans or animals by a fecal–oral route, primarily through a contaminated food and water supply. Over 2.5 billion people worldwide lack basic sanitation, and in the developing world, human-to-human spread is perpetuated by inadequate knowledge of the causes of diarrheal disease and inadequate knowledge of basic hygiene practices.

Similarly, agricultural manure runoff, and consumption of unpasteurized dairy products are sources of zoonotic infections. Flies and insects may be significant vectors to transmit fecal material to food and drink. In the developed world, travelers to endemic areas may become infected and carry organisms home. Widespread outbreaks from contaminated food products also occur with regular frequency.

There are an estimated 2 billion episodes of diarrhea each year worldwide. Precise case counts are unknown as many developing world areas lack reporting systems, and only a minority of nonbloody diarrheal illnesses present for medical attention or have testing to identify an organism.

Table 47.3 Selected summary (bacteria)

Bacteria	Risk factors	Symptoms	Endoscopy
Campylobacter jejuni	Foreign travel	Fever; malaise; abdominal pain; dysentery; hematochezia	Friable colonic mucosa; erythema hemhorrage; aphthoid ulcers (**47.1**)
Clostridium difficile	Hospitalization Antibiotic use	Asymptomatic carrier; mild diarrhea; fulminant colitis	Edematous/hyperemic/ulcerative mucosa; pseudomembrane (left colon > right colon) (**47.2**)
Escherichia coli O157:H7	Contaminated food	Hematochezia	Erythema; friability; longitudinal ulcers; pseudomembranes (right colon > left colon) (**47.4, 47.5**)
Salmonella typhimurium	Contaminated food Foreign travel	Hematochezia; abdominal pain; fever; weight loss	Patchy erythema; exudate; diffuse erythema; ulceration; thickened bowel wall; raised nodules aphthoid ulcers; linear and discoid ulcers (right colon > left colon)
Shigella species	Travel to endemic area	Fever; abdominal pain; watery diarrhea; tenesmus; bloody/mucoid stool	Patchy mucosal edema; pale mucosa; loss of vascular pattern; ulceration (40%); pseudomembranes (20%); lymphoid hyperplasia (8%); patchy hemorrhagic mucosa (left colon > right colon)
Spirochetes	No risk factors identified	Diarrhea; rectal bleeding	Nonspecific findings
Yersinia species	Cold climates Winter months Contaminated food Contaminated water Undercooked pork	Abdominal pain hematochezia	Ileocecal inflammation; erythema; friable mucosa; aphthoid ulcers; fibrinopurulent exudate

DNA: deoxyribonucleic acid; HUS: hemolytic uremic syndrome; IBS: irritable bowel syndrome; PCR: polymerase chain reaction; SMX: sulfamethoxazole; TMP: trimethoprim; TTP: thrombotic thrombocytopenic purpura; UC: ulcerative colitis.

Histology	Dx	Treatment	Complications
Cryptitis; crypt abscesses; surface epithelial damage; neutrophilic infiltrate in lamina propria; edema of lamina propria; capillary congestion	Culture	Ciprofloxacin	Cystitis; Guillain–Barré; pancreatitis; postinfectious IBS; reactive arthritis; toxic megacolon
Patchy necrosis of the superficial lamina propria; massive crypt dilatation; volcano-like exudates of mucus and fibrin streaming neutrophils arranged in single file; pseudomembranous colitis (**47.3**)	Toxin assay	First line for outpatient: metronidazole First line for hospitalized, ill patients, or metronidazole failures: vancomycin	Ileus; toxic megacolon; postinfectious IBS; protein-losing colopathy
Apoptosis of epithelial cells; mucosal apoptosis; combined ischemic, acute infectious & pseudomembranous colitis (**47.6**)	Toxin assay	Supportive care	HUS; ischemic colitis; TTP; toxic megacolon
Hyperplastic Peyer's patches; macrophage invasion of lymphoid follicules; edema; neutrophil infiltrate	Culture:blood, urine, stool	Antibiotics: ciprofloxacin, penicillin, quinolones; supportive care	HUS; toxic megacolon
Mucosal edema; capillary congestion; swelling of endothelial cells focal hemhorrage crypt hyperplasia; depletion of goblet cells; margination and infiltration of neutrophils microulcers with purulant exudate; crypt abscesses; capillary thrombi dilation and branching crypts (**47.7**)	Stool culture PCR; DNA probe; serology	Antibiotics: TMP-SMX, 3rd generation cephalosporins, fluoroquinolones, nalidixic acid; supportive care	HUS; appendicitis; erythema nodosum; leukemoid reaction; meningismus; postinfectious colitis; postinfectious IBS; protein-losing enteropathy; reactive arthritis; TTP; toxic megacolon; colonic perforation
Spirochete attachment to surface absorptive cells but not goblet cells	Warthin-Starry stain of biopsy tissue	Metronidazole	None identified
Early: no chronic changes, mucin depletion, crypt abscesses, neutrophil infiltrate of lamina propria, aphthoid ulcers overlying lymphoid folicles; late: plasma cell and lymphocyte infiltrate of lamina propria, architectural distortion resembling UC	Stool culture; serology	Antibiotics: aminoglycosides; TMP-SMX; supportive care	Erythema nodosum; exudative pharyngitis; glomerulonephritis; carditis; polyarthritis; reactive arthritis; sepsis; toxic megacolon; intestinal perforation; appendicitis

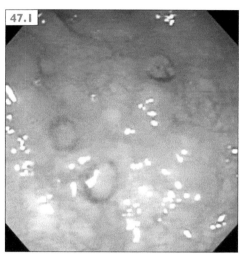

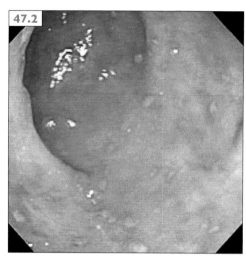

47.1 Endoscopic findings in a patient diagnosed with *Campylobacter jejuni*.

47.2 Endoscopic findings in patient diagnosed with *Clostridium difficile*.

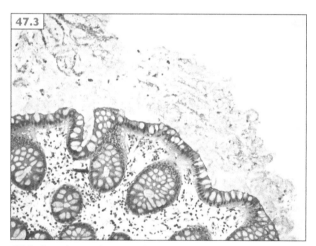

47.3 Pseudomembranous debris containing mixed inflammatory cells overlying colonic mucosa in a 14-year-old patient recovering from *Clostridium difficile* colitis.

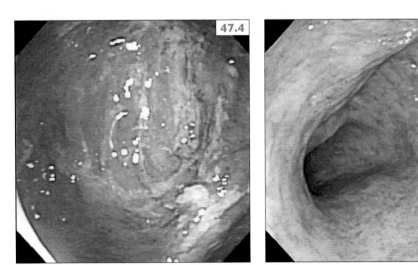

47.4, 47.5 Endoscopic findings in a patient diagnosed with enterohemorrhagic *Escherichia coli*.

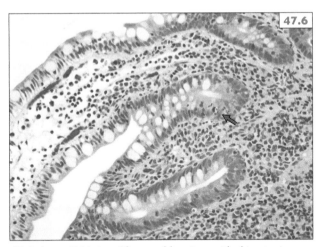

47.6 Acute ileitis in a 10-year-old patient with shiga-toxin producing *Escherichia coli* dysentery. Neutrophilic infiltrate (arrow) is present in the mucosal epithelium.

Table 47.4 Selected summary (virus, protozoa, parasite)

Virus	Risk factors	Symptoms	Endoscopy
Adenovirus (types 11 & 21)	Immunocompromised; AIDS	Dysentery	Nonspecific
Cytomegalovirus	Immunocompromised; IBD	Nonspecific	Discrete ulcerations (right colon > left colon)
Herpes simplex virus	Immunocompromised; anal intercourse transmission	Nonspecific, anorectal discharge	Distal colon affected more than proximal colon; purulent exudate
Protozoa	**Risk factors**	**Symptoms**	**Endoscopy**
Balantidium coli	Food and water contamination with pig excrement	Nonspecific	Terminal ileum and colon especially rectosigmoid friable, edematous mucosa, diffuse erythema covered with mucopurulant exudate
Cryptosporidium spp.	HIV; malnourished; under age 2 years; swimming pools	Often a chronic diarrhea	Focal nonspecific atrophy with small erosions
Entamoeba histolytica	3rd world travel; pregnancy; malnourished; immunosuppression	Dysentery	Deep penetrating ulcers, individual or confluent
Parasite	**Risk factors**	**Symptoms**	**Endoscopy**
Schistosoma mansoni, japonicum, mekongii, intercalatum	Endemic	Rash; fever	Scattered ulceration; inflammatory pseudopolyp
Strongyloides	Living in endemic areas	Upper/lower GI bleeding	Ulcers with ragged margins
Trichuris trichiura	Endemic to tropic and subtropics	Diarrhea; abdominal pain; tenesmus	Cecum/terminal ileum affected more than cecum

AIDS: acquired immunodeficiency syndrome; GI: gastrointestinal; HIV: human immunodeficiency virus; IBD: inflammatory bowel disease; PAS: periodic acid-Schiff; PCR: polymerase chain reaction.

Histology	Dx	Treatment	Complications
Amorphic or basophilic intranuclear inclusion	Viral culture	Supportive	n/a
Intracytoplasmic inclusion bodies; intranuclear inclusion bodies	Urine culture; Immunohistochemistry; PCR	Ganciclovir, valganciclovir	n/a
Intranuclear inclusion bodies	Antibody in formalin fixed tissue	Acyclovir, valacyclovir, famciclovir	n/a

Histology	Dx	Treatment	Complications
Flask shaped ulcer crater covered with purulent necrotic material; adjacent tissue contains lymphocytes and plasma cells	Identification of cysts, precysts, or trophozoites in feces or trophozoites in mucosal biopsy	Tetracycline, iodoquinol	Intestinal perforation; peritonitis
Intracellular but extracytoplasmic position of the parasite bulging from the apical surface of the epithelium	Stool	Paromomycin, metronidazole, nitazoxanide	n/a
PAS-postive staining sharply outlined cell membrane nucleus, central karyosome with concentration of chromatin	Stool for trophozoites; biopsy at margin of ulcer	Metronidazole followed by iodoquinol or paromomycin, nitazoxanide	Amebic appendicitis; perforation scarring/stricture; perianal extension; amebic abscesses

Histology	Dx	Treatment	Complications
Granulomas contain any stage of life cycle, scarred foci with eggs	Stool examination; serologic testing; biopsy	Praziquantel, metrifonate, or oxamniquine	Portal fibrosis
Mononuclear infiltrate of submucosa; edematous enteritis; edema of submucosa; flattened villi; ulcerative enteritis	Stool examination; serologic testing; biopsy	Thiabendazole	Jejunal perforation; emphysematous gastritis; appendicitis
Larvae in tissue samples; edema/eosinophilia in duodenum/jejunum	Eggs in stool	Mebendazole	Weight loss; neurotoxicity

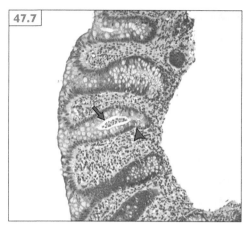

47.7 Acute colitis in a 12-year-old patient with *Shigella* dysentery. Note crypt abscesses (arrow) and acute cryptitis (arrowhead).

DIAGNOSIS

All patients with dysentery should have a complete blood count with microscopic examination for schistocytes as well as serum creatinine and electrolytes, specifically to screen for HUS. Fecal smear for leukocytes, or measurement of fecal calprotectin or lactoferrin level can help differentiate infectious colitis from primarily small bowel disease. However, routine stool cultures lack the sensitivity needed for identification of some organisms known to cause infectious colitis; rather, pathogen-specific stool antigen or toxin assays should be requested based on individual patient risk factors.

Imaging is not routinely necessary. However, a physician is often asked to interpret nonspecific findings from radiographic studies done under suspicion of appendicitis or a surgical abdomen. Patterns of inflammation are generally patchy and may mimic those findings seen in Crohn disease.

Endoscopy is not indicated in the work-up of acute infectious colitis and is normally discouraged. Care should be taken to identify chronic symptoms before undertaking a work-up for inflammatory bowel disease. Biopsy findings are nonspecific. Acute infectious colitis (**47.7**) cannot be distinguished from acute onset inflammatory bowel disease (*Table 47.2*).

TREATMENT

In the otherwise healthy patient, treatment is supportive. Antimotility agents should be avoided. Empiric use of antibiotics is strongly discouraged in most cases and should be limited to high-risk populations and where antibiotic therapy has shown efficacy.

There is little evidence that antimicrobial use will shorten the course of many cases of infectious colitis in any clinically significant way, even with an identified, treatable bacterial pathogen. Empiric use of antibiotics can facilitate antimicrobial resistance. Carrier status may be prolonged, particularly in nontyphoid *Salmonella* infections, which increases the period the patient is contagious. There is evidence that antibiotic use in *E. coli* infections may increase risk of HUS.

All patients need counseling on strict household hygiene to prevent spread of the illness. In any patient with diarrhea, history and physical examination should focus on identification and triage of patients at highest risk of complications. Extensive diagnostic work-ups are low-yield and can generally be replaced with close outpatient observation. Only a small percentage of patients will benefit from antimicrobial therapy.

PROGNOSIS

Most patients who are otherwise healthy will clear their infection without sequelae within 5–7 days. There are recognized postinfectious irritable bowel syndromes described in the literature, however, in which symptoms may persist for months or even years after an acute infectious colitis, despite no evidence of ongoing infection. It is unclear if this finding is distinct from standard irritable bowel syndrome.

CHAPTER 48

Drug, Chemical, and Other Forms of Colitis

Humaira Hashmi

- **Drug-induced colitis**
- **Chemical-induced colitis**
- **Radiation-induced colitis**

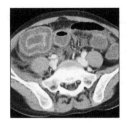
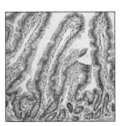
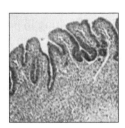

Drug-induced colitis

Pharmacotherapy is often associated with adverse effects in the gastrointestinal (GI) tract ranging from nausea to severe colitis. Many pharmacologic agents can cause drug-induced colitis and only a few such agents are discussed in this chapter.

Neutropenic colitis, frequently referred as necrotizing enteropathy or typhlitis is a serious condition that often occurs in the setting of severe neutropenia. Causes of neutropenia can range from chemotherapeutic agents and radiation exposure to underlying neo-plastic conditions interfering with normal hematopoietic activity. In immunocom-promised patients, severe inflammation that can lead to bowel necrosis can be visualized on abdominal computed tomography (CT) scan or endoscopy. Clinically, a patient can present with severe right lower quadrant pain, bloody diarrhea, and fever indicative of intestinal perforation, sepsis, and peritonitis. Treatment includes aggressive supportive care, antibiotics, and often surgical resection of the involved bowel. Pathology of the affected bowel can have features of transmural edema, significant mucosal inflammation with denuded epithelium, hemorrhage, ulcerations, and necrosis associated with perforation.

Drug-induced hypomotility from various agents, such as anticholinergics, tricyclic antidepressants, and opioids, can disturb intestinal motility through anti-cholinergic activity. Luminal stasis and bacterial overgrowth can further trigger or exacerbate mucosal inflammation. Vin-cristine is a chemotherapeutic agent used in lymphoma and leukemia protocols that has neurotoxic side-effects and interferes with myenteric plexus resulting in paralytic ileus. Concomitant treatment with itraconazole can increase the risk of inflammation through inhibition of cytochrome P450 which is required for breakdown and metabolism of vincristine. Vigilant attention to drug interaction and drug metabolism in patients on chemotherapeutic agents is critical.

Nonsteroidal anti-inflammatory drugs (NSAIDS) can cause severe damage in the stomach, small bowel, and colon including ulceration, stricture, obstruction, bleeding, and perforation. NSAID-induced colitis can mimic clinical and pathologic findings of inflammatory bowel disease. Patients can present with nonspecific abdominal pain and bloody or nonbloody diarrhea. NSAID-induced ulcers and strictures most commonly present in the right colon. Symptomatic relief and mucosal recovery are seen after discon-tinuation of the medication.

Mycophenolate mofetil (MMF), a prodrug of mycophenolic acid, is extensively used in transplant medicine and has known side-effects of diarrhea, nausea, vomiting, gastritis, enterocolitis, and intestinal perforation. Clinical symptoms may improve with dose reduction or discontinuation of MMF. Typhlitis (neutropenic enterocolitis) is a life-threatening necrotizing enterocolitis seen in severely immunocompromised patients. Radiologic findings can support clinical suspicion (**48.1**).

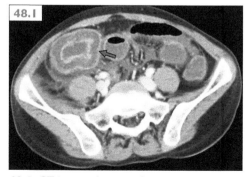

48.1 CT image of a young boy on mycophenolate mofetil with lesions in the colon outlining inflamed and thickened mucosa consistent with typhlitis (arrow).

Alosetron, a targeted serotonin receptor antagonist $(5\text{-}HT_3)$, is approved for patients with irritable bowel syndrome. Ischemic colitis has been reported in patients receiving alosetron in clinical trials as well as during marketed use of the drug.

Dihydroergotamine (DHE), used in cyclic vomiting syndrome, is also associated with intestinal ischemia. DHE has been shown to cause ischemia because of vasospasm or prolonged vasoconstriction. Intestinal ischemia due to ergotamine ingestion is very rare. Multiple cases have been reported in the presence of other risk factors such as tobacco use, thrombophilic factors, Crohn disease, or oral contraceptives; however there are cases of DHE-associated ischemia in adults and children in the absence of any other risk factor.

Docetaxel and vinorelbine are used in metastatic breast cancer. These medications can cause ischemic colitis in 4–10 days following administration. The clinical features mimic neutropenic enterocolitis but not all patients are neutropenic at presentation.

Other medications that can cause ischemic colitis belong to the categories of anti-hypertensive drugs, vasopressors, as well as psychotropic drugs.

Chemical-induced colitis

Common causes of chemical-induced colitis are listed in *Table 48.1*. Chemical-induced colitis can be caused by accidental contamination of the endoscope by disinfecting solution containing glutaraldehyde or hydrogen peroxide. Accidental or intentional exposure to different chemicals, such as alcohol, radiocontrast agents, herbal medications, and formalin, has been associated with the development of colitis.

Patients present with acute abdominal pain, diarrhea, and hematochezia after using enemas with various chemical compounds. History and timing of the onset of symptoms is important in order to identify a likely cause. Onset of severe abdominal pain, fever, and hematochezia 48 hours after a sigmoidoscopy or a colonoscopy could suggest endoscope contamination with glutaraldehyde. Due to inadequate flushing and rinsing, even a small amount of glutaraldehyde can cause colitis. In most cases, damage from chemical irritants is reversible; however, some chemicals, such as soap enemas, can cause significant morbidity. Treatment includes supportive care along with antibiotics, intravenous steroids, and mesalamine agents as clinically indicated.

Table 48.1 Compounds associated with chemical-induced colitis

Glutaraldehyde	Chemical acids and alkali	Herbal medications
Hydrogen peroxide	Sulfuric acid	Potassium permanganate
Alcohol	Acetic acid	Formalin
Radiocontrast agents	Hydrofluoric acid	Soap
Ergotamine	Ammonia	Sodium hydroxide

Radiation-induced colitis

Ionizing radiation is the most common type of radiation used for therapeutic and diagnostic purposes. For clinical settings the quantification of radiation is expressed in Gray (Gy) units with 1 Gy = 100 rad = 1 J/kg. Ionizing radiation encompasses a wide range of radiation including α, β, γ, X-rays and ultraviolet spectrum. High-energy ionizing radiation causes cell death by direct interaction with the deoxyribonucleic acid (DNA) structure, compromising the delicate replication process leading to mitotic cell death. Cellular exposure to ionizing radiation causes disruption in the molecular bonds causing denaturing of proteins and an inflammatory cascade, leading to apoptotic cell death. Injured cells may release free radicals and cause further damage to the surrounding tissues which often is referred to as a 'bystander effect'. The inherent high mitotic index of the GI tract is very susceptible to radiation-induced damage leading to wide cellular destruction and inability to regenerate GI mucosa effectively. Animal models of GI acute radiation syndrome demonstrate significant mucosal changes in the small bowel and colon in response to a range of radiation exposure (**48.2**).

Symptoms can present early during radiation therapy or can appear months to years later. Symptoms depend on:

- Radiation dose.
- Dose rate.
- Dose per fraction.
- Field size.
- Volume of irradiated bowel.
- Concomitant chemotherapy.
- Previous surgery.

Most commonly, acute radiation enteritis presents with vomiting and diarrhea. Symptoms can develop within hours of the first radiation dose, but usually develop gradually during the first few weeks after radiation exposure. Acute radiation syndrome is caused by irradiation of more than 1 Gy to the whole body or part of body in a very short period of time. Its cause is mostly accidental in a nonmedical setting. Endoscopic examination is rarely warranted. Pathologic changes are usually reversible and acute enteritis will resolve 2–3 weeks after the treatment. Treatment is supportive.

Chronic radiation enteritis develops months to years following the completion of the radiation therapy. It is characterized by ulceration, stricture, obstruction, fistula formation, or intestinal perforation. The pathogenesis of chronic radiation enteritis is not clear, but it is thought to be due to chronic up-regulation of transforming growth factor-beta (TGF-β). Diagnosis is based on history, clinical symptoms, and radiologic findings. Treatment includes medical management with antibiotics and nutritional support. Surgical intervention is reserved for strictures, fistulas, abscess formation, and perforations.

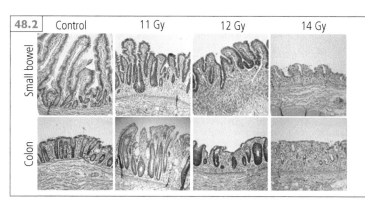

48.2 Small bowel and colon pathology of an animal model of dose-dependent radiation exposure. (Courtesy of MCART, University of Maryland School of Medicine.)

Hirschsprung Disease and Disorders of Intestinal Hypoganglionosis

Adam Paul, Shamila Zawahir

- **Hirschsprung disease**
- **Intestinal hypoganglionosis**

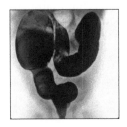
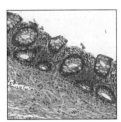
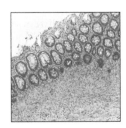

Hirschsprung disease

DEFINITION AND EPIDEMIOLOGY

Hirschsprung disease (HD) results from the failure of migration in the enteric nervous system in the distal bowel during fetal development. It is characterized by an absence of ganglion cells in the myenteric (Auerbach) and submucosal (Meissner) plexus of the affected bowel and extends proximally in variable lengths from the internal anal sphincter. Short segment or classic HD is confined to the rectum and sigmoid colon, whereas, long segment HD can affect the entire length of the bowel. Rarely, the disorder can also affect variable lengths of the small bowel.

HD affects approximately 1 in 5,000 live births. Males are four times more likely than females to have short segment HD; however, as the segment length increases, males and females are more equally affected. There is no racial predilection in HD.

CLINICAL PRESENTATION

Up to 90% patients with HD are diagnosed in the neonatal period. The first sign of HD is failure to pass meconium in the first 24 hours of life; this failure occurs in 60–90% of HD patients. HD patients can also present with constipation, abdominal distention, bilious emesis, thin or normal caliber stools, failure to thrive, and enterocolitis. On examination, the anus is tight, and the rectal vault is typically collapsed and empty. Upon completion of the rectal examination there may be a rapid expulsion of stool and air, due to decompression of the aganglionic segment of bowel allowing for rapid passage of its contents. One should suspect enterocolitis in an HD patient with foul-smelling diarrhea, fever, and abdominal distention which can rapidly progress to toxic megacolon and sepsis.

ETIOLOGY AND PATHOPHYSIOLOGY

HD arises from the failure of migration of the vagal neural crest cells during the 5th–12th weeks of gestation. When mechanoreceptors in the normal rectum are stimulated by distention they activate inhibitory neurons in the myenteric plexus, causing relaxation of the internal anal sphincter (IAS). In HD patients, the affected bowel segment does not relax and peristaltic waves are not propagated. On distention of the rectum, there is no relaxation of the IAS preventing normal defecation. There may also be a variable length of hypoganglionosis proximal to the aganglionic segment called the transition zone.

HD is associated with other conditions such as Down syndrome (trisomy 21), X-linked hydrocephalus, Waardenburg syndrome, Smith–Lemli–Opitz syndrome, multiple endocrine neoplasia type 2, neurofibromatosis, congenital central hypoventilation syndrome, and Bardet–Biedl syndrome. There is a 4% risk for siblings of affected children, and that risk increases as the affected segment length increases. Genetic testing for the *RET* proto-oncogene, the most common susceptibility gene, may be helpful to determine risk for other associated conditions.

DIFFERENTIAL DIAGNOSIS

- Hypo/hyperganglionosis.
- Intestinal neuronal dysplasia.
- Meconium plug syndrome.
- Meconium ileus.
- Anorectal malformations.
- Hypoplastic left colon syndrome.
- Intestinal atresia.
- Intestinal malrotation (volvulus).
- Maternal infection/substance abuse.
- Medications.
- Congenital hypothyroidism.
- Sepsis.

DIAGNOSIS

Evaluation of suspected HD may include a contrast enema done on an unprepared bowel (nothing per rectum for minimum 48–72 hours prior to procedure). It may show a clear delineation between the narrow affected segment and the dilated proximal segment (**49.1**) called a radiographic transition zone, although its absence does not rule out the disorder (sensitivity 76%, specificity 97%).

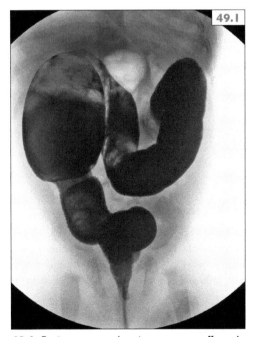

49.1 Barium enema showing a narrow affected segment distal to the transition zone, and proximally dilated bowel.

Anorectal manometry may be used to demonstrate the lack of the rectoanal inhibitory reflex (RAIR), or the relaxation of the IAS when distending the rectum with an air-filled balloon (**49.2, 49.3**). This modality has a sensitivity of 83% and a specificity of 93%.

Rectal suction biopsy involves taking several posterior rectal biopsies 2 cm and 4 cm above the anal verge; however, they may miss the myenteric plexuses. Full thickness rectal biopsy remains the gold standard in diagnosing HD (sensitivity 93%, specificity 100%). Typical pathologic features include the absence of ganglion cells and increased acetylcholinesterase staining with hypertrophic nerve fibers (**49.4, 49.5**). The absence of the calcium-binding protein, calretinin, on immunostaining, is also indicative of an aganglionic segment.

TREATMENT

The primary treatment is surgical resection of the aganglionic segment of bowel and reanastamosis of the ganglionic segment to the anus. Stepwise approach with a decompression ostomy prior to resection may be warranted in some cases.

Postoperative complications include constipation, encopresis, enuresis and, rarely, obstruction, enterocolitis, or fistulae formation. Occasionally obstructive symptoms, such as anal stenosis, IAS dysfunction, and residual aganglionosis, can occur.

Hirschsprung enterocolitis is a potentially life-threatening condition which can occur prior to diagnosis as well as postoperatively. The presentation includes lethargy, fever, abdominal distension, and diarrhea which is characteristically very foul-smelling. Radiographically, these patients show bowel loop

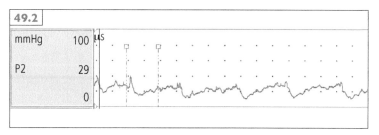

49.2 Normal rectoanal inhibitory reflex as seen during anorectal manometry testing. Peaks in pressure indicate distention of the rectum with the balloon, followed by subsequent normal relaxation of pressures.

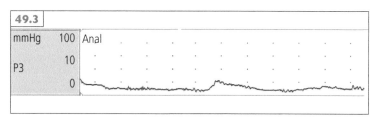

49.3 Abnormal anorectal manometry tracing, demonstrating a failure of the relaxation of the internal anal sphincter following distention with the balloon (the peak in the graph tracing).

distension although it is a nonspecific finding. These children can appear toxic and quickly become septic.

PROGNOSIS

Postoperative prognosis is good, with constipation occurring in approximately 8% of patients following surgery. Postoperative diarrhea and fecal incontinence is a significant morbidity of corrective procedures but tends to improve with time. Enterocolitis occurs in 10–20% of patients postoperatively. However, most patients have normal or near-normal anorectal function following definitive surgery. Though rare, if there is small bowel involvement and the remaining bowel length following surgery is less than 50 cm, there is a high chance of remaining dependent on parenteral nutrition or being considered a candidate for a small bowel transplantation.

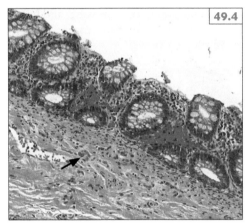

49.4 Arrow showing presence of ganglion cells in the myenteric plexus consistent with normal colonic tissue.

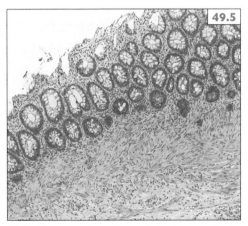

49.5 Absence of ganglion cells in the myenteric plexus consistent with Hirschsprung disease.

Intestinal hypoganglionosis

Hypoganglionosis is a rare entity within the group of disorders resulting from congenital innervation defects in the colon. Anatomically, it typically affects the colon and rectum. It has epidemiologic and clinical correlates with HD, a male-to-female ratio of 3:1, and presents with intractable constipation, ileus, and enterocolitis. The isolated form of hypoganglionosis has two presentations: the first, a severe neonatal form with small bowel involvement and which has a poor prognosis despite surgical intervention, and the second, a milder childhood form with a shorter segment of affected bowel which has a good prognosis with conservative management or surgical intervention.

Hypoganglionsosis is also associated with HD and occurs in the portion of bowel proximal to the aganglionic segment. If it involves a long segment of bowel, there may by residual dysmotility after corrective surgery.

Diagnosis requires a full thickness biopsy of multiple sections of the bowel. Histologically, there is a significant deficiency of nerve cells in the myenteric plexuses, very low acetylcholinesterase activity with staining of tissue, and hypertrophy of the muscularis mucosa.

CHAPTER 50

Constipation

Jose M Garza, Ajay Kaul

DEFINITION AND EPIDEMIOLOGY

Constipation is defined as a delay or difficulty in defecation, present for 2 or more weeks. Beyond the neonatal period, the most common cause of constipation is functional, without objective evidence of a pathologic condition. Constipation has a significant impact on a child's quality of life and on health care costs. The estimated medical care cost of a child with constipation per year is three times that of children without constipation.

Constipation is a very common complaint in childhood and constitutes 3–10% of general pediatric outpatient visits. About 25% of pediatric gastroenterology consultations are related to a perceived defecation disorder.

CLINICAL PRESENTATION

The peak incidence occurs at the initiation of toilet training, but other presentations include the introduction of solid foods and when children start school.

Children with constipation present with infrequent and/or painful passage of hard stools with or without fecal incontinence (passage of stools into underwear in a child older than 4 years of age). Fecal incontinence can be classified into retentive (overflow incontinence) and nonretentive (incontinence with no evidence of fecal retention).

Occasionally, parents may misinterpret stool withholding behavior and report it as 'trying very hard or straining to have a bowel movement'. Abdominal pain, loss of appetite, and urinary frequency or incontinence can coexist.

ETIOLOGY AND PATHOPHYSIOLOGY

The pathophysiology of constipation is multi-factorial; the two major categories are functional and organic. Functional constipation can result from a delay in colonic transit, abnormal sensation, or disordered anorectal function (outlet obstruction). A delay in colonic transit time has been described in a subset of children with chronic constipation and a reduction of interstitial cells of Cajal (**50.1**) and has been demonstrated in colonic biopsies of patients with slow transit constipation. Whether these changes are cause or effect has not been elucidated. Although no definite risk factors have been proven, some studies have identified lower socioeconomic background, living in urban areas, and war-affected zones as risk factors. The most common etiology in children is stool withholding that is triggered by an unpleasant experience having a bowel movement (hard, painful, frightening), leading to a vicious cycle of worsening rectal pain and constipation (**50.2**).

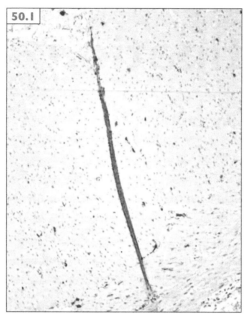

50.1 Normal immunohistochemical stain for c-kit (CD117), highlighting interstitial cells of Cajal in a colonic biopsy.

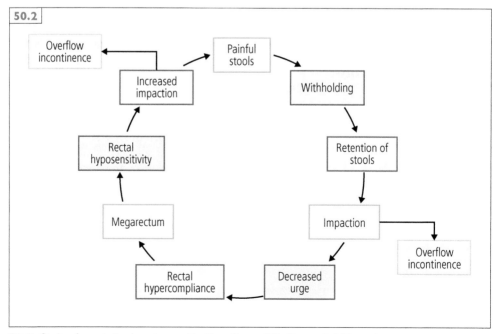

50.2 Cycle of events in chronic constipation after a difficult or painful bowel movement.

DIFFERENTIAL DIAGNOSIS
- Celiac disease.
- Anorectal malformations.
- Hirschsprung disease.
- Spinal cord abnormalities.
- Medications.
- Sexual abuse.
- Cystic fibrosis.
- Protein allergy.
- Electrolyte abnormalities.
- Lead toxicity.
- Hypothyroidism.

DIAGNOSIS
The Rome III committee suggests a symptom-based diagnostic criteria for functional constipation (*Table 50.1*). A thorough history and complete physical examination including rectal examination are usually adequate to diagnose accurately functional constipation. It is important to enquire about defecation frequency, quality, and quantity of feces, pain with defecation, blood in stool, fecal soiling, retentive posturing, and urinary symptoms. The examination should focus on position of the anal sphincter, presence of perianal disease, fissures, stool in the perineum, anal wink reflex, anal sphincter tone, presence of fecal impaction, and neurologic examination of lower extremities. Rectal fecal mass either by abdominal palpation or rectal examination is present in 30–75% of children with constipation.

Testing
Over 95% of children that present with constipation have functional constipation. Testing is indicated when: 1) there are red flags (*Table 50.2*) in the history or examination; 2) when conventional treatment has failed; and 3) to assess better colonic dysfunction and the defecation dynamics. Laboratory tests in the absence of other symptoms are rarely diagnostic. If initial medical management is unsuccessful one can consider celiac screening, sweat test, thyroid studies, serum lead, and electrolyte levels.

Table 50.1 Rome III criteria for functional constipation

Must include 2 or more of the following in a child with a developmental age of at least 4 years with insufficient criteria for diagnosis of IBS:
- Two or fewer defecations in the toilet per week
- At least one episode of fecal incontinence per week
- History of retentive posturing or excessive volitional stool retention
- History of painful or hard bowel movements
- Presence of a large fecal mass in the rectum
- History of large diameter stools which may obstruct the toilet

IBS: irritable bowel syndrome

Table 50.2 Red flags in children presenting with constipation

- Failure to thrive
- Delayed passage of meconium (>48 hours after birth)
- Neurologic symptoms
- Developmental delays
- Vomiting
- Abdominal distention
- Bloody diarrhea
- Anal stenosis
- Tight empty rectum with palpable abdominal mass
- Explosive diarrhea after rectal examination
- Fever
- Spine abnormalities

Radiologic examination

An abdominal X-ray (AXR) should not be used to diagnose constipation. There is no diagnostic correlation between clinical symptoms of constipation and fecal loading on AXR, and image-based fecal load interpretation has high interobserver variability. AXR or transabdominal ultrasound to measure transverse diameter of the rectum should only be used to determine the presence of fecal retention when there is uncertainty about fecal impaction and a rectal examination cannot be performed because of refusal or psychologic factors.

Spine MRI (**50.3**) is indicated when there are neurologic symptoms or symptoms suggestive of spinal cord abnormalities (gluteal cleft deviation or sacral skin lesions).

A contrast enema is useful to identify anatomic abnormalities (**50.4**) and to evaluate the rectosigmoid caliber in patients with chronic constipation with fecal incontinence refractive to medical management (**50.5**).

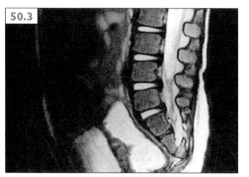

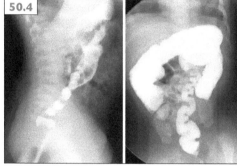

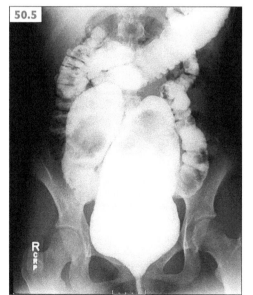

50.3 Lumbosacral MRI in a patient with caudal regression and sacral dysgenesis.

50.4 Contrast enema consistent with Hirschsprung disease in an infant with history of constipation, showing a reduced caliber of rectosigmoid followed by transition to normal caliber colon.

50.5 Contrast enema in teenager with chronic constipation and frequent fecal soiling showing a dilated rectosigmoid colon.

Anorectal manometry

Anorectal manometry quantifies the function of internal and external anal sphincters. In normal individuals distention of the rectum with a balloon results in internal anal sphincter relaxation, referred to as a rectoanal inhibitory reflex (RAIR) (**50.6**). The presence of RAIR excludes Hirschsprung disease but its absence is not diagnostic and indicates the need for a rectal biopsy. Anorectal manometry also assesses rectal sensation and can help diagnose rectosphincteric dyssynergia (**50.7**) which can be treated with biofeedback.

Colonic transit time

Colonic transit can be measured with radiopaque markers. Scintigraphy and wireless motility capsule can also measure colonic transit time but both are still considered research tools in pediatrics. Radiopaque markers are inexpensive and widely available and can classify constipation into anorectal retention (70%), slow colonic transit (20%), and normal transit (10%) (**50.8**). They are also useful in differentiating patients with retentive from those with nonretentive fecal incontinence.

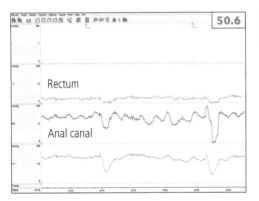

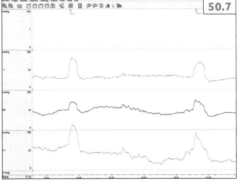

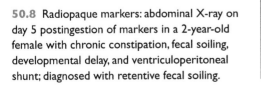

50.6 Anorectal manometry. Presence of rectoanal inhibitory reflex: note distention of a rectal balloon produces a decrease in anal pressure.

50.7 Rectosphincteric dyssynergia: abnormal defecation with increased rectal and anal pressure.

50.8 Radiopaque markers: abdominal X-ray on day 5 postingestion of markers in a 2-year-old female with chronic constipation, fecal soiling, developmental delay, and ventriculoperitoneal shunt; diagnosed with retentive fecal soiling.

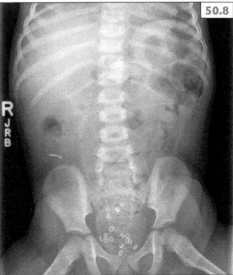

Colonic manometry

Colonic manometry can differentiate between normal colonic motor function and neuromuscular disorders. It can identify children who may benefit from surgery (antegrade continence enema or rectosigmoid resection) (**50.9**).

TREATMENT

To be effective, treatment needs to include education, behavioral modification (sitting program and positive reinforcement), medication (disimpaction and maintenance), and follow-up.

A well-balanced and age-appropriate diet is always encouraged. Advice should include a normal fluid and fiber intake (excessive intake of fiber can result in abdominal pain, gassiness, and worsening of constipation).

A sitting program should be instituted in all children over 4 years of age. They should sit on the toilet for 5–10 minutes: 1) after meals; 2) when they experience cramping; and 3) when parents notice retentive posturing.

An important reason for treatment failure is omitting the initial disimpaction before initiating maintenance therapy. This can result in worsening of incontinence and increase in frustration. Complete bowel evacuation is the first step and can be accomplished by oral, nasogastric, or rectal agents. High-dose polyethylene glycol (PEG) has been proven safe and effective when given at doses of 1–1.5g/kg per day for 3–6 days. For maintenance therapy enough medication should be used to reach a goal of regular, soft, and painless bowel movements and avoid reaccumulation of stool in the rectum. Options include osmotic (PEG, lactulose) or stimulant laxatives (bisacodyl and senna) or a combination of both in certain cases.

Treatment of constipation in children is experience-based and not evidence-based. Little data exist regarding safety profile of laxatives in short- and long-term treatment of constipation. In some instances, this lack of data has led to under-treatment and worsening of constipation and fecal soiling. If patients have retentive fecal incontinence with a dilated rectosigmoid, large doses of osmotic agents often worsen fecal soiling. These patients benefit more from stimulant laxatives that facilitate rectal emptying. Stimulant laxatives can cause cramping which gives a proxy sensation to defecate. These laxatives should be given consistently at the same time every day to foster a pattern of defecation which can be used to time the toilet-sitting regime. Once the vicious cycle (**50.2**) is broken, a regular stool pattern has been established, and there have been no episodes of painful defecation or fecal soiling for a couple of months, the stimulant laxatives can be slowly weaned and transitioned to osmotic laxatives. Patients need close monitoring and families need to be educated and given instructions when to notify their care team so that therapy can be adjusted.

Surgery should be reserved for those patients that have failed aggressive conventional medical therapy.

PROGNOSIS

Constipation is not self-limiting and most children will not grow out of their symptoms without treatment. Persistence of symptoms has been reported in 30–50% of child studies with at least a 5-year follow up. A long-term follow-up study reported that in 25% of children with functional constipation, symptoms persisted into adulthood.

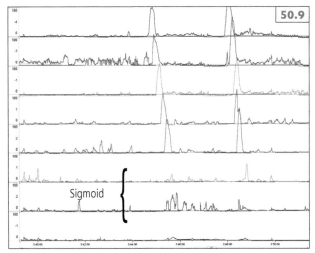

50.9 Colonic manometry tracing showing absence of propagation of high amplitude propagated contractions in the sigmoid colon of the patient in **50.5**.

CHAPTER 51

441

Anorectal Malformations

Ami N. Shah, Saleem Islam

- Introduction
- Imperforate anus in boys
- Imperforate anus in girls

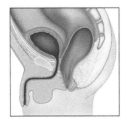
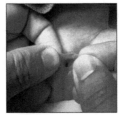
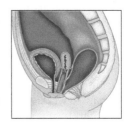

Introduction

Anorectal malformations (ARMs) encompass a class of congenital malformations that range from minor defects to severe defects that can lead to lifelong bowel management difficulties. ARM is a relatively frequent abnormality of hindgut development with an estimated incidence of 1 in 2500 live births. There is a large variation in disorders that ranges from easily correctable disorders to complex cloacal defects or cloacal exstrophy that require significant surgical planning and aftercare. Most patients have good long-term results with approximately a 75% fecal continence rate overall. The most frequent defect in male patients is imperforate anus with a rectobulbar urethral fistula. The most frequent defect in female patients is a rectovestibular fistula.

EMBRYOLOGY

Between 4 and 6 weeks of gestation the cloaca becomes the common depository for the developing urinary, genital, and rectal systems. The cloaca is then divided into the urogenital sinus and posterior intestinal canal by the urorectal septum. The descent of the urorectal septum is associated with simultaneous lateral ingrowths that result in an anterior chamber receiving the allantois and the Wolffian ducts, and a posterior chamber receiving the rectum. Failure of the cloacal membrane to develop posteriorly results in the development of an anteriorly placed hindgut opening. The extent of failure of development of the posterior aspect of the cloacal membrane determines the degree of misplacement of the fistula. A mild failure results in a perineal fistula whereas a severe developmental fistula results in a rectourethral or vestibular fistula. Complete failure of development of the anterior and posterior cloacal membranes may result in a cloaca with a common hindgut and urogenital opening. Associated anomalies may also occur at 7–8 weeks when patency of the anal canal occurs by recanalization.

ASSOCIATED ANOMALIES

Often ARM patients have associated anomalies. Genitourinary tract defects including vesicoureteral reflux which can occur in up to 60% of patients. 10–40% of infants can have significant cardiac defects such as tetralogy of Fallot, ventricular septal defects, or a patent ductus arteriosus. Other abnormalities of the gastrointestinal tract include intestinal atresia, esophageal or duodenal atresia, or malrotation. 25% of infants will also have a tethered cord or other type of spinal cord anomaly detected on spinal ultrasound. The classic 'VACTERL' (vertebral, anal, cardiac, tracheoesophageal, renal, and radial limb anomalies) association occurs in only 15% of patients.

CLASSIFICATION

There have been several classifications of imperforate anus historically. The least accurate is a separation into a 'low' or 'high' lesion. A classification of ARMs is presented in *Table 51.1*.

DIAGNOSIS

When initially faced with a newborn with an anorectal anomaly, it is often best to wait 24 hours to determine the type of anomaly and therefore the type of treatment needed. During those first 24 hours it is important to search for other anomalies. The diagnostic work-up includes an abdominal radiograph, placement of a nasogastric tube, echocardiogram to rule out cardiac disease, a renal ultrasound, a spinal ultrasound, and a radiograph of the entire spine including the sacrum. A urinalysis can be performed to check for meconium, which may suggest a rectourethral fistula in males. After the initial 24 hours, a lateral pelvic X-ray can be obtained with the pelvis propped up in order to determine if there is any air located near the perineum, although this radiograph is not always accurate.

Table 51.1 Classification of anorectal malformations

Male defects
  Perineal fistula
  Rectourethral bulbar fistula
  Rectourethral prostatic fistula
  Rectovesical (bladder neck) fistula
  Imperforate anus without fistula
  Rectal atresia and stenosis

Female defects
  Perineal fistula
  Vestibular fistula
  Rectovaginal fistula
  Imperforate anus without fistula
  Rectal atresia and stenosis
  Cloacal defects

Imperforate anus in boys

Perineal fistula (51.1)

After the initial work-up is complete, a careful physical examination should be repeated at 24 hours. If a 'low lying' or perineal fistula (anal stenosis, bucket handle deformity, midline raphe fistula) is visible, then the infant can undergo a primary repair with an anoplasty without a protective ostomy. If an infant is too ill for surgery, the opening can be dilated with a Hegar dilator until the child is medically stable for a definitive procedure. All operations for infants with anorectal abnormalities begin with electrical stimulation of the muscle complex to determine the location of the sphincters and the anus.

TREATMENT
The first aspect of management is to determine whether or not an infant needs a colostomy or can undergo a primary repair. Decisions about primary repair should never be made immediately after birth because the presence or absence of a perineal fistula is not always established. It takes about 24 hours for the intraluminal pressure of the bowel to increase, forcing the meconium to pass through the fistula.

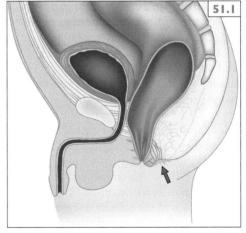

51.1 Rectoperineal fistula in a male anterior to the anal pit (arrow).

If the muscle is located outside of the anal sphincters then operative repair is indicated. The rectum and urethra are located very close together even though there is no fistulous connection. An anoplasty is done by placing a hemostat in the anus and the tissue is cut in the midline to the posterior border of the external sphincter. The mucosa is then sutured to the anoderm with absorbable sutures.

Rectourethral fistulas (51.2)

Classically rectourethral (bulbar and prostatic) fistulas are both treated with a colostomy in the first few days of life at the junction of the descending colon and sigmoid colon. The colon is completely divided with two separate stomas on the abdominal wall. The distal stoma is completely diverted from the fecal stream in order to prevent urinary tract infections or megarectum, and to protect the anastomosis after the corrective surgery as well as to obtain a colostogram to determine the anatomy. A normal appearing perineum suggests a lower fistula (i.e. a bulbar fistula). Flat buttocks with a lack of gluteal folds and an anal dimple suggests a prostatic or higher fistula. A flat bottom portends a worse prognosis for overall long-term bowel control. Usually 1 month after the colostomy the definitive repair can be performed. The operation is a posterior sagittal anorectoplasty (PSARP) and is started by locating the muscle complex with an electrical stimulator. The sphincter muscle is then divided in the midline posteriorly and the rectum is separated from the genitourinary tract and mobilized until it can be brought down to the perineum and an anoplasty is performed.

Some institutions are performing a laparoscopic assisted immediate repair in these infants at the time of birth without a protective ostomy. The laparoscopic approach can identify the fistula allowing it to be ligated with a clip. The rectum is mobilized and the levators can be visualized.

Rectovesical bladder neck fistula (51.3)

This defect accounts for 10% of all anorectal defects in males. These babies have a high incidence of urologic abnormalities and urgent work-up is indicated. A plain kidneys, ureters, bladder X-ray (KUB) may demonstrate air in the bladder, and these infants may urinate meconium. These defects require a combined abdominal and perineal approach to ligate the bladder neck fistula.

Imperforate anus without fistula

Imperforate anus without fistula consists of a spectrum of defects with variable distance between the rectal pouch and perineum. Almost one-half of these patients have trisomy 21. These infants can be treated with a PSARP or a combined laparoscopic and perineal approach.

Rectal atresia and stenosis

Medical staff trying to insert a rectal thermometer often diagnose rectal atresia or stenosis on the initial examination. The outer anus appears normal because the atresia is located 1–2 cm above the anal verge with a dilated rectal pouch above that region. The separation between the anal canal and the rectum may be a thin membrane or a thick fibrous cord; if a thick cord is found these infants will need a colostomy.

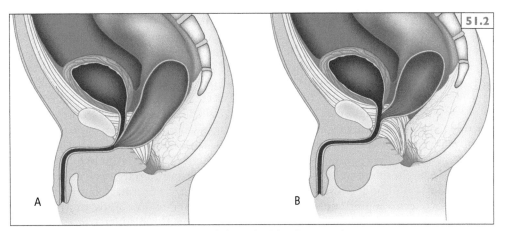

51.2 Rectobulbar (**A**) and rectoprostatic (**B**) urethral fistula in a male.

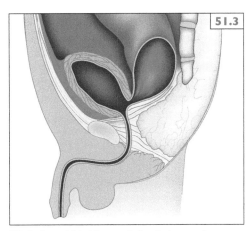

51.3 Rectal bladder neck fistula in a male.

Imperforate anus in girls

Perineal fistulas (51.4)

A perineal fistula is similar to that in boys and the opening is between the anal dimple and the introitus. These fistulas can be variable in size. Some openings may need serial dilation to provide satisfactory evacuation of stool. Some fistulas can be managed with an anoplasty or anal transposition procedure. Normal fecal continence can be possible throughout childhood; however, vaginal delivery may cause significant continence issues.

Vestibular fistulas (51.5)

This is the most common type of fistula seen in females with imperforate anus. The intestine opens into the vestibule located immediately posterior to the vaginal orifice. The vagina and rectum must be completely separated to obtain a favorable result. This dissection can be very difficult as there is no plane of separation between the two structures. The operation can be performed on newborn babies; however, the most conservative measure includes a colostomy at birth followed by a repair in 4–8 weeks. This fistula can often go unrecognized initially and they can present later in life.

Cloaca

A cloaca is a complex malformation in which the urethra, vagina, and rectum all open to one common channel on the perineum. On physical examination a cloaca can be suspected when there is only a single orifice identified on examination (**51.6**). A cloaca is a gynecourologic emergency as there is a high incidence of urinary tract or vaginal obstruction. An abdominal ultrasound evaluating for hydronephrosis or hydroureter is essential. The urinary obstruction may result from hydrocolpos of the vagina obstructing the bladder trigone and the urethra. The obstruction may also cause a palpable abdominal mass. Cloacas range from a spectrum of 'short channel' cloacas to 'long channel' cloacas that need complex reconstruction and may have poor long-term continence (**51.7**). After diagnosing a cloaca a colostomy is indicated to divert stool from the urinary stream. If the vagina is dilated, a vaginostomy may be indicated. Urinary diversion is occasionally needed. After the infant is approximately 6 months old, a total urogenital mobilization is performed that allows for reconstruction of the anatomy.

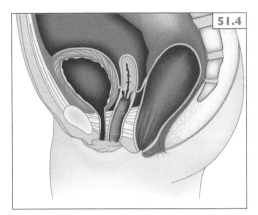

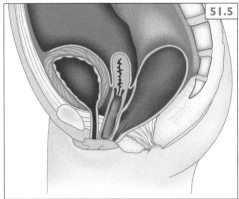

51.4 Rectoperineal fistula in a female.

51.5 Rectovestibular fistula in a female.

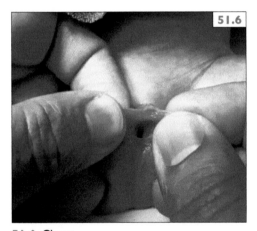

51.6 Cloaca.

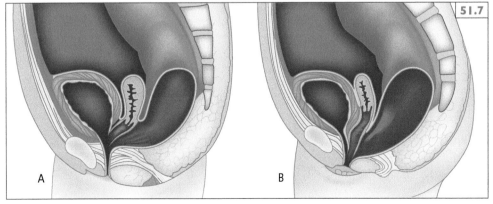

51.7 Cloaca with (**A**) long and (**B**) short common channels.

SECTION 8
GASTROINTESTINAL BLEEDING AND THERAPEUTICS

CHAPTER 52

Esophageal and Gastric Bleeding

Rohit Gupta, Ghassan Wahbeh

- **Introduction**
- **Supraesophageal bleeding sources**
- **Esophageal bleeding sources**
- **Gastric bleeding**

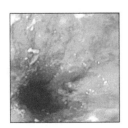
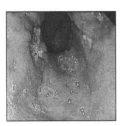
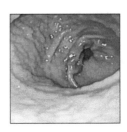
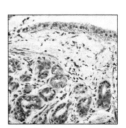

Introduction

Upper gastrointestinal bleeding (UGI) is from a source between the pharynx and the ligament of Trietz. It can present either as hematemesis or melena.

Although rarely severe in the pediatric population, UGI bleeding can be a life-threatening condition.

Esophagogastroduodenoscopy is the initial diagnostic procedure of choice with the benefit of direct access to the bleeding site for diagnosis and management. Swallowed blood from a supraesophageal source can present similar to esophageal and gastric bleeding. A careful nasal and oral examination is important for children with UGI bleeding.

Goals of therapy include:
- Resuscitation, volume and blood replacement.
- Assuring adequate platelets and coagulation factors.
- Identification and control of bleeding source.
- Prevention of future bleeding episodes.

Supraesophageal bleeding sources

NASAL

Bleeding from anterior or posterior nasal passage can happen as a result of allergic and nonallergic rhinitis, trauma, or less frequently vascular tumors. Patients on anticoagulants can bleed profusely even with minor trauma.

ORAL

Bleeding gums or oral mucosa can result from trauma, oral infections, or in the setting of a bleeding diathesis. Local control of the bleeding source is warranted.

THROAT

Infectious laryngitis associated with vigorous coughing as well as pharyngitis and tonsillitis can result in mucosal irritation and bleeding. Hemorrhage following adenoidectomy needs to be considered in the appropriate setting.

Esophageal bleeding sources

FOREIGN BODY

Foreign bodies lodged in the esophagus can erode into the wall although significant bleeding is uncommon. The size, shape, and duration of the foreign body relate to its effect on the mucosa. Objects that can penetrate the esophageal wall, especially button batteries, have been reported to cause catastrophic esophageal bleeding rarely through formation of an aortoesophageal fistula. Timely removal of the foreign body is the definitive treatment. Esophageal button batteries should be treated as emergencies.

PILL ESOPHAGITIS

Direct esophageal mucosal injury can be due to the pressure effect of a lodged pill or direct mucosal cell injury. Common sites are at the physiologic esophageal narrowing regions, e.g. at the aortic arch level or distal most esophagus. Drugs such as doxycycline, tetracycline, clindamycin, ascorbic acid, ferrous sulfate, warfarin, ethinylestradiol, rifampin, and bisphosphonates tend to cause transient, self-limiting esophagitis. Other medications like quinidine, potassium chloride, and nonsteroidal anti-inflammatory drugs (NSAIDs) cause persistent and more severe esophagitis. Management includes prompt identification and removal of the pill. Pill esophagitis can be prevented by taking smaller size pills or capsules and, if permissible, co-ingestion with food.

REFLUX ESOPHAGITIS

Mild, microscopic esophagitis is unlikely to cause significant bleeding (**52.1**). Severe or erosive esophagitis is uncommon and Barrett's esophagus is quite rare in children. Predisposing factors relate to possible abnormal anatomy and function of the gastroesophageal junction allowing more esophageal acid exposure. This is seen in hiatal hernias, repaired esophageal atresia, chronic neuromuscular disorders with anatomic spinal deformities (i.e. kyphoscoliosis), chronically increased abdominal pressure due to hypertonia, and diaphragmatic dysfunction. Treatment consists of effective esophageal acid exposure reduction with medical therapy and possibly surgery to restore the gastroesophageal junction's integrity. Proton pump inhibitors (PPIs) are more effective than H2-blockers in treating erosive esophagitis. Long-term use of acid-reducing medications without a diagnosis has not been advised.

Fundoplication reduces both pathologic and physiologic gastroesophageal reflux but does not correct any underlying esophageal or gastric dysmotility. Children with neuromuscular disorders are more likely to undergo surgery for severe reflux than other children and have a higher rate of surgical complications and repeat procedures.

EOSINOPHILIC ESOPHAGITIS

Bleeding is an uncommon complication of eosinophilic esophagitis (EoE). More commonly children present with dysphagia or feeding aversion in infancy. Esophageal injury can occur due to esophageal dysmotility and foreign body impaction. Specific food or environmental triggers are sometimes but not always identified. Possible treatments include allergen avoidance, esophageal acid reduction, topical steroids, and anti-interleukin-5 antibody.

ESOPHAGEAL VARICES

Patients with esophageal varices typically present with hematemesis with or without melena (**52.2**). Variceal bleeding is caused by portal hypertension which in children is more commonly due to impedance of blood flow in the portal vein than to hepatic cirrhosis, contrary to what is seen in adults. Pediatric data suggest that the underlying liver disease and not variceal hemorrhage predicts survival after variceal bleeding. Risk of bleeding becomes higher as the portal pressures rise (resulting in splenomegaly, endoscopic presence of large esophageal variceal veins and the endoscopic findings of so-called 'red wale' markings on esophageal varices) and the platelet counts and coagulation factor become abnormal. There are no clear pediatric guidelines to suggest the need for screening endoscopy or prophylactic intervention in children with esophageal varices but without a history of bleeding. Priority in acute variceal bleeding is hemodynamic stabilization. Hemodynamically unstable patients should not undergo endoscopy initially.

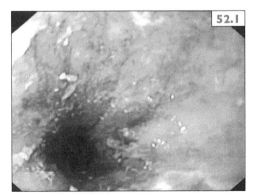

52.1 Reflux esophagitis.

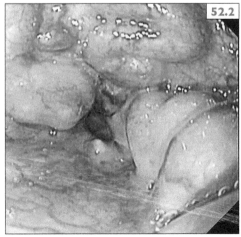

52.2 Esophageal varices.

Medical management includes use of vasopressin, somatostatin, terlipressin (not available in the United States), and octreotide. These medications are thought to work by reducing portal pressure and decreasing the splanchnic blood flow. Octreotide infusion can be associated with disturbances in glucose homeostasis and abdominal pain, but generally is considered both safe and effective. Most patients are also started on PPI therapy to address any concomitant gastric irritation or ulceration. Endoscopic therapy includes endoscopic band ligation or sclerotherapy, both equally efficacious in controlling bleeding. When medical and endoscopic therapies are unsuccessful, a surgical portosystemic shunt can be placed but such procedures are associated with high morbidity and mortality. A transjugular intrahepatic portosystemic shunt is a less invasive but effective procedure to reduce portal pressure. Propranolol, a nonselective beta-blocker that decreases the portal blood flow via constriction of the splanchnic blood supply, has been used extensively in adults for primary and secondary prophylaxis but not in the acute setting.

IATROGENIC

Esophageal instrumentation, for example with nasogastric tube placement or therapeutic endoscopy, can cause mucosal trauma and bleeding. Often this bleeding is self-limited and intervention is not necessary aside from supportive care. Long-term complications can include esophageal stricture formation.

MALLORY–WEISS SYNDROME

This is defined as UGI bleeding from a vomiting-induced mucosal tear at the gastro-esophageal junction. Typically there is history of nonbloody emesis and severe retching eventually resulting in hematemesis. Mallory–Weiss syndrome is rare in children. There are no specific therapies since the bleeding is self-limiting.

Gastric bleeding

GASTRITIS

The correlation of gastric symptoms and macro- or microscopic gastritis is tenuous. Often, gastritis is asymptomatic (e.g. *Helicobacter pylori* gastritis) and does not cause significant UGI bleeding (e.g. Crohn disease of the stomach, cytomegalovirus gastritis in the immunocompromised patient). The following are some causes of more significant gastric bleeding.

NSAIDs

NSAIDs are some of the most commonly used medications in children. Through their effect on prostaglandin metabolism, NSAIDs impair the gastric mucosal healing and are associated with ulcerations that are commonly asymptomatic. In a subset of patients, significant ulceration and bleeding may occur (**52.3**). NSAID ulcers tend to be superficial and diffuse. The presence of *H. pylori* is associated with higher bleeding risk. Moreover, critically ill patients who have a higher risk of gastric bleeding (so called 'stress ulcer') may also be more sensitive to NSAID effects and subsequent bleeding. Although some data suggest that critically ill children may benefit from prophylaxis against UGI bleeding, there remains no high quality evidence to guide clinical practice. Selective cyclo-oxygenase-2 inhibitors may carry a lower risk for bleeding. Patients who are unable to discontinue NSAIDs may decrease the bleeding risk by taking acid-reducing medications concomitantly.

Helicobacter pylori

Bleeding related to *H. pylori* gastritis (**52.4**) can be insidious or acute and profuse due to an ulcer formation. Medical management with *H. pylori* antimicrobial regimen and acid reduction is usually successful. If an ulcer has a visible vessel within the base or an adherent clot is present, there is a higher risk of rebleeding. In adults, endoscopic management reduces that risk more effectively than medical therapy alone. Techniques include thermal coagulation, epinephrine (adrenaline) injection, and endoscopic clip.

Other infections

Acute viral or bacterial infections can rarely cause acute hemorrhagic gastritis. While the presenting symptoms can be severe, the condition is self-limited with low recurrence risk. Severe infections in immunocompromised hosts can cause significant and at times life-threatening gastric bleeding. Examples include *Actinomyces*, and varicella.

VASCULAR LESIONS
Gastric varices

These varices have a similar pathophysiology to esophageal varices. Gastric varices may be more difficult to manage. Cyanoacrylate injection into the varices has been used successfully.

Dieulafoy lesion

In a Dieulafoy lesion, bleeding originates from erosion into a submucosal artery (**52.5**). The bleeding is painless and brisk. Although rare, it is commonly located in the proximal stomach (versus *H. pylori* ulcers which tend to be more distal). To control and prevent bleeding, endoscopic management is necessarily similar to an *H. pylori*-related ulcer.

Vascular ectasia

Gastric antral vascular ectasia (GAVE) is a rare cause of gastric bleeding often associated with systemic illnesses: cirrhosis of the liver, autoimmune connective tissue diseases, and chronic renal failure. It is important to differentiate GAVE from diffuse gastropathy due to portal hypertension. GAVE affects mostly the gastric antrum while portal gastropathy commonly affects the gastric cardia and fundus. GAVE-associated bleeding cannot be controlled with measures that reduce portal pressure. Endoscopic ablation with either Nd:YAG-laser or argon plasma coagulation is the treatment of choice. Partial antrectomy is reserved for severe unresponsive bleeding.

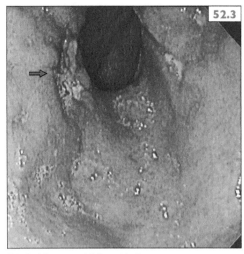

52.3 Nonsteroidal anti-inflammatory drug-related gastric ulcer (arrow).

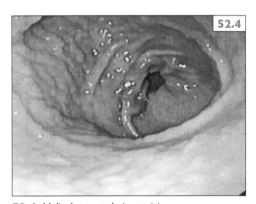

52.4 *Helicobacter pylori* gastritis.

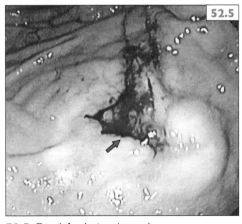

52.5 Dieulafoy lesion (arrow).

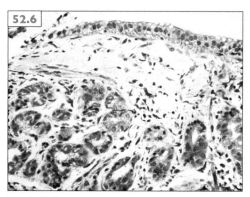

52.6 Collagenous gastritis.

IATROGENIC
Postbiopsy
Usually self-limited, postbiopsy bleeding can result from poor healing of underlying diseased mucosa and can be seen in association with a bleeding disorder.

Gastrostomy device related
Gastric devices can cause bleeding by direct trauma to the gastric wall with gross movements within the stomach such as retching. Bleeding is usually mild and self-limited.

GRAFT VERSUS HOST DISEASE
Bleeding after hematopoietic stem cell transplantation is multifactorial. Severe gastric bleeding from ulceration that occurs with acute graft versus host disease (GvHD) is uncommon. Effective prophylaxis against potential infectious agents that could add to the mucosal injury lowers the bleeding risk. Given the diffuse nature of GvHD injury, endoscopic intervention has little if any role. Supportive measures remain the key management.

COLLAGENOUS GASTRITIS
Pediatric onset collagenous gastritis is rare (**52.6**). Common manifestations are abdominal pain and potentially severe anemia. The histologic hallmark is a thickened irregular subepithelial collagen band. There are no specific standard therapies; management includes symptomatic treatment and iron supplementation.

CHAPTER 53

Small Intestinal Bleeding

David M. Troendle, Bradley A. Barth

- **Introduction**
- **General evaluation and treatment**
- **Congenital and anatomic anomalies**
- **Inflammatory and ulcerative lesions**
- **Polyps, tumors, and vascular anomalies**

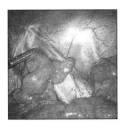
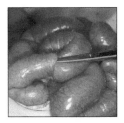
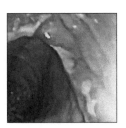
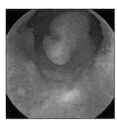

Introduction

Small intestinal bleeding, defined as bleeding occurring between the ampulla of Vater and ileocecal valve, often poses diagnostic and therapeutic challenges in the care of pediatric patients. While the incidence of obscure gastrointestinal (GI) bleeding in children is unknown, it accounts for 5% of all GI bleeding in adult series. This chapter will review the diagnostic modalities most often used for evaluation, and will subsequently discuss etiologies of and therapy for small intestinal bleeding in children.

General evaluation and treatment

Video capsule endoscopy (CE) has replaced radiologic techniques as the primary method for evaluation of small bowel mucosa in children, and it can be safely performed in most patients weighing over 10–12 kg. Small bowel CE has been approved by the United States Food and Drug Administration for use in children 2 years of age and older. The technique utilizes a 26 mm × 11 mm capsule that contains a camera, light source, battery, and transmitter to obtain high quality images of the small bowel mucosa. Ideally the capsule is swallowed voluntarily, but endoscopic placement of the device into the duodenum is easily performed and often required in those less than 6 years of age.

When endoscopic therapy is indicated, antegrade and retrograde balloon assisted enteroscopy has also been successfully performed in children. This technique involves an enteroscope and a soft, flexible overtube which has a pressure controlled balloon at the distal tip. Manipulation of the scope and overtube allows for deep intubation into the mid or distal small bowel. The equipment is somewhat large for younger patients, and the smallest child reported to undergo antegrade single balloon enteroscopy was 13.5 kg. Larger series report routine use in children weighing over 20 kg. In centers where balloon enteroscopy is not readily available, surgically assisted enteroscopy may be performed in children, typically employing laparotomy with a surgeon advancing the small bowel by hand over an orally passed enteroscope or pediatric colonoscope. Laparoscopic assisted enteroscopy can also be performed but is technically more challenging.

Radiologic evaluation of suspected small bowel bleeding is possible with the use of 99mTc pertechnetate scan (Meckel scan), radioisotope bleeding scans (tagged red blood cell scans), or angiography. While tagged red blood cell scans are more sensitive and can reportedly detect lesions bleeding as slowly as 0.1 ml/min, angiography has the benefit of potential therapy at the time of identification.

A proposed algorithm for the evaluation of children with suspected small bowel bleeding is shown in **53.1**.

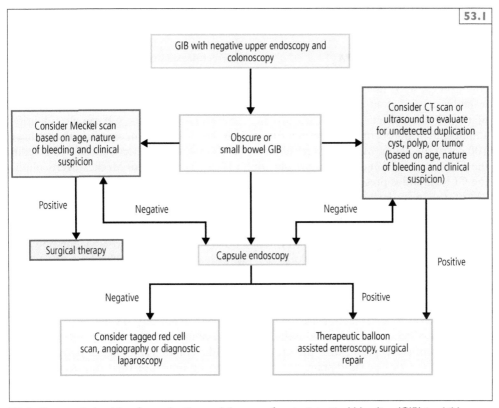

53.1 Proposed algorithm for evaluation and therapy of gastrointestinal bleeding (GIB) in children.
CT: computed tomography.

Congenital and anatomic anomalies

MECKEL DIVERTICULUM

Meckel diverticulum is likely to be the most common cause of small intestinal bleeding in children, and is an anomalous remnant of the vitelline duct. It is found on the antimesenteric border of the bowel in the final 100 cm of the ileum. Meckel diverticulum is the most common congenital abnormality of the GI tract and is present in approximately 2% of the population. While most are asymptomatic, 60% of symptomatic lesions present in children less than 2 years of age, although the adolescent presentation is not uncommon and should not be overlooked.

Bleeding from Meckel diverticulum is the result of mucosal ulceration due to the secretions of ectopic gastric or pancreatic tissue located in the diverticulum itself. Bleeding may also occur secondary to ischemia caused by intussusception, with the Meckel diverticulum serving as a lead point.

The typical presentation involves lower GI bleeding that is often painless. The bleeding may present as occult GI bleeding with iron deficiency anemia or acute massive lower GI bleeding.

Exploratory laparoscopy is the diagnostic modality of choice when clinical suspicion is high or if the patient is experiencing ongoing life threatening bleeding (**53.2**). In the clinically stable patient, 99mTc pertechnetate scan (Meckel scan) can identify ectopic gastric mucosa with a sensitivity of approximately 60–80%. Sensitivity may be greater following the administration of H2 receptor antagonists. CE can also identify a Meckel diverticulum, usually in the setting of evaluating other causes of occult GI bleeding (**53.3**). Treatment of Meckel diverticulum is surgical excision.

INTUSSUSCEPTION

Intussusception occurs when a portion of bowel telescopes onto adjacent bowel. It classically occurs in children aged 4–10 months, with 80% of cases occurring prior to 2 years of age. Usually idiopathic with no identifiable lead point, greater than 80% of intussuceptions are ileocolic in nature. Lead points are more likely to be identified in older children and include polyps, Meckel diverticulum, intestinal duplications, and lymphoma.

Presentation is typically associated with vomiting and colicky abdominal pain, after venous congestion and ischemia have occurred (**53.4**). Rectal bleeding may be noted in the form of a 'currant jelly stool', defined as a dark mixture of mucus, stool, and

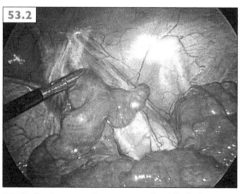

53.2 Exploratory laparotomy for Meckel diverticulum.

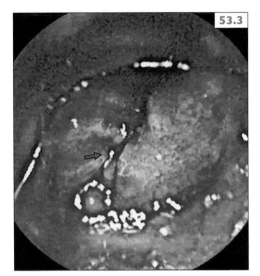

53.3 Capsule endoscopy image of bleeding in Meckel diverticulum (arrow).

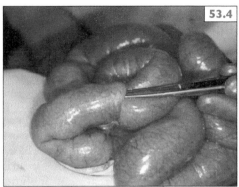

53.4 Intussusception.

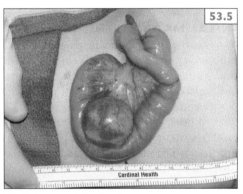

53.5 Intestinal duplication.

blood. Physical examination findings may include a sausage-shaped palpable abdominal mass, or evidence of lethargy and shock if left untreated.

Ultrasound evaluation is quite accurate, but a contrast enema may also be diagnostic and is frequently therapeutic, thus avoiding the need for surgery. Surgery is required for those patients who do not respond to a therapeutic contrast enema. Recurrence of intussusception is reported to occur in 8–15% of patients, typically in the first few days following the initial reduction.

INTESTINAL DUPLICATION

Intestinal duplication cysts arise from the mesenteric border of the bowel, and are typically located in the small intestine, particularly at the terminal ileum. The etiology of duplication cysts is unknown, and they have been identified in approximately 1 in 4,500 autopsies. Several mechanisms may lead to lower intestinal hemorrhage associated with duplication cysts. Ectopic gastric mucosa may lead to peptic ulceration as seen in Meckel diverticulum. Bleeding

may also be secondary to ischemic necrosis secondary to intussusception or from bacterial overgrowth inducing mucosal injury.

Presentation may be similar to that of Meckel diverticulum or intussusception with GI bleeding and abdominal pain of varying intensity, but intestinal obstruction is the more common presentation. On physical examination an abdominal mass may be palpable. Abdominal ultrasound or computed tomography (CT) with oral contrast may identify the duplication, and CE or enteroscopy may also be diagnostic. However, surgical exploration by laparoscopy or laparotomy is definitive (**53.5**) and is the treatment of choice.

Inflammatory and ulcerative lesions

CELIAC DISEASE

One of the less common presentations of gluten sensitivity (celiac disease) includes occult midintestinal bleeding. In this setting, celiac disease is typically discovered during the routine work-up of obscure intestinal bleeding by conventional endoscopy, blood testing, or less commonly by CE or small bowel endoscopy. Treatment includes removal of gluten from the diet. Nutritional deficiencies leading to anemia should also be investigated and are the more common cause of anemia with this disease.

INFLAMMATORY BOWEL DISEASE

Crohn disease presenting primarily with diffuse or scattered involvement of the small intestine is not uncommon, but may go undetected by conventional upper and lower endoscopy. Presentation is typically that of poor growth, delayed puberty, and micronutrient deficiencies. While routine markers of inflammation are variably elevated, stools tend to be positive for occult blood and fecal markers, such as calprotectin or lactoferrin, may be elevated.

Significant intestinal lesions may be identified using imaging modalities such as barium small bowel follow-through, or magnetic resonance enterography. CE however, has a higher sensitivity, particularly for more subtle lesions, and biopsies can be easily obtained from abnormal areas using balloon assisted enteroscopy (**53.6**). Standard therapies for Crohn disease are beyond the scope of this chapter, but it should be noted that dietary therapy (elemental liquid nutritional therapies) is noted to be effective in treating this region of the bowel compared to colonic disease.

HENOCH–SCHÖNLEIN PURPURA

Henoch–Schönlein purpura (HSP) is a small vessel vasculitis that classically affects the skin, joints, and kidneys in addition to the GI tract. The peak age of onset is 3–7 years with an approximate incidence of 4 cases per 100,000 children. Male-to-female ratio is 2:1. The small vessel inflammation associated with HSP may lead to GI mucosal ischemia and ulceration resulting in small intestinal bleeding. GI lesions may also act as a lead point for intussusception with subsequent vascular congestion and ischemia.

Patients may present initially with an urticarial rash on the lower extremities and buttocks that progresses over the course of several days to purpuric lesions, abdominal pain, and large joint involvement. In around 15% of patients, GI bleeding or abdominal pain may precede other signs and symptoms by up to 10 days. Physical examination findings may include palpable purpura on the buttocks and legs, soft tissue edema, arthritis of large joints, abdominal tenderness, scrotal swelling, and occult or frank blood on rectal examination. On laboratory evaluation, inflammatory markers are usually quite elevated. Urinalysis may show hematuria or proteinuria. Standard esophagogastroduodenoscopy or CE is not necessary for diagnosis but can determine the extent of GI involvement.

In general HSP is a benign disorder that is self-limited, even in the setting of significant GI involvement. Symptomatic recurrence is seen in up to 40% of patients, usually around 6 weeks after initial symptoms. Less than 1% of patients suffer end-stage renal failure. Treatment of HSP is supportive, and while corticosteroid use may improve GI symptoms, it is rarely necessary.

ANASTOMOTIC ULCERATIONS

Small intestinal bleeding may occur in children with anastomotic ulcers (**53.7**) resulting from previous small bowel resections. While the etiology remains obscure, the ulcers may occur secondary to vascular compromise at the anastomotic site or bacterial overgrowth. These children typically present several years after their intestinal surgery with gross or occult bleeding, often with significant anemia. Diagnosis can be made with standard endoscopy or colonoscopy, or CE if necessary.

Empiric treatment with stool softeners, low fiber diets, antibiotics, acid suppression, and cholestyramine may be attempted but is rarely successful. Endoscopic intervention is feasible if the lesion can be reached, but long-term benefit of endotherapy for anastomotic ulcerations has yet to be proven.

Surgical resection may be curative, but must be weighed against the negative effects of further bowel resection and risk of recurrence.

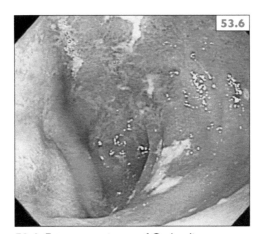

53.6 Enteroscopy image of Crohn disease.

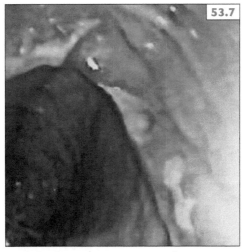

53.7 Small intestine anastamotic ulcer.

Polyps, tumors, and vascular anomalies

SMALL BOWEL ANGIODYSPLASIA

While typically occurring in the colon, vascular ectasias can be found anywhere in the GI tract and may present with obscure GI bleeding. The lesions are often described as red, flat or slightly raised, typically measuring less than 1 cm in diameter. Bleeding may be occult or severe and tends to stop spontaneously, although it is reported to recur in up to one-half of patients. Small intestinal lesions can be identified by mesenteric angiography, or more commonly by CE. Asymptomatic lesions need no therapy, whereas thermal ablation or more rarely surgical resection are treatment options for symptomatic lesions.

DIEULAFOY LESIONS

Dieulafoy lesions refer to abnormally enlarged arterioles coursing within the submucosa which can lead to significant GI bleeding if eroded into. Fewer than 20% of these lesions occur in the small bowel. Presentation may be that of massive GI hemorrhage in an otherwise healthy child. When not found in the stomach by conventional endoscopy, lesions can be detected in the small bowel by mesenteric angiography, CE, or using small bowel endoscopic techniques. First line of treatment is usually endoscopic, and interventions may include epinephrine (adrenaline) injection, thermal ablation, clipping or banding, with surgical resection and selective embolization reserved for refractory cases.

VASCULAR ANOMALIES

Vascular anomalies identified within the GI tract may be idiopathic (**53.8**) or part of a more global systemic disease. Blue rubber bleb nevus syndrome is a rare systemic disorder with both cutaneous and GI venous malformations that can present with occult or life-threatening GI bleeding. Klippel–Trenaunay syndrome is a capillary–lymphaticovenous malformation typically affecting the colon and pelvis but occasionally involving the small bowel as well. Osler–Weber–Rendu disease, or hereditary hemorrhagic telangiectasia, can present initially with obscure GI bleeding, but epistaxis or skin manifestations are more common initial findings.

POLYPS AND TUMORS

Adenomatous polyps (usually as part of familial adenomatous polyposis) and hamartomatous polyps (as part of juvenile polyposis or Peutz–Jeghers syndrome) can present with small intestinal bleeding (**53.9, 53.10**), but frequently the colonic involvement dominates the presentation. Other tumors that have been reported to present with small intestinal bleeding include lipomas, lymphoma, GI stromal tumors, carcinoid tumors, neurofibromas, and metasatic lesions. CE is likely the most accurate method of diagnosing these lesions in the small bowel, but a contrast series or CT scan may also be of benefit. When indicated, polypectomy is possible using balloon assisted enteroscopy or surgically assisted enteroscopy.

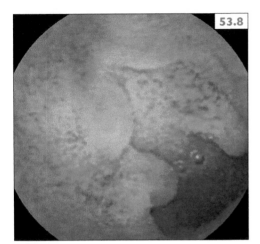

53.8 Small intestine vascular abnormality seen on capsule endoscopy.

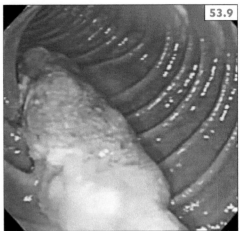

53.9 Polyp seen in a patient with juvenile polyposis.

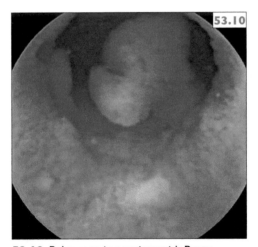

53.10 Polyp seen in a patient with Peutz–Jeghers syndrome.

Colonic Bleeding

Louis Ghanem, Benjamin A Sahn, Petar Mamula

- **Introduction**
- **Constipation**
- **Anal fissure**
- **Hemorrhoids**
- **Solitary rectal ulcer**
- **Infectious enterocolitis**
- **Nodular lymphoid hyperplasia**
- **Polyps**
- **Vascular malformations**
- **Arteriovenous malformation**
- **Blue rubber bleb nevus syndrome**
- **Hemangioma**
- **Hereditary hemorrhagic telangiectasia (Rendu–Osler–Weber syndrome)**
- **Klippel–Trenaunay syndrome**
- **Intestinal ischemia**
- **Other sources of colonic bleeding**

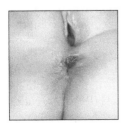
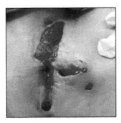
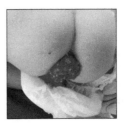
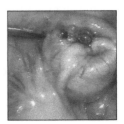

Introduction

Colonic bleeding in infants and children is a common occurrence throughout the world. While infectious disease is the dominant etiology of acute colonic bleeding in the developing world, this chapter will focus on the wide spectrum of underlying pathology. Bleeding originating in the upper gastrointestinal (GI) tract and small intestine, inflammatory bowel disease, allergic colitis, and colonic polyps are important considerations in the differential diagnosis of colonic bleeding and are discussed elsewhere in this volume.

Colonic bleeding has a heterogeneous presentation that can be difficult to localize. Initial clinical management must focus on risk stratification through assessment of volume loss and hemodynamic status. Important distinguishing features include the character and amount of bleeding, stool consistency, stool pattern, systemic signs, the presence or absence of pain, physical findings, and patient age. Hematochezia is highly correlated with colonic bleeding, although it can be seen with brisk upper GI bleeding. Guaiac testing, complete blood count, coagulation measurements, chemistries, and inflammatory markers are useful to gauge bleeding severity and can aid in diagnosis when examination findings and history are equivocal.

Diagnostic colonoscopy in children is a safe, sensitive and often essential means to identify causes of colonic bleeding, mucosal changes, and intraluminal anatomical lesions. Anoscopy and proctosigmoidoscopy have a high diagnostic yield for anal fissures and hemorrhoids, and can detect polyps and colitis, although the preferred diagnostic method for the latter two is full colonoscopy. Wireless capsule endoscopy is an effective adjunct in the diagnosis of endoscopy-negative small bowel GI bleeding.

Cross-sectional imaging, angiography, and barium studies can identify several causes of colonic bleeding. Barium enema may be useful for diagnosis of Hirschsprung disease, enterocolitis, volvulus, intestinal duplication, and nodular lymphoid hyperplasia.

Evaluation of mass and vascular lesions is best done with magnetic resonance imaging (MRI), MR angiography/venography, computed tomography (CT), or CT angiography. Radionuclide tagged red blood cell scanning for occult bleeding is most effective in cases where blood flow is brisk. Direct angiography is a secondary modality usually reserved for selective arterial embolization in the setting of a well-delineated vascular malformation.

Constipation

Chronic constipation is a common predisposing feature of lower intestinal bleeding localizing to the rectum and anus that contributes to the formation of anal fissures, hemorrhoids, solitary rectal ulcers, and rectal prolapse. Straining, prolonged sitting, increased intra-abdominal pressure, and mechanical injury stemming from constipation are frequent triggering or exacerbating factors.

Anal fissure

CLINICAL PRESENTATION AND DIAGNOSIS

Perianal pain with defecation associated with a small amount of red blood streaked on a sentinel hard stool is emblematic of acute anal fissure. In a minority of cases, fissures are visible upon retraction of the buttocks (**54.1**). A posterior midline location is typical. Features of chronic fissuring include fibrosis, skin tags, and anal papilla hypertrophy. Constipation is the most common comorbid finding. Fissures off midline, multiple fissures, and significant perianal disease (**54.2**) are atypical and warrant screening for Crohn disease, systemic infection (human immunodeficiency virus [HIV], tuberculosis [TB]) or other etiologies. Anoscopy may be required for identification of occult fissure. End-viewing endoscopes are of limited value in the diagnosis of anal fissure.

ETIOLOGY AND PATHOPHYSIOLOGY

Anal fissure is a common perianal problem in infants and children that is most often characterized by a linear tear in the anoderm. Trauma by hard stool is thought to be the most frequent precipitating event in children. Several mechanisms have been proposed as potential initiating and exacerbating factors including hypertonicity of the anal sphincters and poor perfusion of the dermal tissue. Pain with defecation often leads to withholding behaviors that can worsen local perfusion and increase sphincter tone.

DIFFERENTIAL DIAGNOSIS

- Constipation.
- Crohn disease.
- Infection (TB, HIV).
- Sexual abuse.
- Leukemia.

TREATMENT

Treatment of acute anal fissure is successful using conservative medical therapy in the majority of cases. Gentle anal dilation can be used in infants and young children to address anal spasm. Medical therapies including topical nitrates, local analgesics (lidocaine, eutectic mixture of local anesthetics [EMLA]) and botulinum toxin injection for chronic anal fissure are effective in children. Recent analysis in adults suggests the benefit of these therapies over placebo is marginal. Surgical sphincterotomy for refractory cases is effective in adults, but can be complicated by incontinence in rare instances. Sphincterotomy in children has been reported with similar complication rates, though its contemporary use is rare.

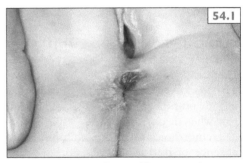

54.1 Anterior anal fissure. (Courtesy of M. Nance, MD; Department of Surgery, The Children's Hospital of Philadelphia.)

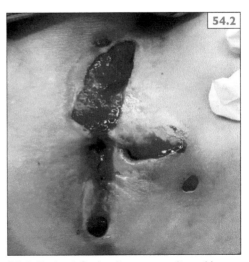

54.2 Perianal Crohn disease complicated by severe pyoderma gangrenosum.

Hemorrhoids

CLINICAL PRESENTATION AND EPIDEMIOLOGY

Painless bleeding with bowel movements is a hallmark of hemorrhoids. Other symptoms include pruritus, prolapse, soilage, and acute pain when thrombosis occurs.

Hemorrhoids arising in children in the absence of portal hypertension are rare, although the incidence increases during adolescence. Up to 35% of children with portal hypertension will develop colonic or anorectal varices, or external hemorrhoids.

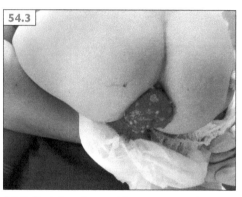

54.3 Rectal prolapse with numerous polyps.

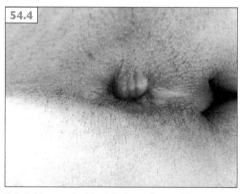

54.4 Hemorrhoid with thrombosis. (Courtesy of S. Tharakan, MD; Department of Surgery, The Children's Hospital of Philadelphia.)

ETIOLOGY AND PATHOPHYSIOLOGY

This network of vessels is in direct communication with the portal system. Straining, chronic constipation, and portal hypertension are risk factors for hemorrhoid formation in children. Rectal prolapse (**54.3**) is an uncommon cause of lower intestinal bleeding that is often mistaken for hemorrhoids. Because the incidence of isolated hemorrhoids in young children is low, rectal prolapse must be considered in the differential diagnosis of perianal mass lesions in this population. If rectal prolapse is confirmed, sweat testing to rule out cystic fibrosis is essential. Rectal prolapse may be confused with a prolapsed rectal polyp.

DIFFERENTIAL DIAGNOSIS

- Anal fissure.
- Rectal prolapse.
- Crohn disease.
- Portal hypertension.
- Skin tags.

DIAGNOSIS

External hemorrhoids are easily visualized nontender, bluish, compressible, soft masses. Clotted blood may be present and associated with tenderness (**54.4**). Anoscopy or flexible sigmoidoscopy can identify internal hemorrhoids. A thorough evaluation for portal hypertension in the preadolescent with hemorrhoids is indicated.

TREATMENT AND PROGNOSIS

Patients receiving supplemental fiber show significant reductions in hemorrhoid-associated bleeding. Hemorrhoid thrombosis is typically self-limited, but pain can be acutely ameliorated by surgical evacuation of clotted blood. Rubber-band ligation and surgical hemorrhoidectomy are effective for internal or refractory hemorrhoids. Sclerotherapy and infrared coagulation are less effective but are associated with less postoperative pain.

Solitary rectal ulcer

CLINICAL PRESENTATION AND EPIDEMIOLOGY

Symptoms of constipation or alternating diarrhea with straining, rectal bleeding, abdominal or rectal pain and tenesmus are common. There are no specific symptoms for solitary rectal ulcer making diagnosis challenging and often delayed from the onset of symptoms.

Solitary rectal ulcer occurs in 1 in 100,000 adults and is rare in children with an undefined pediatric incidence. The condition may present as a true solitary rectal ulcer; however, the syndrome may also present with multiple areas of ulceration or no ulcer at all, and only localized erythema. This variable presentation adds to the challenge in defining the true incidence and prevalence.

ETIOLOGY AND PATHOPHYSIOLOGY

Impaired defecation dynamics and straining leads to elevated proximal rectal pressure, which in turn causes internal prolapse of the anterior rectal wall resulting in mucosal irritation and ulceration. The cycle of straining leading to irritation leading to withholding or more straining ultimately worsens ulceration and bleeding.

DIFFERENTIAL DIAGNOSIS
• Constipation.
• Anal fissure.
• Hemorrhoids.
• Inflammatory bowel disease (IBD).
• Polyp.
• Sexual abuse or anal digital manipulation.

DIAGNOSIS

Typically, laboratory evaluation is normal. Rectal bleeding is commonly present, but anemia is an unusual finding. Endoscopic evaluation with mucosal biopsy is diagnostic. An ulcer often is found within 10–15 cm of the anal verge (**54.5, 54.6**). Retroflexion of the colonoscope in the rectum is an important technique if no ulcer is visualized upon initial insertion. Biopsies must be taken to distinguish between other conditions such as IBD. Microscopy reveals smooth muscle

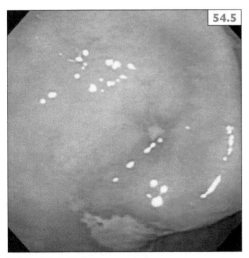
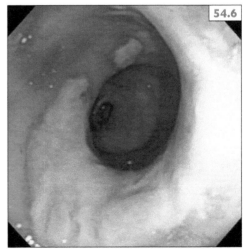

54.5, 54.6 Solitary rectal ulcer.

hyperplasia in the lamina propria, hyperplasia of the muscularis mucosae, mucosal surface ulceration, crypt distortion, and superficial capillary ectasia. The condition can occur in conjunction with IBD and overlap of histologic findings may be present.

TREATMENT AND PROGNOSIS

Nonpharmacologic approaches to treatment include biofeedback to improve defecation dynamics, structured toilet sitting to minimize time spent straining, and decreased overall frequency at bowel movement attempts. Medication regimens may include laxatives, stool softeners, and rectal mesalamine preparations. Endoscopic thermocoagulation may be useful, and, if available, argon plasma coagulation (APC) is becoming a favorable modality. Surgical resections are reserved for refractory cases; however, postsurgical recurrence is high if the underlying problem of straining and mucosal prolapse is not addressed.

Infectious enterocolitis

CLINICAL PRESENTATION AND EPIDEMIOLOGY

Diarrhea containing a small to moderate amount of frank blood and mucus in the stools is typical of infectious colitis. Abdominal pain and fever may be present, although these symptoms often are absent and may not reflect the severity of mucosal injury. The occurrence and timing of upper GI tract symptoms, such as nausea and vomiting, may aid in diagnosis of food-borne illness or systemic infection, although these are often nonspecific findings.

Infectious gastroenteritis is among the most common causes of intestinal bleeding and a major cause of morbidity and death on a global scale. Significantly, worldwide nontyphoidal *Salmonella* species alone cause approximately 94 million cases of acute gastroenteritis, with >150,000 fatalities. The incidence of community-acquired *Clostridium difficile* colitis in the United States has risen sharply over the last decade with estimates of 7–46 cases per 100,000 person-years. Cases of hospital-acquired disease are increasing in prevalence.

ETIOLOGY AND PATHOPHYSIOLOGY

Contaminated food, antibiotic exposure, and immunodeficient states are all associated with increased risk of infectious enterocolitis. Common bacterial pathogens that result in hemorrhagic colitis include *Escherichia coli* O157:H7, *Shigella* and *Salmonella* spp., *Campylobacter jejuni*, *Yersinia enterocolitica*, and *Clostridium difficile*. *Entamoeba histolytica* is responsible for the highest incidence of parasitic infection in children worldwide. Hemorrhagic cytomegalovirus (CMV) colitis occurs more frequently in patients with congenital or acquired immunodeficiency, most notably underlying chronic colitis in children on long-term therapy with steroids for IBD. Pediatric cases of hemolytic uremic syndrome (HUS) result from shiga toxin-producing enterohemorrhagic *Escherichia coli* (EHEC) and *Shigella* in most cases, with pathology predominant in the left and transverse colon. Pseudomembranes, mucosal necrosis, and vascular thrombosis are colonic features of acute and severe HUS.

DIFFERENTIAL DIAGNOSIS

- Amebic (*Entamoeba histolytica*).
- *Clostridium difficile*.
- Hemorrhagic *Escherichia coli* strains.
- Salmonella.
- Schistosomiasis.
- *Shigella* spp.
- Trichuriasis.
- *Balantidium coli*.
- Cytomegalovirus.
- *Yersinia enterocolitica*.
- *Campylobacter jejuni*.
- *Aeromonas hydrophilia*.
- *Klebsiella oxytoca*.
- *Neisseria gonorrheae*.

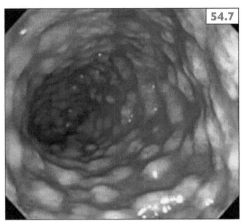

54.7 Descending colon pseudomembranous *Clostridium difficile* colitis.

DIAGNOSIS

Stool culture and examination of stool for ova and parasites are essential. Elevated fecal leukocyte tests are supportive but not specific. *C. difficile* testing with rapid antigen assay or polymerase chain reaction (PCR) is of particular importance in the hospital setting.

The endoscopic appearance of infectious enterocolitis is characterized by patchy or diffuse erythema, edema, small foci of hemorrhage, ulcerations of variable size and morphology, and mucosal friability. Early endoscopy (<7 days) when an offending pathogen is not identified may reveal patchy distal colitis and help distinguish between infection and a coalescent inflammation more characteristic of ulcerative colitis. Rectal sparing is a common feature in early phases of bacterial infection. *C. difficile* colitis is highly correlated with the presence of colonic pseudomembranes (**54.7**). Acute inflammation is typical of infectious enterocolitis on histologic examination. Tissue biopsies may demonstrate viral cytopathic effect or parasitic infection.

TREATMENT AND PROGNOSIS

Bacterial enterocolitis is a self-limited disease in most instances. Targeted antimicrobial therapy is often necessary for immunocompromised patients, CMV colitis, and in cases of parasitic infection. *C. difficile* colitis mandates antibiotic therapy and may require chronic antibiotic prophylaxis for frequent recurrence. Endoscopic administration of fecal transplantation therapy for intractable *C. difficile* infection has shown promise, though standardized protocols have not been adopted.

Nodular lymphoid hyperplasia

CLINICAL PRESENTATION AND EPIDEMIOLOGY

Isolated colonic nodular lymphoid hyperplasia (NLH) is found in patients undergoing colonoscopy for chronic or recurrent abdominal pain, constipation, diarrhea, bloody diarrhea, growth retardation, and chronic vomiting. A self-reported food intolerance or history of food hypersensitivity is often present.

NLH is found in up to 32% of children undergoing colonoscopy and is most common in children under 7 years of age.

ETIOLOGY AND PATHOPHYSIOLOGY

Though common, the etiology of NLH remains a subject of active debate. In the majority of cases, NLH is a benign condition. Allergic response to food is the most often cited pathologic mechanism. Infection and immunoglobulin deficient states are other suspected causes. Akin to Peyer's patches of the terminal ileum, NLH consists of lymphoid follicles that arise within the mucosa or span the mucosa and submucosa. NLH can distort the surface architecture of the colonic mucosa and increase the risk of localized bleeding. NLH can act as a lead point in cases of ileocolonic or colocolonic intussusception.

DIFFERENTIAL DIAGNOSIS

- Benign finding.
- Food hypersensitivity (cow's milk protein).
- Immunoglobulin (Ig) A deficiency.
- Common variable immunodeficiency.
- Viral infection:
  - CMV.
  - Epstein–Barr virus.
  - HIV
  - Human T-lymphotropic virus.
- *Yersinia enterocolitica*.
- Giardiasis.
- Juvenile idiopathic arthritis.

DIAGNOSIS

The endoscopic appearance of NLH is clusters of extruding mucosal lymphoid follicles, pale to yellow in color with each up to 2 mm in diameter (**54.8**) (at least half the diameter of a fully open biopsy forceps). Mucosal thinning with ulceration above lymphoid clusters on histology can be seen in the setting of hematochezia. NLH may be evident on barium enema or small bowel series.

TREATMENT

Evaluation for infection and immunodeficiency is justified in cases where allergic testing and elimination diet with antigen challenge has not implicated NLH as a cause of colonic bleeding.

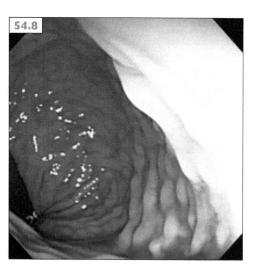

54.8

54.8 Rectal nodular lymphoid hyperplasia, retroflexed view.

Polyps

Polyps are covered in greater detail in Chapter 45. Briefly, colonic polyps have been found in approximately 6% of children undergoing colonoscopy for any indication and 12% for those with lower GI bleeding. Solitary juvenile polyps do not carry increased risk for malignant transformation. The hamartomatous polyposis syndromes, such as juvenile polyposis syndrome, Peutz–Jeghers syndrome, and Cowden syndrome, involve multiple polyps with genetic mutations underlying their development and carry an increased risk of malignancy. Adenomatous polyps are present in familial adenomatous polyposis which carries 100% risk of malignancy by the fifth decade of life (**54.9**). Children with colonic polyps are typically well appearing, with a complaint of painless rectal bleeding. Other symptoms may include abdominal pain or rectal prolapse of the polyp. Bleeding occurs from the friability of the polyp mucosa or from the base after the polyp outgrows its blood supply and auto-amputates (**54.10**). Colonoscopy should be performed if a polyp is suspected for diagnostic and therapeutic purposes. Flexible sigmoidoscopy is inadequate as a significant minority of polyps will be in the right colon. A solitary juvenile polyp carries an excellent prognosis, as polypectomy is often curative. The prognosis is variable for the polyposis syndromes, as each carries its own malignant transformation risk over time and the need for serial colonoscopic evaluations.

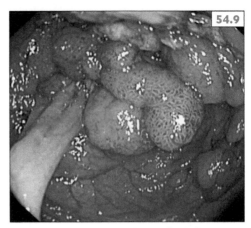

54.9 Multiple colonic polyps in familial adenomatous polyposis. (Courtesy of Z. Djuric, MD; Department of Gastroenterology, Children's Hospital, Nis, Serbia.)

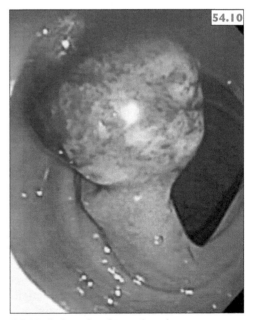

54.10 Pedunculated juvenile polyp.

Vascular malformations

Vascular lesions of the colon are uncommon and can occur as isolated malformations or in association with several well-described syndromes. Comprehensive classification schemes distinguish vascular lesions based upon vessel subtype (capillary, lymphatic, venous, arterial) and more broadly as tumors or malformations.

Esophagogastroduodenoscopy, colonoscopy, and video capsule endoscopy are an effective means of visualizing GI lesions. Endoscopic ultrasound can characterize the extent of bowel wall involvement. The endoscopic appearance of colonic vascular lesions is heterogeneous, and biopsy is not recommended. Flat or slightly raised lesions ranging from punctate to several centimeters in diameter can be arborized and vary in shade from red to venous blue. Mass lesions are most frequently associated with hemangiomas. The appearance of concurrent cutaneous lesions should raise suspicion for syndromes that affect both the skin and GI tract such as hereditary hemorrhagic telangiectasia, blue rubber bleb nevus syndrome, and others.

Endoscopic classification systems have been proposed. MRI sequences for angiography and venography with contrast are the most sensitive imaging modalities. Once identified, direct angiography of lesions provides optimal spatial resolution that can guide selective vessel embolization or complement surgical approaches. Thermal coagulation is the primary endoscopic treatment modality. Bipolar, laser, and argon plasma-based devices are effective (**54.11**), though comprehensive studies are limited by the low incidence of GI vascular lesions. Dieulafoy and other arteriolar or pulsatile lesions may require clipping or banding. Medical management is variable and etiology driven. Antiangiogenic therapy is of limited value in most instances. Surgical resection is frequently required for definitive treatment.

Arteriovenous malformation

DEFINITION AND EPIDEMIOLOGY

An arteriovenous malformation (AVM) is an anomaly of vascular morphology that shunts blood directly from the arterial to venous system. Congenital and acquired AVMs are described. Determining the incidence of intestinal AVM in children is difficult as many lesions remain asymptomatic or only become symptomatic in adulthood. A Dieulafoy lesion is a unique arteriole malformation characterized by a large tortuous submucosal arteriole that does not divide into a normal capillary bed, and may erode through a defect in the overlying mucosa. The lesion is classically found in the lesser curvature of the stomach (**54.12**), but has been described in the small intestine and colon.

CLINICAL PRESENTATION

AVMs are often clinically silent until lower GI hemorrhage occurs. Occult bleeding and anemia, intussusception, and intestinal obstruction are potential outcomes depending on the location of the lesion. AVMs may occur in the stomach (**54.13**), small bowel, or colon. In adults, the most common location is the cecum and right colon. In children, AVMs are found in increased frequency in the small bowel, stomach, and rectum. On physical examination, a bruit may be audible on auscultation. A palpable abdominal mass is unlikely. Of importance, Turner syndrome is associated with intestinal vascular ectasias (incidence ~7%). Therefore, colonic bleeding in female patients with phenotypic stigmata of Turner syndrome (short stature, webbed neck, broad-based chest, and pubertal delay) mandate referral for further genetic evaluation.

ETIOLOGY AND PATHOPHYSIOLOGY

The pathogenesis of AVMs is unknown. Congenital lesions are hypothesized to stem from aberrant vascular endothelial growth

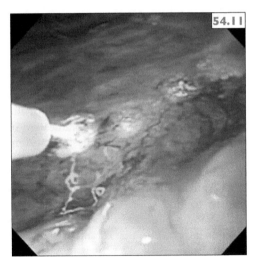

54.11 Argon plasma coagulation of diffuse radiation proctitis. (Courtesy of M. Kochman, MD; Department of Medicine, Hospital University of Pennsylvania.)

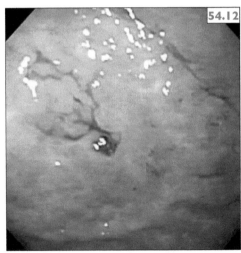

54.12 Gastric Dieulafoy lesion. (Courtesy of M. Kochman, MD; Department of Medicine, Hospital University of Pennsylvania.)

factor (VEGF) and transforming growth factor-beta (TGF-β) signaling events that result in a disordered vascular network and underdeveloped capillary bed. Alternatively, acquired lesions may develop from initially normal vessels inappropriately responding to hormonal changes during puberty or during faulty repair following local trauma. In contrast to slow-flow venous or capillary malformations, an AVM is a high-flow lesion at much higher risk for severe hemorrhage. AVMs may increase in size as children grow, infiltrating the mucosa prior to an acute bleed.

DIFFERENTIAL DIAGNOSIS

- Other vascular ectasias: venous or capillary malformations.
- Intestinal hemangioma.
- Blue rubber bleb nevus syndrome.
- Hereditary hemorrhagic telangiectasia.
- Meckel diverticulum.
- Polyarteritis nodosa.
- Fibromuscular dysplasia.
- Turner syndrome.

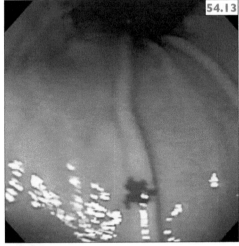

54.13 Gastric arteriovenous malformation. (Courtesy of M. Kochman, MD; Department of Medicine, Hospital University of Pennsylvania.)

DIAGNOSIS

Cross-sectional imaging is often diagnostic. Both CT angiogram and MR angiogram provide the necessary vascular details to make the diagnosis. Angiography remains the gold standard to confirm the diagnosis, but is more invasive with increased risk of complication. Colonoscopy may be used to confirm after a lesion is defined with an imaging study or as the primary test of choice for diagnosis and treatment in a patient with active lower GI bleeding.

TREATMENT

Management is often determined by the location and size of the AVM and if active bleeding is causing hemodynamic instability. Gastric and colonic AVMs are more amenable to endoscopic injection therapy, thermocoagulation, and/or hemostatic clips. Small bowel lesions may be treated endoscopically if single or double balloon enteroscopy is available. Angiographic embolization carries greater risk of bowel necrosis and is generally less preferred if an endoscopic treatment is feasible. Lesions too large for endoscopic therapy or those that cannot be reached by standard endoscopy may need surgical resection (**54.14**). Case series support the use of estrogen supplementation therapy for bleeding vascular ectasias in children with Turner syndrome.

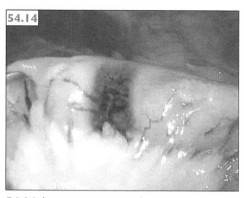

54.14 Laparoscopic view of arteriovenous malformation in the distal jejunum. (Courtesy of T. Blinman, MD; Department of Surgery, The Children's Hospital of Philadelphia.)

Blue rubber bleb nevus syndrome

ETIOLOGY, EPIDEMIOLOGY, AND PATHOPHYSIOLOGY

The cause of blue rubber bleb nevus syndrome (BRBNS) is unknown, with the majority of cases occurring sporadically. An aberrant process in angiogenesis including VEGF dysregulation is thought to play a central role. The condition is characterized by venous malformations of various sizes mostly found in the skin and GI tract, but BRBNS can affect other organs. The skin lesions have a bluish color and are soft and compressible giving its rubbery appearance. The skin lesions are typically of cosmetic importance and do not bleed or cause pain. The upper and lower GI tract can harbor the venous malformations that frequently cause occult or frank chronic rectal bleeding. Severe hemorrhage is less common.

BRBNS is rare with an undefined incidence. Over 200 cases are reported in the literature.

DIFFERENTIAL DIAGNOSIS
- Vascular anomalies:
  - Hemangiomas.
  - Klippel–Trenaunay syndrome.
  - Proteus syndrome.
  - Hereditary hemorrhagic telangiectasia (Rendu–Osler–Weber syndrome).
- Meckel diverticulum.
- Polyposis syndromes.

DIAGNOSIS

The diagnosis is made on clinical grounds based on detection of the characteristic blue lesions in the skin and GI tract on endoscopy and colonoscopy, supported by the finding of anemia (**54.15–54.17**). Cross-sectional imaging may be a useful adjunct in detecting the vascular lesions in the GI tract and other organs, with MRI being more sensitive than CT for detection of venous malformations.

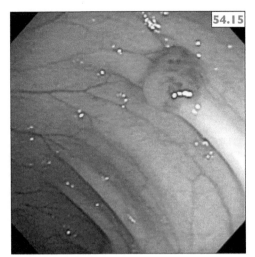

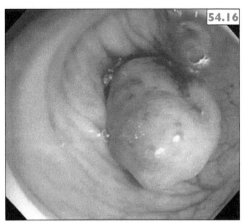

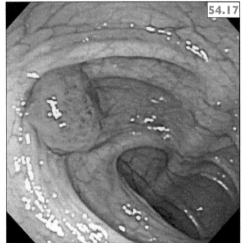

54.15–54.17 Characteristic venous lesions of blue rubber bleb nevus syndrome. (52.15, 52.17 courtesy of M. Kochman, MD; Department of Medicine, Hospital University of Pennsylvania.)

TREATMENT

Management of BRBNS depends on symptom severity. Iron deficiency anemia is commonplace and chronic iron supplementation with periodic red blood cell transfusions may be enough to maintain clinical stability for many years. If transfusion requirements are frequent, endoscopic treatment of individual vascular lesions is often necessary to slow the rate of bleeding. Electrocoagulation with APC is a useful technique in treatment of vascular lesions. APC delivers a monopolar current of argon gas without making probe contact with the tissue, leading to tissue coagulation and hemostasis. However, some of these lesions are deep enough to go through the bowel wall, increasing the risk of perforation. Some authors advocate definitive and complete surgical resection of these lesions regardless of their number, sometimes needing to be done in multiple staged surgeries. Laser photocoagulation is being actively studied in treatment of vascular ectasia, but is not yet a standard therapy in pediatrics. Recent reports suggest oral siroliums (rapamycin) may have a beneficial effect as an antiangiogenic agent that slows the development of progressive venous malformations. Corticosteroids have not been shown to be of benefit in this condition.

Hemangioma

CLINICAL PRESENTATION AND EPIDEMIOLOGY

When located in the GI tract, hemangiomas are often isolated to an intestinal segment, rather than consisting of disseminated lesions along a great length of bowel which is a characteristic of intestinal hemangiomatosis. When clinically apparent, the presentation is invariably lower GI bleeding and anemia, both of which can be profound. Rarely, hemangiomas can cause obstruction, perforation, or act as an intussusception lead point.

Intestinal hemangiomas are rare and usually occur in conjunction with a large segmental cutaneous hemangioma or PHACE (posterior fossa abnormalities, hemangioma of the cervical facial region, arterial cerebrovascular anomalies, cardia defects, eye anomalies) syndrome rather than as isolated bowel lesions. Due to inconsistent vascular tumor and malformation nomenclature, estimating the incidence is challenging. A true hemangioma refers to the infantile hemangioma, which is the most common tumor of infancy, with the vast majority being cutaneous. A cavernous hemangioma represents a separate vascular malformation characterized by large blood-filled sinuses lined by endothelium and is not a true hemangioma.

ETIOLOGY AND PATHOPHYSIOLOGY

The cause of infantile hemangiomas is unclear. Current hypotheses suggest that disordered *in utero* signaling of angiogenic factors, such as fibroblast growth factor (FGF) and VEGF, leads to abnormal endothelial proliferation. Most will proliferate during infancy and involute toward the end of the first year of life. Those that do not self-resolve continue to proliferate, eventually becoming symptomatic.

DIFFERENTIAL DIAGNOSIS

- Other vascular malformations in the GI tract.
- Meckel diverticulum.
- Bleeding esophageal or rectal varices.
- Polyp.
- Dieulafoy lesion.

DIAGNOSIS

The diagnosis is suspected when a child with a current or past history of a cutaneous hemangioma presents with GI bleeding. Cross-sectional imaging with CT or MR angiography will detail a vascular mass within the bowel wall. Upper and lower endoscopy may locate the lesion; however, the most common location for an intestinal infantile hemangioma is the jejunum out of the reach of standard endoscopes, with the rectosigmoid region being the most common colonic location. When bleeding is active, a technetium labeled red blood cell scan may be useful in localizing an isolated vascular lesion.

TREATMENT AND PROGNOSIS

Propanolol is becoming the treatment of choice for cutaneous hemangiomas. Its use in intestinal hemangiomas is not well studied but may be considered in appropriate settings. Thermocoagulation and endoscopic clips may be considered to address active bleeding. Segmental bowel resection is often required and is curative if the lesion can be completely removed.

Hereditary hemorrhagic telangiectasia (Rendu–Osler–Weber syndrome)

DEFINITION AND EPIDEMIOLOGY
Also known as Rendu–Osler–Weber syndrome, hereditary hemorrhagic telangiectasia (HHT) is an autosomal dominant vascular dysplasia associated with gene defects in endoglin (type I) and activin receptor–like kinase-1 (ALK1) (type 2). Fragile vessel walls are prone to hemorrhage and range in presentation from dilated microvasculature to AVMs. HHT is more prevalent than previously thought, and current evidence suggests an incidence of 1:5000–1:16,500, with the highest incidence in the Afro-Caribbean populations. Penetrance is age-related.

CLINICAL PRESENTATION
Telangiectasias on the upper torso, mouth, tongue, or nasal passages are central features. Recurrent epistaxis is an early manifestation, often by age 10 years. HHT must be considered in patients presenting with colonic bleeding who carry a history of recurrent epistaxis. Anemia and colonic bleeding are more common in adults, though may be significant in children. Intestinal telangiectasias occur throughout the GI tract with most found in the upper GI tract and small bowel. Stigmata of portal hypertension and cirrhosis are rare in children.

ETIOLOGY AND PATHOPHYSIOLOGY
Telangiectasias involve the skin, mucosa and viscera. Skin, nasal passages and the GI mucosa (10–25% of cases) are most commonly involved. Hepatic lesions occur and can progress to fibrosis and cirrhosis. Patients with both juvenile polyposis and HHT have been linked to SMAD4 mutations.

DIFFERENTIAL DIAGNOSIS
- AVM.
- BRBNS.
- Collagen vascular disorders (telangiectasia of scleroderma).
- Hemangioma.
- Telangiectasia.

DIAGNOSIS
Diagnostic criteria are established and require three of the following: epistaxis, telangiectasia, visceral lesions, and an affected first-degree relative. Diffuse, small, and tortuous telangiectasias can be seen as flat, red anomalies within the intestinal mucosa on endoscopy (**54.18**). Video-capsule endoscopy is effective at identifying active bleeding and diffuse telangiectasia in patients with HHT. Mesenteric angiography may be required when a focus of intestinal bleeding remains occult. Genetic testing is available if HHT is suspected. There is no consensus on screening for cerebral, hepatic, intestinal, or pulmonary AVMs in asymptomatic children.

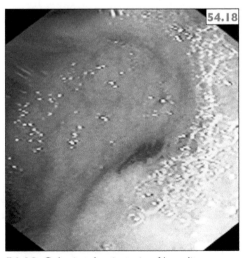

54.18 Colonic telangiectasia of hereditary hemorrhagic telangiectasia. (Courtesy of M. Kochman, MD; Department of Medicine, Hospital University of Pennsylvania.)

TREATMENT AND PROGNOSIS

Endoscopic treatment by thermocoagulation with argon plasma coagulator, bipolar probe, and laser coagulation are effective means to address acute colonic bleeding in patients with HHT. Serial transfusion often is required in cases of extensive intestinal involvement. Medical therapy is aimed at reducing the frequency of transfusions and based on combination estrogen and progesterone preparations. Prognosis is dependent upon the severity of disease penetrance.

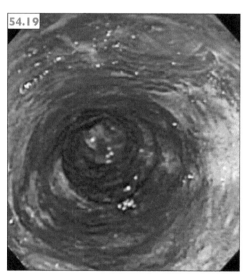

54.19 Extensive colonic involvement of Klippel–Trenaunay vascular malformation.

Klippel–Trenaunay syndrome

DEFINITION AND EPIDEMIOLOGY

Klippel–Trenaunay syndrome (KTS) is a rare disorder associated with venous and lymphoid malformations, and soft tissue and bone overgrowth. Its global incidence is estimated at 1 in 100,000 people.

CLINICAL PRESENTATION

Cutaneous port-wine stains are nearly universal and varicose veins may be present in children. Single limb hypertrophy is typical and progressive. Vascular lesions can infiltrate the colonic wall and present as painless rectal bleeding or hematochezia (**54.19**). Deep vein thrombosis (DVT) or tissue ischemia should be suspected when bleeding is associated with abdominal pain. Hematuria suggests additional pelvic infiltration.

ETIOLOGY AND PATHOPHYSIOLOGY

The genetic underpinnings of the disease remain unknown. Pathology stems from slow-flow capillary lymphovenous malformations, usually of the lower limbs and pelvis, which arise in the embryonic period. Limb and soft tissue hypertrophy is present and spatially connected to vascular anomalies in most instances, though a mechanistic link between abnormal vessels and tissue hypertrophy has not been established. Vascular malformations and hypertrophy, usually of a single limb, progress with growth. Colorectal localization of malformations is the dominant GI feature. Malformations may be complicated by DVT.

DIFFERENTIAL DIAGNOSIS

• Sturge–Weber syndrome.
• AVM.
• Portal hypertension with varicosities.
• Proteus syndrome.
• HHT (Rendu–Osler–Weber syndrome).
• BRBNS.

DIAGNOSIS

Endoscopic features of KTS lesions include bluish, pale or mixed discoloration, sessile or cavernous projection from the mucosal surface, and foci of bleeding or ulceration. Angiography and MRI are important primary studies when the clinical syndrome is already established. Capsule endoscopy is warranted to evaluate the small bowel.

TREATMENT AND PROGNOSIS

When bleeding is not life-threatening, the extent of venous malformations should be well delineated by angiography in advance of endoscopic therapy. Preoperative embolization of lesions may be required. Obliteration with APC is effective for venous malformations in stable patients. Bipolar or heater probe coagulation can be used when APC is not available.

Intestinal ischemia

Colonic ischemia with mucosal injury results from obstruction of the inferior mesenteric artery, portions of the superior mesenteric artery or its branches, and can lead to colonic bleeding. Necrotizing enterocolitis and malrotation with midgut volvulus (**54.20**) arise most often in the neonatal period and early childhood. Bleeding is frequently absent, but when present, is often occult or presenting as melena. Sigmoid volvulus is rare in infants and young children. Other sources of childhood colonic ischemia include incarcerated hernia, ileocolonic (**54.21**) or colocolonic intussusception, and mesenteric thrombosis.

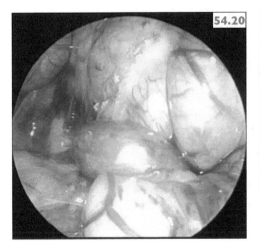

54.20 Neonatal midgut volvulus with ischemia, laparoscopic view. (Courtesy of T. Blinman, MD; Department of Surgery, The Children's Hospital of Philadelphia.)

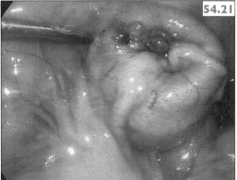

54.21 Ileocolonic intussusception, laparoscopic view. (Courtesy of T. Blinman, MD; Department of Surgery, The Children's Hospital of Philadelphia.)

Other sources of colonic bleeding

Other sources of colonic bleeding have been described in children. Diversion colitis, intestinal duplication, eosinophilic colitis, allergic colitis (**54.22**), Hirschsprung enterocolitis, neoplasia (**54.23**), post-operative complications such as ileocolonic anastomotic ulceration (**54.24**), and graft versus host disease (**54.25**) are included in a comprehensive differential diagnosis, although these diseases are not often encountered.

Blood vessel fragility due to connective tissue disease (Ehlers–Danlos), and vasculitides can result in colonic bleeding. Henoch–Schönlein purpura is a vasculitic autoimmune syndrome that presents with cutaneous lesions (purpura), joint involvement, glomerulonephritis, and colonic bleeding. Abdominal pain and bleeding may precede cutaneous symptoms or co-exist with other immunopathology including inflammatory bowel disease (**54.26**). Intestinal bleeding from other systemic vasculitides occurs but is uncommon in children.

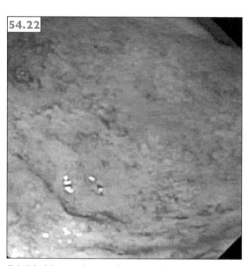

54.22 Hemorrhagic allergic colitis.

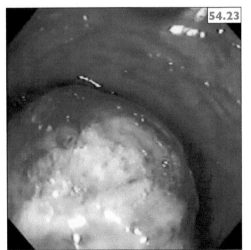

54.23 Colonic mass lesion of Burkitt lymphoma.

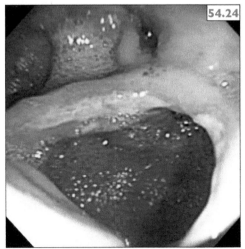

54.24 Ileocolonic anastomotic ulceration.

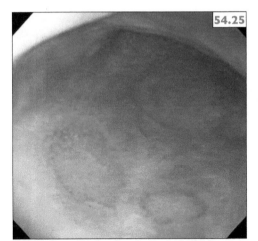

54.25 Superficial and well-circumscribed rectal ulcers characteristic of intestinal graft versus host disease.

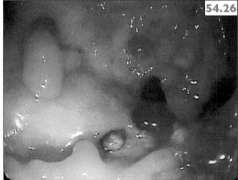

54.26 Ischemic purpura from Henoch–Schönlein purpura on a background of colonic pseudopolyps in Crohn disease.

MISCELLANEOUS CONDITIONS

CHAPTER 55

Ascites and Peritonitis

Candi Jump, Douglas Moote, Wael N. Sayej

DEFINITION AND EPIDEMIOLOGY

Ascites is of Greek derivation ('askos') and refers to a bag or sack. Ascites is the pathologic accumulation of fluid within the peritoneal cavity. Peritonitis is inflammation of the peritoneum and peritoneal cavity, usually caused by a localized or generalized infection. Primary peritonitis results from bacterial or fungal infection in the absence of perforation of the gastrointestinal (GI) tract, whereas secondary peritonitis occurs in the setting of GI perforation.

In the pediatric population, liver and kidney disease are the most frequently encountered etiologies for ascites. In adults with compensated cirrhosis, the prevalence is approximately 10%, and over a 10-year period 50% of patients with previously compensated cirrhosis are expected to develop ascites. In pediatric liver disease ascites can be the presenting sign of portal hypertension in up to 20% of patients. The true incidence of ascites in pediatrics is unknown.

ETIOLOGY AND PATHOPHYSIOLOGY

The etiologies of ascites are variable and are highly dependent on the age of the patient. Fetal ascites most commonly occurs in the setting of hydrops fetalis, a condition characterized by fluid collection in at least two body cavities, or fluid collection in a single cavity plus diffuse subcutaneous edema. Isolated ascites is much less common and accounts for approximately 30% of fetal cases. In a case series of 79 infants, ascites was idiopathic in 15%, associated with an organic malformation in 57%, and of infectious origin in 16%. Meconium peritonitis resulting

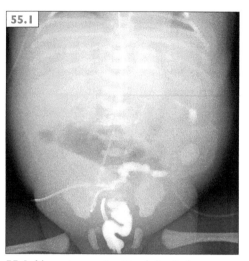

55.1 Meconium peritonitis: abdominal roentogram.

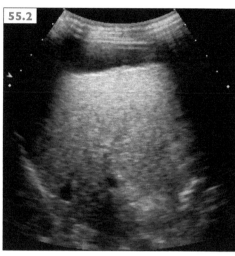

55.2 Abdominal ultrasound: portal hypertension with associated ascites.

from *in utero* bowel perforation is the most frequent reported cause (**55.1**). The most common infectious agent causing neonatal ascites is parvovirus. The etiology of neonatal ascites is similar to that of fetal ascites and the majority of the literature is limited to case reports or small case series. Uroascites in neonates can arise secondary to iatrogenic bladder perforation or complex genitourinary anatomy. Liver disease is a rare cause of ascites in the first month of life but there have been reports of biliary ascites from extrahepatic biliary perforation.

The most common cause for ascites in children is portal hypertension resulting from chronic liver disease (**55.2, 55.3**) or, less commonly, obstruction of hepatic vein outflow (as in Budd–Chiari syndrome) (*Table 55.1*). Other more common causes include pancreatitis, lymphatic obstruction, or trauma. Lymphatic disruption either from abdominal surgery, trauma, or neoplasms leads to chylous ascites (**55.4, 55.5**). Older children may also have traumatic extrahepatic perforation of the bile tree causing biliary ascites (**55.6, 55.7**). There have also been patients with ascites secondary

Table 55.1 Common causes of pediatric ascites

- Hepatobiliary
  - Hepatitis
  - Cirrhosis
  - Budd–Chiari syndrome
  - Alpha-1-antitrypsin deficiency
  - Congenital hepatic fibrosis
  - Perforated common bile duct
- Bowel perforation (meconium peritonitis)
- Pancreatic
- Chylous
  - Congenital
  - Post-traumatic
  - Nontraumatic
- Urinary tract
  - Nephrotic syndrome
  - Peritoneal dialysis
- Heart failure
- Ventriculoperitoneal shunts
- Liver transplantation
- Neoplasm
- Serositis
  - Henoch–Schönlein purpura
  - Eosinophilic gastroenteritis

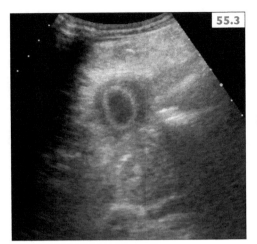

55.3 Abdominal ultrasound: thickened gallbladder.

55.4 Congenital chylous ascites: roentogram.

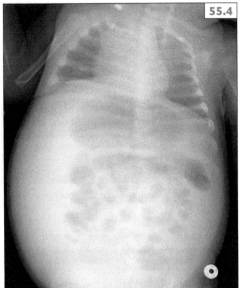

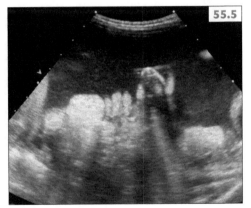

55.5 Congenital chylous ascites: abdominal ultrasound.

55.6 Perforated gallbladder (star): CT with peritoneal ascites (arrows).

55.7 Perforated gallbladder: intraoperative image.

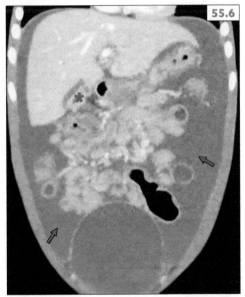

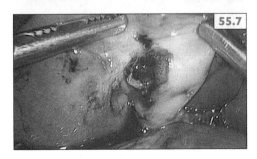

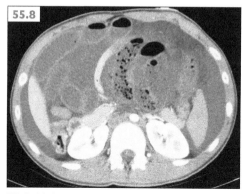

55.8 Midgut volvulus leading to intestinal necrosis and ascites.

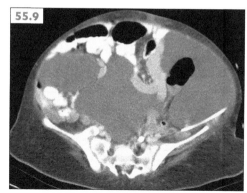

55.9 Loculated ascites: CT.

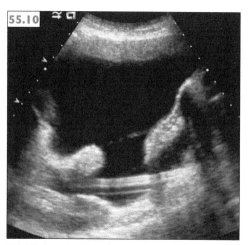

55.10 Loculated ascites: abdominal ultrasound.

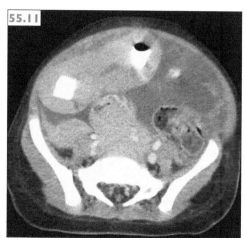

55.11 Abdominal lymphoma.

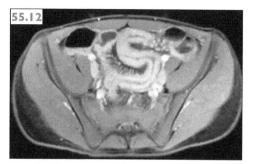

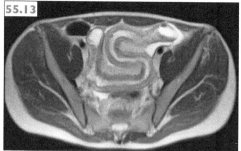

55.12, 55.13 MRI of Crohn disease with ascites. **55.12**: T1-weighted image; **55.13**: T2-weighted image.

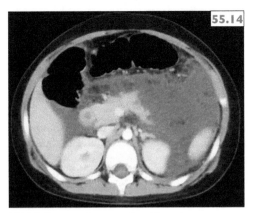

55.14 Pancreatic necrosis with ascites.

to the following causes: right heart failure, constrictive pericarditis, intestinal necrosis (**55.8**), ventriculoperitoneal shunts (**55.9, 55.10**), intra-abdominal neoplasms such as lymphoma (**55.11**), Henoch–Schönlein purpura, Crohn disease (**55.12, 55.13**), and vitamin A toxicity.

The current model for pathogenesis of ascites accredits peripheral arterial vasodilation. This is a combination of the preceding two models that hypothesized underfilling and overflow of the arterial circulation as the proposed mechanisms. Cirrhotic ascites is secondary to a complex interaction of portal hypertension, vasodilation, and renal retention of sodium and water. In cirrhosis there is activation of vasodilators such as nitric oxide, which facilitate splachnic arterial bed vasodilation. Volume overload in the splachnic circulation causes an increase in the splachnic capillary pressure. In early advanced fibrosis, the body is able to compensate for arterial underfilling with an increase in cardiac output, but with advanced fibrosis, the heart can no longer compensate and the kidneys subsequently sense hypovolemia. When 'underfilling' is present, the renin–angiotensin–aldosterone (RAA) system is activated in an attempt to maintain arterial pressure which triggers the retention of sodium and water through antidiuretic hormone to facilitate expansion of the plasma volume. The increase in splanchnic capillary pressures and expanded plasma volume produces a rate of lymph formation that exceeds the rate of lymph return and fluid accumulates in the peritoneal cavity.

There are variable methods of ascitic fluid accumulation in children without cirrhosis. In noncirrhotic ascites secondary to nephrotic syndrome and congestive heart failure, there is a low arterial blood volume and secondary activation of the RAA, leading to sodium and water retention. Budd–Chiari syndrome, a blockage of hepatic venous outflow, can cause portal hypertension and eventual ascites without the presence of liver cirrhosis. Chylous ascites accumulates secondary to trauma in the setting of surgical transection of the abdominal lymphatics, retroperitoneal lymph node dissection, or can be atraumatic in the setting of congenital lymphatic anomalies. Infectious ascites as seen in tuberculosis or coccidioidomycosis is caused by the secretion of proteinaceous fluid from the peritoneum. A proposed mechanism for ascites in pancreatitis is the disruption of the pancreatic duct leading to spillage of pancreatic secretions in the peritoneum and resultant chemical peritonitis (**55.14**).

DIAGNOSIS

The diagnosis of ascites as well as the underlying etiology and screening for complications of ascites can be accomplished with thorough history gathering, physical examination, imaging studies, and laboratory analysis of the ascitic fluid.

A history focused on the accumulation of ascites should include questions on recent weight gain, ankle edema, and change in abdominal girth. The most obvious sign of ascites is a full and bulging abdomen. Experienced clinicians can note physical signs of abdominal ascites by appreciating dullness on percussion and fluid wave. In adults, approximately 1.5 liters of fluid must be present before dullness can be detected by percussion. Signs of underlying liver disease including palmar erythema, spider angiomata, abdominal wall collateral veins, and jaundice will give clues about underlying liver pathology.

Ultrasound remains the most sensitive imaging for the detection of ascites. Fluid is easily detectable in the dependent areas of the hepatorenal recess and the pelvic cul-de-sac. Abdominal ultrasound can also aid in differentiating ascites from obesity, can look for signs of portal hypertension, such as an enlarged spleen or portal vein, and can assess hepatic vasculature flow with Doppler imaging. Computed tomography is a sensitive method to evaluate for ascites, but because of the risk of radiation exposure, it is only indicated when further information is needed such as in intraperitoneal bleeding. Magnetic resonance imaging (MRI) can also be used as a modality to detect ascites and has the benefit of no radiation exposure, but it can require sedation in young children secondary to the length of the examination as well as the associated sound of the MRI.

Paracentesis is recommended in the setting of an initial diagnosis of ascites, rapid accumulation of ascitic fluid, abdominal pain, fever, or any other clinical deterioration. Typical location for the procedure is the area two fingerbreadths both cephalad and medial to the anterior superior iliac spine. This region is chosen because of larger accumulation of fluid and smaller depth of the abdominal wall. The technique is accomplished using a 'Z tract' which allows the skin displaced prior to needle insertion to seal the needle pathway. Complications are uncommon with a paracentesis procedure. Most patients who require paracentesis are coagulopathic, and although bleeding can be seen occasionally, there is no contraindication with a prolonged prothrombin time, unless there is evidence of fibrinolysis or disseminated intravascular coagulation.

At the initial diagnostic paracentesis, fluid can be analyzed to help identify the etiology of the ascites. For example, a triglyceride concentration greater than 200 mg/dl (0.23 mmol/l) and a milky appearance is indicative of chylous ascites. An elevated amylase level, usually greater than fivefold the serum level, can be seen in instances of acute pancreatitis or intestinal perforation. When ascitic bilirubin concentration is greater than 6 mg/dl (103 μmol/l) and is greater than the serum bilirubin, one can expect biliary or proximal small intestinal perforation as a cause of ascites.

The serum-ascites albumin gradient (SAAG) divides ascites into low and high gradient categories. The gradient is simply the difference between the serum and ascitic fluid albumin concentrations and gives an index of portal pressure. A high gradient (>1.1 g/dl [>11 g/l]) is caused by an abnormally high hydrostatic pressure between the portal bed and ascitic fluid and is secondary to portal hypertension. A low gradient (<1.1 g/dl [<11 g/l]) is unlikely to be caused by portal hypertension and can be seen in nephrotic syndrome, biliary ascites, pancreatic ascites, and serositis. A falsely low SAAG can be seen in patients with chylous ascites. The exudate/ transudate classification is inferior to the SAAG method, and therefore, the total protein concentration is rarely used to determine etiology of ascites.

A fluid cell count and differential is required in evaluating bacterial infection or inflammation of the ascites. The most common cause of an elevated white count in ascitic fluid is spontaneous bacterial peritonitis (SBP), but any inflammatory process will increase the count. Bloody fluid is usually a result of a traumatic tap.

To detect bacterial peritonitis, a fluid culture is obtained via bedside inoculation of blood culture bottles. This type of testing is done because the estimated bacterial burden of SBP is as low as 1 organism per milliliter. It is unusual to document bacterial ascites on a Gram stain, and the older method of using agar plates is not sensitive for bacterial peritonitis. A study in adults showed that using bedside inoculation of culture bottles versus the conventional culture method increases sensitivity from 43% to 93%. A culture that identifies a polymicrobial infection is worrisome for intestinal perforation.

COMPLICATIONS
Spontaneous bacterial peritonitis
SBP is a potentially fatal cause of deterioration in patients with ascites and is characterized by the spontaneous infection of ascitic fluid in the absence of an intra-abdominal source of infection. One pediatric study showed the prevalence of SBP to be 19.5% among patients with ascites secondary to portal hypertension, but SBP is likely much higher among patients in fulminant liver failure. The proposed mechanism for the development of SBP involves bacterial translocation from the gut into the mesenteric lymph nodes. Patients with cirrhosis are thought to have impaired GI motility which leads to altered gut microflora; such patients also have a weakened immune system that does not promote clearance and opsonization of encapsulated bacteria from the lymph nodes. In adults, a low total protein concentration of ascitic fluid is thought to predispose patients to the development of SBP, but this observation is not supported by pediatric studies.

The diagnosis of SBP requires the presence of at least 250 polymorphonuclear (PMN) cells per milliliter of ascitic fluid. It can be classified as culture-positive neutrocytic or culture-negative neutrocytic (the less severe variant of SBP). A patient with a PMN count greater than 250 cells/ml and a negative culture is assumed to have had a false-negative culture and should be treated for SBP. Traditionally, gram-negative bacteria such as *Escherichia coli* were the most common isolates but gram-positive isolates have become more common. In a recent small pediatric series, the organisms identified from culture in patients with SBP were: *Streptococcus pneumoniae* (38.5%), *E. coli* (15.3%), *S. viridans* (15.3%), and *Klebsiella pneumoniae*, *Haemophilus influenzae*, enterococci, and nontypeable *Streptococcus* spp. in one patient each. Only a small percentage of patients show the typical features of acute peritoneal infection with diffuse abdominal pain, rebound tenderness, and reduced bowel sounds. It is important to consider a diagnostic paracentesis in any pediatric patient who presents with an initial episode of ascites or any signs of clinical deterioration in a patient with ascites. SBP can also manifest as hepatic encephalopathy or worsening of liver or renal function.

Hepatorenal syndrome
Hepatorenal syndrome (HRS) is a unique form of renal failure that complicates advanced liver disease, hepatic failure, or portal hypertension. The injury to the kidneys is secondary to vasodilation and reduction of effective arterial blood volume, which causes maximum activation of the RAA system leading to extreme renal vasoconstriction and eventual renal failure. HRS can occur spontaneously with worsening liver function or can be secondary to a precipitating event such as bleeding, large volume paracentesis without albumin administration, or SBP. Type I HRS is characterized by progressive oliguria and a rapid rise of the serum creatinine. Type II HRS occurs when the serum creatinine rise is moderate over time

and has less tendency to progress, although patients can develop a clinical picture of refractory ascites.

TREATMENT

Children are especially vulnerable to the complications of ascites, which can lead to extrahepatic organ dysfunction, including compromise of GI, renal, and pulmonary function. Treatment of ascites should be tailored to each patient based upon their level of extrahepatic dysfunction, discomfort, as well as the potential for complications of treatment. The mainstay of therapy is sodium restriction and diuretic therapy, which together work to create a negative sodium balance and mobilization of fluid. Patients with resistant ascites or tense ascites causing discomfort or respiratory compromise should be treated with a therapeutic paracentesis, have a more invasive shunting procedure performed, or have a liver transplantation. Other interventions for ascites include: antimicrobials (coverage for tuberculosis, bacterial, fungal, *Chlamydia*), endoscopic surgery for portal or biliary etiologies, dialysis or kidney transplant for nephrogenic etiologies, and treatment of underlying liver diseases such as chronic or autoimmune hepatitis.

Sodium and water restriction

The SAAG should be calculated to determine if sodium and/or water restriction may be beneficial. The SAAG is calculated as the difference between the serum and ascitic fluid albumin values and helps guide the appropriate management of ascites. If the SAAG is less than 1.1, sodium restriction and diuretics may be ineffective. Many pediatric hepatologists will suggest a low sodium diet as a first-line, noninvasive intervention for ascites. Diets with <10 mEq of sodium per day can prevent ascites formation but are not well tolerated, especially in pediatric patients. The current suggestion is to restrict sodium to <2 mEq/kg/d or to place on a 'no salt added' diet. In adults, the recommendation

for salt restriction is <2000 mg or 88 mEq per day. Water restriction is usually not needed unless the patient becomes profoundly hyponatremic (<125–130 mEq/l or less).

Diuretics

Diuretic therapy must be carefully titrated and monitored as patients with ascites have low effective arterial blood volume. It is titrated to achieve optimal weight loss without complications of the diuretic therapy. In adults, response to diuretic therapy is measured by tracking daily weights with a goal of 1% weight loss or up to 500 grams. In adults, only 750–900 ml of fluid can be mobilized from the abdomen to the general circulation per day; therefore, weight loss of 900 grams or greater can be associated with prerenal azotemia. Response can also be monitored by following urine sodium levels. The most commonly used diuretics are spironolactone and furosemide. Some physicians will start both drugs together and maintain a consistent ratio of spironolactone to aldosterone while others will start spironolactone first and add furosemide later. Spironolactone is an aldosterone antagonist that is used as a first-line therapy because it counters the tubular resorption of sodium activated by the RAA system. If there is no response to spironolactone, oral furosemide can be added to the regimen. Furosemide works through preventing sodium and chloride reabsorption in the ascending loop of Henle.

Cirrhotic patients on diuretic therapy must be diligently monitored for side-effects, namely alteration in serum potassium, metabolic acidosis or alkalosis, hyponatremia, and renal failure secondary to prerenal etiology. If furosemide and spironolactone are used in combination the patient is less likely to have these acid–base and electrolyte disorders.

Albumin

Albumin is a plasma volume expander that improves arterial hypotension. Patients with hepatic impairment can be albumin deficient secondary to loss of the liver's synthetic function. The use of intravenous albumin has been shown to improve diuretic response, decrease the need for paracentesis, and reduce the length of hospital stay and need for readmission in patients with ascites. Traditionally, 5% albumin infusions are used to expand the intravascular volume and to provide albumin. Studies have shown that hemodynamic instability, which is usually seen in large volume paracentesis, is uncommon, and thus volume expansion is usually not necessary. The use of 25% albumin infusions (0.5–1.0 g/kg dry weight) has become the standard of care for both adult and pediatric patients. An alternative plasma volume expander is dextran 70 which has been shown to have similar efficacy to albumin infusions.

Therapeutic paracentesis
Refractory ascites is unresponsive to sodium restriction and maximally tolerated diuretics. Refractory ascites often requires frequent large-volume paracentesis. Multiple studies have demonstrated the safety and efficacy of this procedure in adults, but only a single study has been done in pediatrics. There is the concern that repeated removal of large volumes of ascites may cause protein and complement depletion and the possibility of hemodynamic side-effects from contraction of blood volume. For this reason, pediatric patients undergoing therapeutic paracentesis should have adequate oral protein intake and albumin infusions to prevent further losses.

Portosystemic shunts
Portosystemic shunts divert portal blood flow and decrease portal pressure, which in turn decreases the rate of ascitic fluid accumulation and increases the effective arterial volume. The transjugular intrahepatic portosystemic shunt (TIPS) procedure is a portocaval shunt that was initially used to treat refractory variceal bleeding and is now used to treat ascites and to serve as a bridge to liver transplant. A hepatologist or interventional radiologist places the shunt via an angiographic technique in a transjugular manner under local anesthesia in adults and under general anesthesia in children. In adults the procedure is indicated when large-volume paracentesis fails, but no guidelines exist for implementation in children with ascites. The use of this procedure in the pediatric population is limited by vascular malformations and patient size. In a recently published study of 13 children who had TIPS placed (five with ascites), the shunt was successful in reducing the portosytemic gradient in 11 patients with only one patient having a related complication and three patients requiring revision of the shunt. Less common complications are secondary to shunting blood away from the liver and include portosystemic encephalopathy and worsening liver failure.

The peritoneal–venous shunt was developed to create a conduit for ascitic fluid to flow back into the central circulation. It has a much higher complication rate than TIPS including shunt obstruction, coagulopathy, superior vena cava thrombosis and obstruction, pulmonary embolism, and sepsis. For this reason, this shunt is primarily used in patients whom are not candidates for liver transplantation, TIPS, or therapeutic paracentesis.

Treatment of spontaneous bacterial peritonitis
If ascitic fluid yields a diagnosis of SBP then appropriate antibiotic therapy should be initiated. Broad-spectrum coverage is needed to cover gram-negative bacteria (*E. coli* and *Klebsiella* spp.) as well as emerging gram-positive bacteria (*Pneumococcus* spp.). In adults, cefotaxime has been the initial drug of choice because of its coverage spectrum and lack of nephrotoxic properties. Recently, there has been emergence of nosocomial-acquired organisms resistant to cefotaxime with 40% of adult patients requiring a switch

to a different antibiotic. It has been suggested that a change in the PMN count after 2 days of antibiotic treatment is the best marker of therapeutic response, and in adults, it is recommended to do at least one follow-up paracentesis to confirm response.

The use of prophylaxis antibiotics in nonbleeding cirrhotic patients with ascites has been studied, although no pediatric trials exist. The International Ascites Club recommends continued administration of norfloxacin for cirrhotic patients recovering from an episode of SBP.

PROGNOSIS

Most of the data regarding the specific prognosis of patients with ascites are specific to adults, as pediatric patients with ascites secondary to liver disease typically undergo liver transplant. In adult patients with ascites secondary to cirrhosis the 2-year mortality rate is about 50%. After the first occurrence of SBP the 1-year survival rate is 38%. Once HRS is diagnosed, the probability of 3-month survival is 15%.

Approach to Pediatric Diarrhea

Karolina Maria Burghardt, Tanja Gonska

DEFINITION

Diarrheal illnesses are among the most important contributors to the morbidity and mortality of children of all ages worldwide. In most instances, the onset of diarrhea is self-limited and patients recover with vigilant oral rehydration therapy. Less commonly, diarrhea can be severe, protracted, and may result in hospitalization or serious sequelae such as death, hemolytic uremic syndrome, or Guillain–Barre syndrome. Rarely, diarrhea presents in the first days of life with progressive decompensation and heralds a severe neonatal onset congenital diarrhea. Thus, it is of utmost importance to have an organized approach to assess pediatric patients, to determine the likely etiology, and to manage the illness efficiently and effectively.

Diarrhea is characterized by the passage of more than three watery stools per day of variable volume and description. Most importantly, defining whether the diarrheal episode is acute or persistent will guide the investigations and the treatment plan. Acute diarrhea refers to an episode lasting fewer than 14 days. Protracted diarrhea is defined as a diarrheal episode that lasts for 14 days or more, often associated with more severe weight loss or growth failure. Management of protracted diarrhea often requires nutritional rehabilitation.

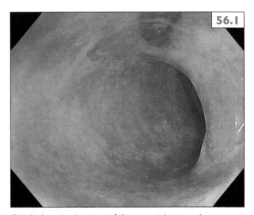

56.1 Luminal view of ileum with complete shedding of the mucosa (nude intestine).

CLINICAL PRESENTATION
Acute diarrhea

The clinical course of a sudden onset of diarrheal symptoms will depend on the etiology and the host. Most episodes are benign and are attributed to an infectious agent. However, when the host is immuno-compromised, such as in postorgan transplant recipients, infections with normally innocuous agents such as cytomegalovirus may cause a life-threatening diarrheal illness with intestinal inflammation (**56.1, 56.2**). Furthermore, the site of infection and

56.2 Luminal view of inflamed colon in a patient with cytomegalovirus enterocolitis.

the pathogenic mechanism deployed will determine the clinical features. For instance, rotavirus affects the proximal small intestine and produces watery diarrhea with vomiting that lead to mild to moderate dehydration and lactose malabsorption. *Salmonella* and *Shigella* spp. infect the small intestine, producing frequent small volume stools that may be bloody and associated with abdominal pain and fever. *Campylobacter* and *Yersinia* spp. have preponderance for the distal ileum and colon where they cause significant water loss leading to dehydration. Enteropathogenic *Escherichia coli* and *Clostridium difficile* infect the colon and present primarily with abdominal pain, fever, and bloody loose stools.

Persistent diarrhea

Watery, frequent stools that continue beyond 14 days are called persistent diarrhea. The clinical course will vary according to the etiology and host factors. In some cases the onset of diarrhea is in the neonatal period due to a congenital defect of electrolyte transport in the intestinal mucosa. In other cases, the onset is acute and the illness becomes protracted.

ETIOLOGY AND PATHOPHYSIOLOGY

The etiology of a diarrheal illness varies greatly and it is useful to divide these etiologies into broader categories based on similar mechanisms of disease.

Secretory diarrhea

In secretory diarrhea, the epithelial cells are actively releasing ions causing a net loss of key electrolytes in the body. Characteristically, the diarrhea is independent of food intake and persists in the fasting state. Early assessment of stool electrolytes may be very helpful in distinguishing the pathophysiology.

Infectious agents

The most common cause of secretory diarrhea is bacterial infection, whereby adherence or invasion of the pathogens stimulates a state of active secretion through the action of intracellular second messengers and recruitment of inflammatory cells. Consequently, sodium chloride (NaCl) reabsorption is impeded on villous enterocytes and/or the chloride secretion is increased in crypt cells. Other pathogens may trigger increased NaCl secretion via direct activation of the epithelial chloride channel

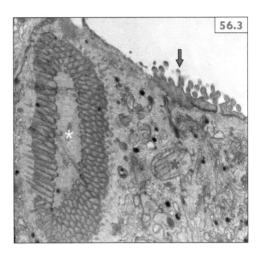

56.3 Transmission electron microscopy of a small intestine biopsy from a patient with microvillus inclusion disease. Cytoplasmic microvillus inclusion (white star), basolateral microvillus inclusion (red star), and shortness or complete loss of microvilli (arrow) are shown. (Courtesy of Ernest Cutz, MD; The Hospital for Sick Children, Toronto, Canada.)

(cystic fibrosis transmembrane conductance receptor) in the presence of enterotoxins such as those produced by *Vibrio cholerae*. The volume of stool tends to be large, unresponsive to fasting, and with a stool ion gap of <50 mOsm/kg.

A multitude of pathogens have the potential to infect the intestinal tract and cause a diarrheal illness. These pathogens may be viruses (rotavirus and calicivirus), bacteria (*Campylobacter jejuni*, *Salmonella* spp., *E. coli*) or parasites (*Cryptosporidium* spp. and *Giardia lamblia*). Bacterial pathogens may use various pathways to interfere with intestinal homeostasis: invasion, channel blocking, modulation of tight junctions, and induction of inflammatory responses with mucosal sloughing and dissemination.

Electrolyte channel defects

Inherited defects within the intestinal epithelium include diseases such as congenital chloride diarrhea, which is caused by a defective chloride and bicarbonate exchanger (mutation of *SLC26A3*). The consequence is diarrhea, severe chloride loss in the stool, metabolic alkalosis, and acidification of stool. A similar presentation is noted in congenital sodium diarrhea, but with a characteristic high sodium concentration in the fecal effluent instead.

Structural enterocyte defects

Neonatal enteropathies present early with severe onset of diarrhea and a rapid loss of electrolytes in the stool. Some of these enteropathies are caused by structural enterocyte defects, while for others the molecular pathogenesis is still to be refined. An early clue to this pathology is often found in the maternal history of polyhydramnios during the pregnancy. Two examples of this pathology are tufting enteropathy and microvillous inclusion disease. In microvillous inclusion disease, the net reduction of absorptive surface area is due to a disorganization and loss of microvilli within the brush border (**56.3**). In tufting enteropathy, the epithelial layer is disorganized with focal aggregation of villi into 'tufts'. In addition there is an abnormal distribution of laminin and integrins that leads to disturbances in the cell–matrix interactions (**56.4**).

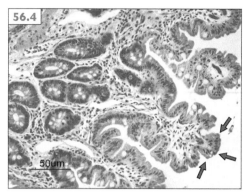

56.4 Small intestine biopsy from a patient with tufting enteropathy. Charactertistic 'tufts' of villi are noted in the lumen of the small intestine (arrows). (Courtesy of Cornelia Thoeni and Ernest Cutz, MD; The Hospital for Sick Children, Toronto, Canada.)

Short gut
Individuals with short bowel syndrome have a decreased surface available for absorption due to a functional or anatomic loss of bowel. Moreover, some patients lack an ileocecal valve, which increases the transit time across the gastrointestinal tract leading to malabsorption.

Osmotic diarrhea
In osmotic diarrhea, an increasing osmotic force is created within the lumen of the intestine when the intestinal mucosa cannot digest and/or absorb certain nutrients or when the abundance of the nutrient exceeds the absorptive capacity of the mucosa. Characteristically, the diarrhea resolves when the specific offending nutrients are eliminated or when a patient undergoes a fasting state. Stool investigations show high osmolality, normal electrolytes, high fecal fat or low fecal elastase (if associated with pancreatic insufficiency), the presence of reducing substances (due to carbohydrate malabsorption), and rarely inflammatory markers in stool (i.e. elevated stool lactoferrin and calprotectin).

Malabsorption/maldigestion
Classic examples are lactose intolerance (congenital or acquired) and toddler's diarrhea (functional diarrhea). In the former, the accumulation of undigested lactose reaches the colon where it is fermented by the microflora to short-chain organic acids, which creates an osmotic gradient that retains water in the lumen. In the latter case, toddler's diarrhea results from the consumption of sugar or sorbitol-containing fluids, such as fruit juices and carbonated drinks, in amounts that exceed the absorptive capacity of the intestine. The diarrhea is characterized by an increased stool ion gap of >100 mOsm/kg.

Fat and protein malabsorption are the cause of persistent diarrhea noted in patients with pancreatic insufficiency such as cystic fibrosis, Shwachman–Diamond syndrome, and protein losing enteropathy. Similarly, cholestatic disorders of the liver also lead to fat malabsorption as a result of a reduction in bile acids available for digestion. Patients whose terminal ileum has been resected or diseased (e.g. Crohn disease) are unable to reabsorb bile salts and may experience bile acid loss with similar consequences.

Motility-related diarrhea
Patients with hypomotile peristalsis, as in the case of disorders of the enteric nervous system (Hirschsprung colitis and chronic intestinal pseudo-obstruction), or individuals with dysmotility stemming from short bowel syndrome are at increased risk for small intestinal bacterial overgrowth (SIBO), which is accompanied by maldigestion and/or malabsorption. SIBO causes diarrhea as a result of an increased number of bacteria (>10^5 bacterial colony forming units per milliliter of duodenal fluid) and/or the presence of anaerobic bacteria species in the proximal bowel. These bacteria may interfere directly with enzymatic, absorptive, and metabolic processes at the brush border of enterocytes. In addition, the pathogens may contribute to the deconjugation/dehydroxylation of

bile salts and hydroxylation of fatty acids leading to diarrheal symptoms. In contrast, individuals with hypermotile peristalsis experience a rapid transit time of luminal contents due to hyperactive peristalsis and decreased opportunity for digestion and absorption.

Immune-mediated diarrhea

The intestinal barrier that is needed to regulate nutrient absorption can be defective and/or have increased permeability as a result of immunologic processes. Autoimmune enteropathy is characterized by immunoglobulin (Ig) G antibodies specific for components of the enterocyte brush border that initiate a cell-mediated immune dysregulation and damage of the epithelial barrier. Similarly, children with a mutation of the transcription factor FoxP3 (scurfin) which modulates CD4+ T cell proliferation have a propensity for having antienterocyte antibodies resulting in immune dysregulation polyendocrinopathy, enteropathy syndrome. Moreover, the state of inflammation that waxes and wanes in the intestine of patients with inflammatory bowel disease (IBD), ulcerative colitis (**56.5**), or Crohn disease (**56.6**) leads to a fluctuating degree of diarrhea.

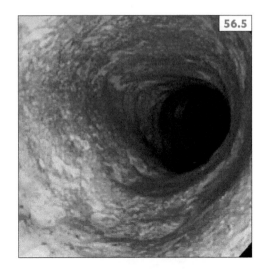

56.5 Luminal view of inflamed colonic mucosa typical of colitis in a patient with ulcerative colitis. (Courtesy of Thomas Walters, MD; The Hospital for Sick Children, Toronto, Canada.)

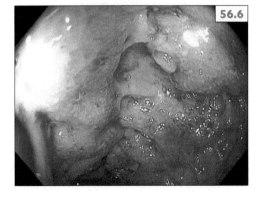

56.6 Luminal view of ulcerated colonic mucosa in a patient with Crohn disease. (Courtesy of Thomas Walters, MD; The Hospital for Sick Children, Toronto, Canada.)

Similarly, in celiac disease (**56.7, 56.8**) the consequence of the (auto)immune onslaught is intraepithelial accumulation of lymphocytes, loss of villous height, and decreased absorptive surface area with variable diarrheal symptoms. IBD and celiac disease are discussed in detail elsewhere. Other disorders of immune activation and function, such as agammaglobulinemia, isolated IgA deficiency, and acquired immunodeficiency syndrome, are also characterized by bouts of persistent diarrhea.

Food allergies and intolerance

Food allergic enteropathies, the most common example is cow's milk protein enteropathy (CMPE), are characterized by an infiltration of lymphocytes and plasma cells in response to an offending food antigen resulting in impaired absorption. In classic CMPE, children have any combination of symptoms of diarrhea, irritability, variable degree of blood in the stool (none to gross bleeding), growth failure (after a period of normal growth), abdominal distention, and perianal rash. Typically in these cases, skin-prick testing may be negative and specific IgE can be undetectable. Among these children, up to 40% also react to soy protein. The condition is self-limited and after a period of dietary exclusion, the cow milk antigen is tolerated well in most children by the age of 2–3 years. The majority of cases of CMPE are mild to moderate. However, in rare instances

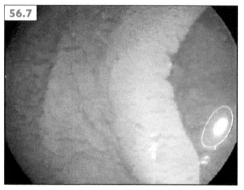

56.7 Luminal view of duodenum with scalloping in a patient with celiac disease.

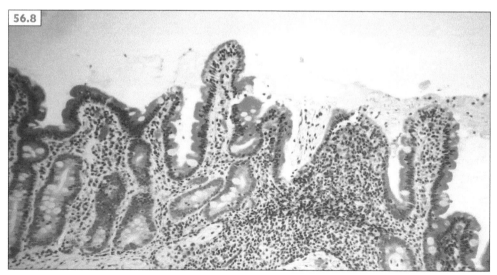

56.8 Small intestinal biopsy histology of celiac disease, showing intraepithelial lymphocyte accumulation with loss of villous height.

severe reactions and life-threatening mucosal food hypersensitivity reactions develop as an expression of a food protein-induced enterocolitis. Although cow's milk and soy are the most common triggers, other food antigens include egg, nuts, shellfish, wheat, rice, oat, barley, vegetable, or poultry. Children with food allergies have endoscopic evidence of intestinal lymphoid hyperplasia or even eosinophilia. In a minority of cases, exposure to the food allergen is immediate, often concurrent with positive IgE-mediated skin-prick test, and persists life-long.

Diarrhea related to micronutrients and trace elements

Micronutrient deficiencies may exacerbate persistent diarrhea. In particular it has been shown that diarrhea caused by vitamin A deficiency or zinc deficiency (acrodermatitis enteropathica) resolve with appropriate supplementation. Likewise, poor folate status and niacin deficiency (pellagra) in children from developing countries has been reported to be an independent predictor of persistent diarrhea.

Epidemiologic studies have reported that certain heavy metals have the propensity to cause diarrhea. Copper-induced liver cirrhosis is well documented and copper intoxication in drinking water has also been linked to persistent diarrhea.

DIFFERENTIAL DIAGNOSIS AND DIAGNOSIS

Differential diagnosis is presented in *Table 56.1*. In most instances, the proposed etiology of the diarrheal episode is elaborated from the history of presenting illness and then confirmed with a careful selection of laboratory investigations and radiologic imaging.

Laboratory studies

In most episodes of acute diarrhea, the laboratory tests are focused on assessing the serum electrolyte status (in view of dehydration), stool electrolytes (in view of a possible electrolyte channel defect), stool osmolality, and screening for common infectious pathogens. For example, most laboratories target bacterial screening for *Salmonella*, *Shigella*, *Campylobacter* spp., and *E. coli* O157:H7. A detailed history including travel, extracurricular activities (e.g. lake swimming) and sick contacts will define the scope of the infectious panel of organisms to be investigated. In the large majority of cases, the pathogen is not identified.

Emphasis should always be placed on a careful diet history and associated timeline of the appearance of symptoms. In considering toddler's diarrhea, diet history along with benefit noted from reduction of sorbitol/fructose intake is sufficient to make the diagnosis.

CMPE is often entertained as a possibility when an infant has loose stools accompanied by rectal bleeding. Rectal bleeding by itself is usually benign and self-limited. CMPE is the most common cause of rectal bleeding in infants accompanied by a variable degree of anorexia, vomiting, eczema and, in a minority of cases, peripheral blood eosinophilia. Resolution of symptoms with an elimination diet and recurrence of rectal bleeding with reintroduction of cow's milk is diagnostic. Intestinal biopsies usually are not indicated.

In persistent diarrhea, most of the 'acute' investigations have already been performed initially without success in elucidating the etiology. Further tests are necessary and are tailored to the clinical presentation and personal history of the child. If considering an immune-mediated disorder, more specific laboratory tests, such as inflammation markers (in serum and in stool), albumin, hemoglobin, and iron studies, may already raise suspicion for autoimmune enteropathy or IBD. In these cases, obtaining tissue histology by gastroscopy or ileocolonoscopy is the diagnostic standard.

If considering celiac disease it may be useful to screen using a quantitative serology assay for IgG and IgA to tissue transglutaminase and endomysium. The

Table 56.1 Differential diagnosis of diarrhea according to age group and duration of illness

	Acute	Persistent
Infant	Infectious diarrhea	Toddler's diarrhea
	Systemic infection	Postinfectious lactase deficiency
	Hirschsprung toxic colitis	Cow's milk protein enteropathy
	Primary disaccharidase deficiency	Celiac disease
	Antibiotic-associated diarrhea	Immune deficiencies
		Glucose–galactose malabsorption
		Electrolyte channel defect
		Microvillus inclusion disease
		Tufting enteropathy
		Hirschsprung toxic colitis
		Cystic fibrosis
		Shwachman syndrome
		Acrodermatitits enteropathica
		Intestinal lymphangiectasia
		Eosinophilic gastroenteritis
		Short bowel syndrome
		Autoimmune enteropathy
		Inflammatory bowel disease
Child	Infectious diarrhea	Toddler's diarrhea
	Systemic infection	Postinfectious lactase deficiency
	Toxin ingestion (food poisoning, heavy metals)	Irritable bowel syndrome
		Celiac disease
	Intussusception	Giardiasis
	Antibiotic-associated diarrhea	Inflammatory bowel disease
		Immune deficiencies
		Sucrase–isomaltase deficiency
		Lactase deficiency
		Eosinophilic gastroenteritis
Adolescent	Infectious diarrhea	Postinfectious lactase deficiency
	Systemic infection	Irritable bowel syndrome
	Toxin ingestion (food poisoning, heavy metals)	Celiac disease
		Giardiasis
	Intussusception	Inflammatory bowel disease
	Antibiotic-associated diarrhea	Lactose intolerance
	Appendicitis	Sucrase–isomaltase deficiency
		Eosinophilic gastroenteritis
		Constipation with encopresis
		Addison disease
		Vasoactive intestinal protein-producing tumors

screening test is useful in cases with a high pretest probability in view of typical symptomatology, growth failure/pubertal delay, family history, and/or high-risk population. The gold standard diagnostic test for celiac disease is histology analysis of intestinal biopsies from an upper endoscopy while on a gluten-containing diet (**56.8**). If considering pancreatic insufficiency, informative tests include fecal elastase or stool quantification for fecal fat.

Imaging studies
Most patients with diarrhea do not require radiologic imaging. In specific instances, patients having diarrhea associated with an acute abdomen or severe abdominal pain should undergo an abdominal radiograph to rule out perforation or obstruction. Various imaging modalities can help delineate inflammatory lesions, anatomical problems, or extraintestinal complications. For example, ultrasound imaging, magnetic resonance imaging, or computed tomography imaging of the abdomen may be required. Notably, some pathogens such as *Yersinia* spp. have a propensity for causing focal inflammation of the terminal ileum with associated lymphadenitis, which makes stool cultures an important prerequisite before committing patients to endoscopic studies.

TREATMENT
The first priority in the treatment of any child with diarrhea is hydration to re-establish a normal electrolyte balance. There are no clinically significant differences between oral rehydration therapy (ORT) and intravenous fluid resuscitation. The major advantages in ORT are in the ease of delivery and avoidance of complications of intravenous use (phlebitis and pain). Since 1975, the World Health Organization has been refining their formulation of ORT. There is no evidence to suggest that restricting a child's diet is of any benefit. Early refeeding as tolerated by the child does not increase the risk of intravenous fluid need, episodes of vomiting, or likelihood for persistent diarrhea.

Zinc supplementation is the only adjunct therapy that has proven benefit in reducing the severity and duration of non-cholera diarrheal illnesses. Various strains of probiotics have been studied for the treatment of acute onset diarrhea. Reports in the literature suggest a moderate clinical improvement of diarrhea with strains of *Lactobacillus* GG and *Saccharomyces boulardii* with no adverse effects attributed to probiotic treatments. The efficacy is strain- and dose-dependent. Further research is needed to establish specific treatment guidelines for the use of probiotics in the pediatric population.

PROGNOSIS
The majority of acute diarrheal illness will resolve with supportive care and without sequelae. Prognosis is largely dependent on the underlying disease. Nonetheless, a few important key points are worthy of mention. Judicious use of antibiotic therapy is essential since viruses cause most episodes of acute diarrhea. Given that 40% of children younger than 5 years old are hospitalized due to a rotavirus-related diarrheal episode, rotavirus vaccines are widely recommended by pediatricians across Canada, Europe, and the United States. Moreover, there is good evidence for advocating breastfeeding to lessen the burden of diarrheal disease. An organized and multifaceted approach to diarrhea prevention, diagnosis, and treatment is needed to improve the morbidity and mortality of children worldwide.

CHAPTER 1 THE PEDIATRIC GASTROINTESTINAL PHYSICAL EXAMINATION

1 Balas A, Jaffrey F, Kuperman GJ, *et al*. Electronic communication with patients: evaluation of distance medical technology, *JAMA* 1997;**278**(2):152–159.
2 Chandran L, Chitkara M. Vomiting in children: reassurance, red flag or referral? *Pediatr Rev* 2008;**29**(6):183–192.
3 DeGowin R, Brown D. *DeGowin's Diagnostic Examination*. MGraw-Hill, London, 2000.
4 Liederman E, Morefield C. Web messaging: a new tool for patient–physician communication. *J Am Med Assoc Inform* 2003;**10**:260–270.
5 Ross A, LeLeiko N. Acute abdominal pain. *Pediatr Rev* 2010;**31**(4):135–144.
6 Walker WA, Durie PR, Hamilton JR, Walker-Smith AW (eds). *Pediatric Gastrointestinal Disease: Pathophysiology, Diagnosis, Management*, 2nd edn. Mosby Elsevier, London, 1996.

Section 1 Mouth and Phyarynx

CHAPTER 2 ORAL PROBLEMS ASSOCIATED WITH GASTROINTESTINAL DISEASE

1 Amir J, Harel L, Smetana Z, Varsano I. The natural history of primary herpes simplex type 1 gingivostomatitis in children. *Pediatr Dermatol* 1999;**16**:259–263.
2 Assimakopoulos D, Patrikakos G, Fotika C, Elisaf M. Benign migratory glossitis or geographic tongue: an enigmatic oral lesion. *Am J Med* 2002;**113**:751–755.
3 Barton DH, Spier SK, Crovello TJ. Benign migratory glossitis and allergy. *Pediatr Dent* 1982;**4**:249–250.
4 Buchner A, Hansen LS. Pigmented nevi of the oral mucosa: a clinicopathological study of 36 new cases and review of 155 cases from the literature. Part I: A clinicopathological study of 36 new cases. *Oral Surg Oral Med Oral Pathol* 1987;**63**:566–572.
5 Buchner A, Hansen LS. Pigmented nevi of the oral mucosa: a clinicopathological study of 36 new cases and review of 155 cases from the literature. Part II: Analysis of 191 cases. *Oral Surg Oral Med Oral Pathol* 1987;**63**:676–682.
6 Chang LC, Haggstrom AN, Drolet BA, *et al*. Growth characteristics of infantile hemangiomas: implications for management. *Pediatrics* 2008;**122**:360–367.
7 Eisen D, Lynch DP. *Oral Manifestations of Systemic Diseases. The Mouth: Diagnosis and Treatment*. Mosby, St. Louis, 1998, pp. 212–236.
8 Gupta G, Williams RE, Mackie RM. The labial melanotic macule: a review of 79 cases. *Br J Dermatol* 1997;**136**:772–775.
9 Haraszthy VI, Hariharan G, Tinoco EM, *et al*. Evidence for the role of highly leukotoxic *Actinobacillus actinomycetemcomitans* in the pathogenesis of localized juvenile and other forms of early-onset periodontitis. *J Periodontol* 2000;**71**:912–922.
10 Hebert AA, Lopez MD. Oral lesions in pediatric patients. *Adv Dermatol* 1997;**12**:169–193.
11 Kaban LB, Troulis MJ (eds). *Pediatric Oral and Maxillofacial Surgery*. Suanders, Philadelphia, 2004.
12 King DL, Steinhauer W, Garcia-Godoy F, *et al*. Herpetic gingivostomatitis and teething difficulty in infants. *Pediatr Dent* 1992;**14**:82–85.
13 Langlais RP, Miller CS, Nield-Gehrig JS. *Color Atlas of Common Oral Diseases*, 4th edn. Lippincott Williams & Wilkins, Philadelphia, 2009.

14 Leggott PJ. Oral manifestations of HIV infection in children. *Oral Surg Oral Med Oral Pathol* 1992;**73**:187–192.

15 Mueller DT, Callanan VP. Congenital malformations of the oral cavity. *Otolaryngol Clin North Am* 2007;**40**:141–160.

16 Neville B, Damm DD, White DH. *Lymphoreticular and Hematopoietic Diseases. Color Atlas of Clinical Oral Pathology*, 2nd edn. BC Decker, Ontario, 2003; pp. 313–332.

17 Neville D, Allen B. *Oral and Maxillofacial Pathology*, 3rd edn. WB Saunders, Philadelphia, 2009.

18 Pappas PG, Kauffman CA, Andes D, *et al*. Clinical practice guidelines for the management of candidiasis: 2009 update by the Infectious Diseases Society of America. *Clin Infect Dis* 2009;**48**:503–535.

19 Roberts MW, Atkinson JC. Oral manifestations associated with leukocyte adhesion deficiency: a five year case study. *Pediatr Dent* 1990;**12**:107–111.

20 Ship JA. Recurrent aphthous stomatitis: An update. *Oral Surg Oral Med Oral Pathol* 1996;**81**:141–147.

Section 2 Esophagus

CHAPTER 3 ABNORMAL ANATOMY OF THE ESOPHAGUS

1 Arbona JL, Fazzi JG, Mayoral J. Congenital esophageal cysts: case report and review of literature. *Am J Gastroenterol* **79**:177–182, 198.

2 Burkhard H, von Rahden A, Stein HJ, *et al*. Heterotopic gastric mucosa of the esophagus: literature review and proposal of clinicopathologic classification. *Am J Gastroenterol* 2004;**99**:543–551.

3 Carr M, Clarke K, Webber E, Giacomantonio M. Congenital laryngotracheoesophageal cleft. *J Otolaryngol* 1999;**28**:112–117.

4 Eichmann D, Engler S, Oldigs HD, Schroeder H, Partsch CJ. Radiological case of the month. Denouement and discussion: congenital esophageal duplication cyst as a rare cause of neonatal progressive stridor. *Arch Pediatr Adolesc Med* 2001;**155**:1067–1068.

5 Kleinman RE, Goulet O-J, Mieli-Vergani G, Sanderson IR, Sherman PM, Shneider BL (eds). *Walker's Pediatric Gastrointestinal Disease; Physiology, Diagnosis, Management*, 5th edn. McGraw-Hill, New York, 2008.

6 Kluth D, Steding G, Seidl W. The embryology of foregut malformations. *J Pediatr Surg* 1987;**22**:389–393.

7 Stocker TJ, Dehner LP, Hussain AN. *Stocker Dehner Pediatric Pathology*. Lippincott Williams & Wilkins, Philadelphia, 2011.

8 Tobin RW. Esophageal rings, webs, and diverticula. *J Clin Gastroenterol* 1998;**27**(4):285–295.

9 Wyllie R, Hyams J, Kay M (eds). *Pediatric Gastroenterology and Liver Disease*, 3rd edn. Saunders Elsevier, London, 2006.

CHAPTER 4 GASTROESOPHAGEAL REFLUX DISEASE AND ESOPHAGITIS

1 Fiedorek S, Tolia V, Gold BD, *et al*. Efficacy and safety of lansoprazole in adolescents with symptomatic erosive and non-erosive gastroesophageal reflux disease. *J Pediatr Gastroenterol Nutr* 2005;**40**:319–327.

2 Geagea A, Cellier C. Scope of drug-induced, infectious and allergic esophageal injury. *Curr Opin Gastroenterol* 2008;**24**:496–501.

3 Gilger MA, El-Serag HB, Gold BD, *et al*. Prevalence of endoscopic findings of erosive esophagitis in children: a population-based study. *J Pediatr Gastroenterol Nutr* 2008;**47**:141–146.

4 Nelson SP, Chen EH, Syniar GM, Christoffel KK. One-year follow-up of symptoms of gastroesophageal reflux during infancy. *Pediatrics* 1998;**102**:E67.

5 Sherman PM, Hassall E, Fagundes-Neto U, *et al*. A global, evidence-based consensus on the definition of gastroesophageal reflux disease in the pediatric population. *Am J Gastroenterol* 2009;**104**:1278–1295.

6 Vandenplas Y, Rudoph CD, Di Lorenzo C, *et al*. Pediatric gastroesophageal reflux practice guidelines: joint recommendations of the North American Society for Pediatric Gastroenterology, Hepatology and Nutrition (NASPGHAN) and the European Society for Pediatric Gastroenterology, Hepatology and Nutrition (ESPGHAN). *J Pediatr Gastroenterol Nutr* 2009;**49**:498–547.

7 van der Pol RJ, Smits MJ, van Wijk MP, *et al*. Efficacy of proton-pump inhibitors in children with gastroesophageal reflux disease: a systematic review. *Pediatrics* 2011;**127**:925–935.

CHAPTER 5 EOSINOPHILIC ESOPHAGITIS

1 Franciosi JP, Liacouras CA. Eosinophilic esophagitis. *Immunol Allergy Clin North Am* 2009;**29**(1):19–27.
2 Franciosi JP, Tam V, Liacouras CA, Spergel JM. A case-control study of sociodemographic and geographic characteristics of 335 children with eosinophilic esophagitis. *Clin Gastroenterol Hepatol* 2009;**7**:415–419.
3 Furuta GT, Atkins D. Eosinophilic gastrointestinal diseases. *Immunol Allergy Clin North Am* 2009;**29**(1):110–115.
4 Furuta GT, Liacouras CA, Collins MH. First International Gastrointestinal Eosinophil Research Symposium (FIGERS). Eosinophilic esophagitis in children and adults: a systematic review and consensus recommendations for diagnosis and treatment. *Gastroenterology* 2007;**133**(4):1342–1363.
5 Guajardo JR, Plotnick LM, Fende JM, Collins MH, Putnam PE, Rothenberg ME. Eosinophil-associated gastrointestinal disorders: a world-wide-web based registry. *J Pediatr* 2002;**141**: 576–581.
6 Kagalwalla AF, Shah A, Li BU, *et al.* Identification of specific foods responsible for inflammation in children with eosinophilic esophagitis successfully treated with empiric elimination diet. *J Pediatr Gastroenterol Nutr* 2011;**53**:145–149.
7 Kapel RC, Miller JK, Torres C, *et al.* Eosinophilic esophagitis: a prevalent disease in the United States that affects all age groups. *Gastroenterology* 2008;**134**:1316–1321.
8 Liacouras CA, Furuta GT, Hirano I, *et al.* Eosinophilic esophagitis: Updated consensus recommendations for children and adults. *J Allergy Clin Immunol* 2011;**128**(1):2–20.
9 Noel RJ, Putnam PE, Rothenberg, ME. Eosinophilic esophagitis. *N Engl J Med* 2004;**351**:940–941.
10 Rothenberg ME. Reviews in basic and clinical gastroenterology: biology and treatment of eosinophilic esophagitis. *Gastroenterology* 2009;**137**:1238–1249.
11 Shah A, Kagalwalla AF, Gonsalves N, Melin-Aldana H, Li BU, Hirano I. Histopathologic variability in children with eosinophilic esophagitis. *Am J Gastroenterol* 2009;**104**:716–721.
12 Spergel JM, Rothenberg ME, Collins MH, *et al.* Reslizumab in children and adolescents with eosinophilic esophagitis: results of a double-blind, randomized, placebo-controlled trial. *J Allergy Clin Immunol* 2012;**129**(2):456–63, 463.e1–3.
13 Winter HS, Madara JL, Stafford RJ, *et al.* Intraepithelial eosinophils: a new diagnostic criterion for reflux esophagitis. *Gastroenterology* 1982;**83**:818–823.

CHAPTER 6 ESOPHAGEAL MOTILITY: MEASURES AND DISORDERS OF ESOPHAGEAL MOTOR FUNCTION

1 Boeckxstaens GE. Achalasia. *Best Pract Res Clin Gastroenterol* 2007;**21**:595–608.
2 Castell DO. In the diagnosis of achalasia, 'classic' might be 'atypical'. *Clin Gastroenterol Hepatol* 2012;**10**(7):821–822.
3 Chuah SK, Hsu PI, Wu KL, *et al.* 2011 update on esophageal achalasia. *World J Gastroenterol* 2012;**18**(14):1573–1578.
4 Clouse RS, Staiano A, Alrakawi A, Haroian L. Application of topographical methods to clinical esophageal manometry. *Am J Gastroenterol* 2000;**95**:2720–2730.
5 Bredenoord AJ, Fox M, Kahrilas PJ, *et al.* Chicago classification criteria of esophageal motility disorders defined in high resolution esophageal pressure topography. *Neurogastroenterol Motil* 2012;**24**(Suppl 1):57–65.
6 Gockel I, Muller M, Schumacher J. Achalasia – a disease of unknown cause that is often diagnosed too late. *Dtsch Arztebl Int* 2012;**109**(12):209–214.
7 Kahrilas PJ, Sifrim D. High-resolution manometry and impedance-pH/manometry: valuable tools in clinical and investigational esophagology. *Gastroenterology* 2008;**135**:756–769.
8 Pandolfino JE, Kahrilas PJ. AGA technical review on the clinical use of esophageal manometry. *Gastroenterology* 2005;**128**:209–224.
9 Pandolfino JE, Kahrilas PJ. New technologies in the gastrointestinal clinic and research: impedance and high-resolution manometry. *World J Gastroenterol* 2009;**15**:131–138.
10 Pandolfino JE, Kwiatek MA, Nealis T, Bulsiewicz W, Post J, Kahrilas PJ. Achalasia: a new clinically relevant classification by high-resolution manometry. *Gastroenterology* 2008;**135**: 1526–1533.

11 Rohof WO, Boeckxstaens GE. New insights in pathophysiology and management of achalasia. *J Pediatr Gastroenterol Nutr* 2011;**53**(Suppl 2):S17–S19.

12 Richter JE. Update on the management of achalasia: balloons, surgery and drugs. *Expert Rev Gastroenterol Hepatol* 2008;**2**:435–445.

13 Richter JE. Achalasia – an update. *J Neurogastroenterol Motil* 2010;**16**:232–242.

14 Richter JE, Boeckxstaens GE. Management of achalasia: Surgery or pneumatic dilation. *Gut* 2011;**60**:869–876.

CHAPTER 7 ESOPHAGEAL VARICES

1 Fagundes E, Ferreira A, Roquete M, *et al.* Clinical and laboratory predictors of esophageal varices in children and adolescents with portal hypertension syndrome. *J Pediatr Gastroenterol Nutr* 2008;**46**:178–183.

2 Garcia-Tsao G, Sanyal A, Grace N, Carey W, and the Practice Guidelines Committee of the American Association for the Study of Liver Diseases, the Practice Parameters Committee of the American College of Gastroenterology. Prevention and management of gastroesophageal varices and variceal hemorrhage in cirrhosis. *Hepatology* 2007;**46**:922–938.

3 Ling SC. Should children with esophageal varices receive beta-blockers for the primary prevention of variceal hemorrhage? *Can J Gastroenterol* 2005;**19**:661–666.

4 Ling SC, Walters T, McKiernan P, Schwarz K, Garcia-Tsao G, Shneider B. Primary prophylaxis of variceal hemorrhage in children with portal hypertension: a framework for future research. *J Pediatr Gastroenterol Nutr* 2011;**52**:254–261.

5 McKiernan P, Beath S, Davison SA. Prospective study of endoscopic esophageal variceal ligation using a multiband ligator. *J Pediatr Gastroenterol Nutr* 2002;**34**:207–211.

6 Senyüz O, Osman Faruk, Yesildag E, *et al.* Sugiura procedure in portal hypertensive children. *J Hepatobiliary Pancreat Surg* 2001;**8**:245–249.

CHAPTER 8 ESOPHAGEAL INFECTIONS

1 Kofla G, Ruhnke M. Pharmacology and metabolism of anidulafungin, caspofungin, and micafungin in the treatment of invasive candidosis: review of the literature. *Eur J Med Res* 2011;**16**(4):159–166.

2 Marsh WW. Infectious diseases of gastrointestinal tract in adolescents. *Adolesc Med* 2000;**11**(2):263–278.

3 Pace F, Pallotta S, Antinori S. Nongastroesophageal reflux disease-related infectious, inflammatory, and injurious disorders of the esophagus. *Curr Opin Gastroenterol* 2007;**23**(4):446–451.

4 Sutton FM, Graham DY, Goodgame RW. Infectious esophagitis. *Gastrointest Endosc Clin N Am* 1994;**4**(4):713–729.

5 Wilcox CM, Karowe MW. Esophageal infections: etiology, diagnosis, and management. *Gastroenterologist* 1994;**2**(3):188–206.

6 Yee J, Wall SD. Infectious esophagitis. *Radiol Clin North Am* 1994;**32**(6):1135–1145.

CHAPTER 9 ESOPHAGEAL FOREIGN BODIES

1 Brumbaugh DE, Colson SB, Sandoval JA, *et al.* Management of button battery-induced hemorrhage in children. *J Pediatr Gastroenterol Nutr* 2011;**52**(5):585–589.

2 Gmeiner D, von Rahden BH, Meco C, Hutter J, Oberascher G, Stein HJ. Flexible versus rigid endoscopy for treatment of foreign body impaction in the esophagus. *Surg Endosc* 2007;**21**(11):2026–2029.

3 Hurtado CW, Furuta GT, Kramer RE. Etiology of esophageal food impactions in children. *J Pediatr Gastroenterol Nutr* 2010;**52**(1):43–46.

4 Kay M, Wyllie R. Pediatric foreign bodies and their management. *Curr Gastroenterol Rep* 2005;**7**(3):212–218.

5 Larsson H, Bergquist H, Bove M. The incidence of esophageal bolus impaction: is there a seasonal variation? *Otolaryngol Head Neck Surg* 2011;**144**(2):186–190.

6 Litovitz T, Whitaker N, Clark L, White NC, Marsolek M. Emerging battery-ingestion hazard: clinical implications. *Pediatrics* 2010;**125**(6):1168–1177.

7 Louie JP, Alpern ER, Windreich RM. Witnessed and unwitnessed esophageal foreign bodies in children. *Pediatr Emerg Care* 2005;**21**(9):582–585.

8 Mehta DI, Attia MW, Quintana EC, Cronan KM. Glucagon use for esophageal coin dislodgement in children: a prospective double-blind, placebo-controlled trial. *Acad Emerg Med* 2001;**8**(2):200–203.

9 Miller SM, Willging JP, Rutter MJ, Rookkapan K. Chronic esophageal foreign bodies in pediatric patients: a retrospective

review. *Int J Pediatr Otorhinolaryngol* 2004;**68**(3):265–272.

10 Morrow SE, Bickler SW, Kennedy AP, Snyder CL, Sharp RJ, Ashcraft KW. Balloon extraction of esophageal foreign bodies in children. *J Pediatr Surg* 1998;**33**(2):266–270.

11 Waltzman ML. Management of esophageal coins. *Curr Opin Pediatr* 2006;**18**(5):571–574.

CHAPTER 10 ESOPHAGEAL BURNS

1 Dogan Y, Erkan T, Cokugras F C, Kutlu T. Caustic gastroesophageal lesions in childhood: an analysis of 473 cases. *Clin Pediatr* 2006;**45**:435–438.

2 Kay M, Wyllie R. Caustic ingestions in children. *Curr Opin Pediatr* 2009;**21**:651–654.

3 Kikendall JW. Pill esophagitis. *J Clin Gastroenterol* 1999;**28**(4):298–305.

4 Kimball SJ, Park AH, Rollins II MD, Grimmer JF, Muntz H. A review of esophageal disc battery ingestions and a protocol for management. *Arch Otolaryngol Head Neck Surg* 2010;**136**(9):866–871.

5 Litovitz T, Whitaker N, Clark L, White NC, Marsolek M. Emerging battery-ingestion hazard: clinical implications. *Pediatrics* 2010;**125**:1168–1177.

6 Pace F, Antinori S, Repici A. What is new in esophageal injury (infection, drug-induced, caustic, stricture, perforation)? *Curr Opin Gastroenterol* 2009;**25**:372–379.

7 Salzman M, O'Malley RN. Updates on the evaluation and management of caustic exposures. *Emerg Med Clin North Am* 2007;**25**:459–476.

8 Zargar SA, Kochhar R, Mehta S, Mehta SK. The role of fiberoptic endoscopy in the management of corrosive ingestion and modified endoscopic classification of burns. *Gastrointest Endosc* 1991;**37**:165–169.

Section 3 Stomach and Duodenum

CHAPTER 11 GASTRITIS AND GASTRIC ULCERS

1 Azevedo N, Huntington J, Goodman K. The epidemiology of *Helicobacter pylori* and Public Health implications. *Helicobacter* 2009;**14**(Supplement):s1:1–7.

2 Chey W, Wong B. American College of Gastroenterology Guideline on the management of *Helicobacter pylori* infection. *Am J Gastroenterol* 2007;**102**:1808–1825.

3 Dohil R, Hassall E. Gastritis, gastropathy and ulcer disease. In: Wyllie R, Hyams J, Kay M (eds). *Pediatric Gastrointestinal and Liver Disease*, 3rd edn. Saunders Elsevier, London, 2006; Ch. 25, pp. 373–407.

4 Gold B, Colletti R, Abbott M, *et al*. *Helicobacter pylori* infection in children: recommendations for diagnosis and treatment. *J Pediatr Gastroenterol Nutr* 2000;**31**:490–497.

5 Guarner J, Kalach N, Elitsur Y, Koletzko S. *Helicobacter pylori* diagnostic tests in children: review of the literature from 1999 to 2009. *Eur J Pediatr* 2010;**169**:15–25.

6 Koletzko S, Jones N, Goodman K, Gold B, Rowland M, *et al*. Evidence-based guidelines from ESPGHAN and NASPGHAN for *Helicobacter pylori* infection in children. *J Pediatr Gastroenterol Nutr* 2011;**53**:230–243.

7 Walters T, Jones N. *Helicobacter pylori* in childhood. In:, Kay M R, Hyams J (eds). *Pediatric Gastrointestinal and Liver Disease*, 3rd edn. Saunders Elsevier, London, 2006; Ch. 26, pp. 409–437.

CHAPTER 12 ABNORMAL ANATOMY OF THE STOMACH AND DUODENUM

1 Kealey WDC, McCallion WA, Brown S, Potts SR, Boston VE. Midgut volvulus in children. *Br J Surg* 1996;**83**:105–106.

2 Kleinman RE, Goulet O-J, Mieli-Vergani G, Sanderson IR, Sherman PM, Shneider BL (eds). *Walker's Pediatric Gastrointestinal Disease: Physiology, Diagnosis, Management*, 5th edn McGraw-Hill, New York, 2008.

3 Long FR, Kramer SS, Markowitz RI, Taylor GE. Radiographic patterns of intestinal malrotation in children. *Radiographics* 1996;**16**:547–556.

4 Merrill Karrer F, Cuffari C. Pediatric Duodenal Atresia. Medscape. March 5, 2012.

5 Parish A, Cuffari C. Intestinal malrotation. Clinical Presentation. Medscape. April 20, 2010.

6 Stringer MD, Pablot SM, Brereton RJ. Paediatric intussusception. *Br J Surg* 1992;**79**:867–876.

CHAPTER 13 EOSINOPHILIC GASTROENTERITIS

1 Chehade M, Magid MS, Mofidi S, Nowak-Wegrzyn A, Sampson HA, Sicherer SH. Allergic eosinophilic gastroenteritis with protein-losing enteropathy: intestinal pathology, clinical course, and long-term follow-up. *J Pediatr Gastroenterol Nutr* 2006;**42**(5):516–521.

2 Metcalfe DD, Sampson HA, Simon RA. Eosinophilic esophagitis, gastroenteritis (gastroenterocolitis) and colitis. In: Franciosi JP, Markowitz JE, Liacouras CA (eds). *Food Allergy: Adverse Reactions to Foods and Food Additives*, 4th edn. Wiley Blackwell, UK, 2008.

3 Justinich C, Katz A, Gurbindo C, *et al*. Elemental diet improves steroid-dependent eosinophilic gastroenteritis and reverses growth failure. *J Pediatr Gastroenterol Nutr* 1996;**23**(1):81–85.

4 Khan S, Orenstein SR. Eosinophilic gastroenteritis masquerading as pyloric stenosis. *Clin Pediatr* 2000;**39**(1):55–57.

5 Siewert E, Lammert F, Koppitz P, Schmidt T, Matern S. Eosinophilic gastroenteritis with severe protein-losing enteropathy: successful treatment with budesonide. *Dig Liver Dis* 2006;**38**(1):55–59.

CHAPTER 14 GASTRIC INFECTIONS

1 Gold BD, Colletti RB, Abbott M, *et al*. Medical Position Statement: The North American Society for Pediatric Gastroenterology and Nutrition. *Helicobacter pylori* infection in children: recommendations for diagnosis and treatment. *J Pediatr Gastroenterol Nutr* 2000;**31**:490–497.

2 Koletzko S, Jones NL, Goodman KJ, *et al*. Evidence-based Guidelines from ESPGHAN and NASPGHAN for *Helicobacter pylori* infection in children. *J Pediatr Gastroenterol Nutr* 2011;**53**:230–243.

3 Oderda G, Shcherbakov P, Bontems P, *et al*. Results from the pediatric European register for treatment of *Helicobacter pylori* (PERTH). *Helicobacter* 2007;**12**(2):150–156.

4 Ozen A, Ertem D, Pehlivanoglu E. Natural history and symptomatology of *Helicobacter pylori* in childhood and factors determining the epidemiology of infection. *J Pediatr Gastroenterol Nutr* 2006;**42**:398–404.

CHAPTER 15 GASTROPARESIS

1 Parkman HP, Yates K, Hasler WL, *et al*. National Institute of Diabetes and Digestive and Kidney Diseases Gastroparesis Clinical Research Consortium. Clinical features of idiopathic gastroparesis vary with sex, body mass, symptom onset, delay in gastric emptying, and gastroparesis severity. *Gastroenterology* 2011;**140**(1):101–115.

2 Pasricha PJ, Colvin R, Yates K, *et al*. Characteristics of patients with chronic unexplained nausea and vomiting and normal gastric emptying. *Clin Gastroenterol Hepatol* 2011;**9**(7):567–576.e1–4.

3 Rao SS, Camilleri M, Hasler WL, *et al*. Evaluation of gastrointestinal transit in clinical practice: position paper of the American and European Neurogastroenterology and Motility Societies. *Neurogastroenterol Motil* 2011;**23**(1):8–23.

4 Rodriguez L, Rosen R, Manfredi M, Nurko S. Endoscopic intrapyloric injection of botulinum toxin A in the treatment of children with gastroparesis: a retrospective, open-label study. *Gastrointest Endosc* 2012;**75**(2):302–309.

5 Tang DM, Friedenberg FK. Gastroparesis: approach, diagnostic evaluation, and management. *Dis Mon* 2011;**57**(2):74–101.

CHAPTER 16 GASTRIC FOREIGN BODIES

1 ASGE Standards of Practice Committee, Ikenberry SO, Jue TL, Anderson MA, *et al*. Management of ingested foreign bodies and food impactions. *Gastrointest Endosc* 2011;**73**(6):1085–1091.

2 ASGE Technology Committee, Tierney WM, Adler DC, Conway JD, *et al*. Overtube use in gastrointestinal endoscopy. *Gastrointest Endosc* 2009;**70**(5):828–834.

3 Kay M, Wyllie R. Techniques of foreign body removal in infants and children. *Tech Gastrointest Endosc* 2002;**4**(4):188–195.

4 Kay M, Wyllie R. Pediatric foreign bodies and their management. *Curr Gastroenterol Rep* 2005;**7**(3):212–218.

5 Li SZ, Sun ZX, Zou DW, Xu GM, Wu RP, Liao Z. Endoscopic management of foreign bodies in the upper-GI tract: experience with 1088 cases in China. *Gastrointest Endosc* 2006;**64**(4):485–492.

6 Smith MT, Wong RK. Foreign bodies. *Gastrointest Endosc Clin North Am* 2007;**17**(2):361–382.

7 Uyemura M. Foreign body ingestion in children. *Am Fam Physician* 2005;**72**(2):287–291.

CHAPTER 17 DUODENAL ULCER

1 Elitsur Y, Lawrence Z. Non-*Helicobacter pylori* related duodenal ulcer disease in children. *Helicobacter* 2001;**6**(3):239–243.
2 Kalach N, Bontems P, Koletzko S, Mourad-Baars P, *et al*. Frequency and risk factors of gastric and duodenal ulcers or erosions in children: a prospective 1-month European multicenter study. *Eur J Gastroenterol Hepatol* 2010;**22**(10):1174–1181.
3 Mones RL, Mercer GO. Ulcerative duodenitis in a child with celiac disease. *J Pediatr* 2011;**158**(5):857.
4 Tam YH, Lee KH, To KF, Chan KW, Cheung ST. *Helicobacter pylori*-positive versus *Helicobacter pylori*-negative idiopathic peptic ulcers in children with their long-term outcomes. *J Pediatr Gastroenterol Nutr* 2009;**48**(3):299–305.
5 Urganci N, Ozcelik G, Kalyoncu D, Geylani Gulec S, Akinci N. Serum gastrin levels and gastroduodenal lesions in children with chronic renal failure on continuous ambulatory peritoneal dialysis: a single-center experience. *Eur J Gastroenterol Hepatol* 2012;**24**(8):924–928.

CHAPTER 18 PEDIATRIC FUNCTIONAL GASTROINTESTINAL DISORDERS

1 Apley J, Naish N. Recurrent abdominal pains: a field survey of 1,000 school children. *Arch Dis Child* 1958;**33**(168):165–170.
2 Campo JV, Perel J, Lucas A, *et al*. Citalopram treatment of pediatric recurrent abdominal pain and comorbid internalizing disorders: an exploratory study. *J Am Acad Child Adolesc Psychiatry* 2004;**43**(10):1234–1242.
3 Chiou E, Nurko S. Functional abdominal pain and irritable bowel syndrome in children and adolescents. *Therapy* 2011;**8**(3):315–331.
4 Di Lorenzo C, Colletti RB, Lehmann HP, *et al*. Chronic abdominal pain in children: a technical report of the American Academy of Pediatrics and the North American Society for Pediatric Gastroenterology, Hepatology and Nutrition. *J Pediatr Gastroenterol Nutr* 2005;**40**(3):249–261.
5 Francavilla R, Miniello V, Magistà AM, *et al*. A randomized controlled trial of *Lactobacillus*

GG in children with functional abdominal pain. *Pediatrics* 2010;**126**(6):1445–1452.
6 Gawronska A, Dziechciarz P, Horvath A, Szajewska H. A randomized double-blind placebo-controlled trial of *Lactobacillus* GG for abdominal pain disorders in children. *Aliment Pharmacol Ther* 2006;**25**(2):177–184.
7 Horvath A, Dziechciarz P, Szajewska H. Meta-analysis: *Lactobacillus rhamnosus* GG for abdominal pain-related functional gastrointestinal disorders in childhood. *Aliment Pharmacol Ther* 2011;**33**(12):1302–1310.
8 Rasquin A, Di Lorenzo C, Forbes D, *et al*. Childhood functional gastrointestinal disorders: child/adolescent. *Gastroenterology* 2006;**130**(5):1527–1537.
9 Saps M, Seshadri R, Sztainberg M, Schaffer G, Marshall BM, Di Lorenzo C. A prospective school-based study of abdominal pain and other common somatic complaints in children. *J Pediatr* 2009;**154**(3):322–326.
10 Walker LS, Sherman AL, Bruehl S, Garber J, Smith CA. Functional abdominal pain patient subtypes in childhood predict functional gastrointestinal disorders with chronic pain and psychiatric comorbidities in adolescence and adulthood. *Pain* 2012;**153**(9):1798–1806.

Section 4 Jejunum and Ileum

CHAPTER 19 MALABSORPTION

1 Ammoury RF, Croffie JM. Malabsorptive disorders of childhood. *Pediatr Rev* 2010;**31**(10):407–415.
2 Brasitus TA, Sitrin MD. Intestinal malabsorption syndromes. *Ann Rev Med* 1990;**41**:339–347.
3 Finkel Y, Goulet O. Short bowel syndrome. In: Kleinman RE, Goulet OJ, Mieli-Vergani G, Sanderson IR, Sherman PM, Shneider BL (eds). *Walker's Pediatric Gastrointestinal Disease; Physiology, Diagnosis, Management*, 5th edn. McGraw-Hill, New York, 2008; Ch. 22.1.
4 Guandalini S. Pediatric malabsorption. Emedicine.medscape.com/article/931041. Accessed Sept 8, 2012.
5 Hofmann AF. Chronic diarrhea caused by idiopathic bile acid malabsorption: an explanation at last. *Expert Rev Gastroenterol Hepatol* 2009;**3**(5):461–464.

6 Schulzke JD, Troger H, Amasheh M. Disorders of intestinal secretion and absorption. *Best Pract Res Clin Gastroenterol* 2009;**23**(3):395–406.

7 Semrad CE, Poweel DW. Approach to the patient with diarrhea and malabsorption. In: Goldman L, Ausiello D (eds). *Cecil Medicine*, 23rd edn. Saunders Elsevier, Philadelphia, 2007; Ch. 143.

8 Shatnawei A, Parekh NR, Rhoda KM, *et al.* Intestinal failure management at the Cleveland Clinic. *Arch Surg* 2010;**145**(6):521–527.

CHAPTER 20 CELIAC DISEASE

1 Fasano A, Berti I, Gerarduzzi T, *et al.* Prevalence of celiac disease in at-risk and not-at-risk groups in the United States: a large multicenter study. *Arch Intern Med* 2003;**163**(3):286–292.

2 Hill ID, Dirks MH, Liptak GS, *et al.* Guideline for the diagnosis and treatment of celiac disease in children: recommendations of the North American Society for Pediatric Gastroenterology, Hepatology and Nutrition. *J Pediatr Gastroenterol Nutr* 2005;**40**(1):1–19.

3 Husby S, Koletzko S, Korponay-Szabo IR, *et al.* European Society for Pediatric Gastroenterology, Hepatology, and Nutrition Guidelines for the diagnosis of coeliac disease. *J Pediatr Gastroenterol Nutr* 2012;**54**(1):136–160.

4 Ivarsson A, Hernell O, Stenlund H, Persson LA. Breast-feeding protects against celiac disease. *Am J Clin Nutr* 2002;**75**(5):914–921.

5 Lagerqvist C, Dahlbom I, Hansson T, *et al.* Antigliadin immunoglobulin A best in finding celiac disease in children younger than 18 months of age. *J Pediatr Gastroenterol Nutr* 2008;**47**(4):428–435.

6 Norris JM, Barriga K, Hoffenberg EJ, *et al.* Risk of celiac disease autoimmunity and timing of gluten introduction in the diet of infants at increased risk of disease. *JAMA* 2005;**293**(19):2343–2351.

7 Oberhuber G, Granditsch G, Vogelsang H. The histopathology of coeliac disease: time for a standardized report scheme for pathologists. *Eur J Gastroenterol Hepatol* 1999;**11**(10):1185–1194.

8 Sellitto M, Bai G, Serena G, *et al.* Proof of concept of microbiome-metabolome analysis and delayed gluten exposure on celiac disease autoimmunity in genetically at-risk infants. *PloS One* 2012;**7**(3):e33387.

CHAPTER 21 SMALL BOWEL INFECTIONS

1 Chalmers RM, Davies AP. Minireview: clinical cryptosporidiosis. *Exp Parasitol* 2010;**124**(1):138–146.

2 Chao HC, Chen CC, Chen SY, Chiu CH. Bacterial enteric infections in children: etiology, clinical manifestations and antimicrobial therapy. *Expert Rev Anti Infect Ther* 2006;**4**(4):629–638.

3 Guerrant RL, Hughes JM, Lima NL, Crane J. Diarrhea in developed and developing countries: magnitude, special settings, and etiologies. *Rev Infect Dis* 1990;**12**(Suppl 1):S41–50.

4 Marsh WW. Infectious diseases of gastrointestinal tract in adolescents. *Adolesc Med* 2000;**11**(2):263–278.

5 Ochoa TJ, Salazar-Lindo E, Cleary TG. Management of children with infection-associated persistent diarrhea. *Semin Pediatr Infect Dis* 2004;**15**(4):229–236.

CHAPTER 22 SHORT BOWEL SYNDROME

1 Colomb V, Jobert-Giraud A, Lacaille F, Goulet O, Fournet JC, Ricour C. Role of lipid emulsions in cholestasis associated with long-term parenteral nutrition in children. *J Parenter Enteral Nutr* 2000;**24**:345–350.

2 Duro D, Kamin D, Duggan C. Overview of pediatric short bowel syndrome. *J Pediatr Gastroenterol Nutr* 2008;**47**(Supplement 1):S33–36.

3 Duro D, Jaksic T, Duggan C. Multiple micronutrient deficiencies in a child with short bowel syndrome and normal somatic growth. *J Pediatr Gastroenteroland Nutr* 2008;**46**:461–464.

4 Goulet O, Baglin-Gobet S, Talbotec C, *et al.* Outcome and long-term growth after extensive small bowel resection in the neonatal period: a survey of 87 children. *Eur J Pediatr Surg* 2005;**15**:95–101.

5 Jones BA, Hull MA, Richardson DS, *et al.* Efficacy of ethanol locks in reducing central venous catheter infections in pediatric patients with intestinal failure. *J Pediatr Surg* 2010;**45**(6):1287–1293.

6 Kim HB, Lee PW, Garza J, Duggan C, Fauza D, Jaksic T. Serial transverse entero-

plasty for short bowel syndrome: a case report. *J Pediatr Surg* 2003;**38**:881–885.

7 Modi BP, Langer M, Ching YA, *et al*. Improved survival in a multidisciplinary short bowel syndrome program. *J Pediatr Surg* 2008;**43**:20–24.

8 Yang CF, Duro D, Zurakowski D, Lee M, Jaksic T, Duggan C. High prevalence of multiple micronutrient deficiencies in children with intestinal failure: a longitudinal study. *J Pediatr* 2011;**159**(1):39–44.

CHAPTER 23 PROTEIN-LOSING ENTEROPATHY

1 Braamskamp MJ, Dolman KM, Tabbers MM. Clinical practice. Protein-losing enteropathy in children. *Eur J Pediatr* 2010;**169**(10):1179–1185.

2 Maloney J, Nowak-Wegrzyn A. Educational clinical cases series for pediatric allergy and immunology: allergic proctocolitis, food protein induced enterocolitis syndrome and allergic eosinophilic gastroenteritis with protein-losing gastroenteropathy as manifestations of non-IgE-mediated cow's milk allergy. *Pediatr Allergy Immunol* 2007;**18**:360–367.

3 Proujansky R. Protein-losing enteropathy. In: Walker WA, Durie PR, Hamilton JR, Walker-Smith JA, Watkins JB (eds). *Pediatric Gastrointestinal Disease, Pathophysiology, Diagnosis, and Management*, 3rd edn. BC Decker, Philadelphia, 2000; pp. 195–200.

4 Rychik J. Protein-losing enteropathy after Fontan operation. *Congenit Heart Dis* 2007;**2**(5):288–300.

5 Umar SB, DiBaise JK. Protein-losing enteropathy: case illustrations and clinical review. *Am J Gastroenterol* 2010;**105**(1):43–47.

CHAPTER 24 CROHN DISEASE

1 Bentsen B S, Moum B, Ekbom A. Incidence of inflammatory bowel disease in children in southeastern Norway: a prospective population-based study 1990–94. *Scand J Gastroenterol* 2002;**37**(5):540–545.

2 Bonen, DK, Cho JH. The genetics of inflammatory bowel disease. *Gastroenterology* 2003;**124**:521–536.

3 Cosnes J, Gower–Rousseau C, Seksik P, Cortot A. Epidemiology and natural history of inflammatory bowel diseases. *Gastroenterology* 2011;**140**(6):1785–1794.

4 Cuthbert AP, Fisher SA, Mirza MM, *et al*. The contribution of NOD2 gene mutations to the risk and site of disease in inflammatory bowel disease. *Gastroenterology* 2002;**122**:876–874.

5 Day AS, Whitten KE, Sidler M, *et al*. Systematic review: nutritional therapy in paediatric Crohn's disease. *AlimentPharmacol Ther* 2008;**27**:293–307.

6 De Cruz P, Kamm MA, Prideaux L, Allen PB, Moore G. Mucosal healing in Crohn's disease: a systematic review. *Inflamm Bowel Dis* 2013;**19**(2):429–444.

7 Economou M, Trikalinos TA, Loizou KT, Tsianos EV, Ioannidis JP. Differential effects of NOD2 variants on Crohn's disease risk and phenotype in diverse populations: a meta-analysis. *Am J Gastroenterol* 2004;**99**(12):2393–2404.

8 Gower-Rousseau C, Dauchet L, Vernier-Massouille G, *et al*. The natural history of pediatric ulcerative colitis: a population-based cohort study. *Am J Gastroenterol* 2009;**104**(8):2080–2088.

9 Griffiths AM. Crohn's disease. In: Kleinman RE, Goulet O-J, Mieli-Vergani G, Sanderson IR, Sherman PM, Schneider BL (eds). *Walker's Pediatric Gastrointestinal Disease: Physiology, Diagnosis, Management*, 5th edn. McGraw-Hill, New York, 2008; pp. 519–539.

10 Halfvarson J, Bodin L, Tysk C, Lindberg E, Järnerot G. Inflammatory bowel disease in a Swedish twin cohort: a long-term follow-up of concordance and clinical characteristics. *Gastroenterology* 2003;**124**(7):1767–1773.

11 Hou JK, Abraham B, El-Serag H. Dietary intake and risk of developing inflammatory bowel disease: a systematic review of the literature. *Am J Gastroenterol* 2011;**106**(4):563–573.

12 Kugathasan S, Judd RH, Hoffmann RG, *et al*. Epidemiologic and clinical characteristics of children with newly diagnosed inflammatory bowel disease in Wisconsin: a statewide population-based study. *J Pediatr* 2003;**143**(4):525–531.

13 Lesage S, Zouali H, Cézard JP, *et al*. CARD15/NOD2 mutational analysis and genotype-phenotype correlation in 612 patients with inflammatory bowel disease. *Am J Hum Genet* 2002;**70**(4):845–857.

14 Levine A, Griffiths A, Markowitz J. Pediatric modification of the Montreal

classification for inflammatory bowel disease: the Paris classification. *Inflamm Bowel Dis* 2011;**17**(6):1314–1321.

15 Levine JS, Burakoff R. Extraintestinal manifestations of inflammatory bowel disease. *Gastroenterol Hepatol* 2011;**7**(4):235–241.

16 Lichtenstein GR, Abreu MT, Cohen R, Tremaine W, American Gastroenterological Association. American Gastroenterological Association Institute technical review on corticosteroids, immunomodulators, and infliximab in inflammatory bowel disease. *Gastroenterology* 2006;**130**(3):940–987.

17 Mack DR, Langton C, Markowitz J, *et al*. Laboratory values for children with newly diagnosed inflammatory bowel disease. *Pediatrics* 2007;**119**(6):1113–1119.

18 Orholm M, Binder V, Sørensen TI, Rasmussen LP, Kyvik KO. Concordance of inflammatory bowel disease among Danish twins. Results of a nationwide study. *Scand J Gastroenterol* 2000;**35**(10):1075–1081.

19 Polito JM, Childs B, Mellits ED, Tokayer AZ, Harris ML, Bayless TM. Crohn's disease: influence of age at diagnosis on site and clinical type of disease. *Gastroenterology* 1996;**111**(3):580–586.

20 Roth MP, Petersen GM, McElree C, Vadheim CM, Panish JF, Rotter JI. Familial empiric risk estimates of inflammatory bowel disease in Ashkenazi Jews. *Gastroenterology* 1989;**96**(4):1016–1020.

21 Sawczenko A, Sandhu BK. Presenting features of inflammatory bowel disease in Great Britain and Ireland. *Arch Dis Child* 2003;**88**:995–1000.

22 Sawczenko A, Sandhu BK, Logan RFA, *et al*. Prospective survey of childhood inflammatory bowel disease in the British Isles. *Lancet* 2001;**357**:1093–1094.

23 Van Limbergen J, Russell RK, Drummond HE, *et al*. Definition of phenotypic characteristics of childhood-onset inflammatory bowel disease. *Gastroenterology* 2008;**135**(4):1114–1122.

CHAPTER 25 BACTERIAL OVERGROWTH

1 Collins BS, Lin HC. Double-blind, placebo-controlled antibiotic treatment study of small intestinal bacterial overgrowth in children with chronic abdominal pain. *J Pediatr Gastroenterol Nutr* 2011;**52**:382–386.

2 Husebye E. The pathogenesis of gastrointestinal bacterial overgrowth. *Chemotherapy* 2005;**51**(Suppl 1):1–22.

3 Jones HF, Davidson GP, Brooks DA, Butler RN. Is small-bowel bacterial overgrowth an underdiagnosed disorder in children with gastrointestinal symptoms? *J Pediatr Gastroenterol Nutr* 2011;**52**:632–634.

4 Khoshini R, Dai SC, Lezcano S, *et al*. A systematic review of diagnostic tests for small intestinal bacterial overgrowth. *Dig Dis Sci* 2008;**53**:1443–1454.

5 Kleinman RE, Goulet O-J, Mieli-Vergani G, Sanderson IR, Sherman PM, Schneider BL (eds). *Walker's Pediatric Gastrointestinal Disease; Physiology, Diagnosis, Management*, 5th edn. McGraw-Hill, New York, 2008.

6 Wylllie R, Hyams JS. *Pediatric Gastrointestinal and Liver Disease*, 4th edn. Saunders Elsevier, Philadelphia, 2011.

CHAPTER 26 NEOPLASMS OF THE ABDOMEN AND GASTROINTESTINAL TRACT

1 Ehrlich PF. Wilms tumor: progress and considerations for the surgeon. *Surg Oncol* 2007;**16**(3):157–171.

2 Glick RD, Pashankar FD, Pappo A, Laquaglia MP. Management of pancreatoblastoma in children and young adults. *J Pediatr Hematol Oncol* 2012;**34**(Suppl 2):S47–50.

3 Goldberg J, Furman WL. Management of colorectal carcinoma in children and young adults. *J Pediatr Hematol Oncol* 2012;**34**(Suppl 2):S76–79.

4 Janeway KA, Pappo A. Treatment guidelines for gastrointestinal stromal tumors in children and young adults. *J Pediatr Hematol Oncol* 2012;**34**(Suppl 2):S69–72.

5 Kassira N, Pedroso FE, Cheung MC, Koniaris LG, Sola JE. Primary gastrointestinal tract lymphoma in the pediatric patient: review of 265 patients from the SEER registry. *J Pediatr Surg* 2011;**46**(10):1956–1964.

6 Malogolowkin MH, Katzenstein HM, Krailo M, Meyers RL. Treatment of hepatoblastoma: the North American cooperative group experience. Front Biosci (Elite Edn) 2012;**4**:1717–1723.

7 Molyneux EM, Rochford R, Griffin B, *et al*. Burkitt's lymphoma. *Lancet* 2012;**379**(9822):1234–1244.

8 Pappo AS, Janeway K, Laquaglia M, Kim SY. Special considerations in pediatric gastrointestinal tumors. *J Surg Oncol* 2011;**104**(8):928–932.
9 Subbiah V, Varadhachary G, Herzog CE, Huh WW. Gastric adenocarcinoma in children and adolescents. *Pediatr Blood Cancer* 2011;**57**(3):524–527.

CHAPTER 27 BOWEL OBSTRUCTION
1 Carlyle BE, Borowitz DS, Glick PL. A review of the pathophysiology and management of fetuses and neonates with meconium ileum for the pediatric surgeon. *J Pediatr Surg* 2012;**47**:772–781.
2 Cuenca AG, Ali AS, Kays DW, Islam S. Pulling the Plug – management of meconium plug syndrome in neonates. *J Surg Res* 2012;**175**:e43–46.
3 Haricharan RN, Georgeson KE. Hirschprung disease. *Semin Pediatr Surg* 2008;**17**:266–275.
4 Juang D, Snyder CL. Neonatal bowel obstruction. *Surg Clin North Am* 2012;**92**:685–711.

CHAPTER 28 NECROTIZING ENTEROCOLITIS
1 Hunter CJ, Ford HR, Camerini V. Necrotizing enterocolitis. In: Puri P, Höllwarth M (eds). *Pediatric Surgery: Diagnosis and Management*. Springer-Verlag, Berlin Heidelberg, 2009.
2 Lin PW, Stoll BJ. Necrotizing enterocolitis. *Lancet* 2006;**368**:1271–1283.
3 Moss RL, Dimmitt RA, Barnhart DB, *et al.* Laparotomy versus peritoneal drainage for necrotizing enterocolitis and perforation. *N Engl J Med* 2006;**354**:2225–2234.
4 Warner BW, Saito JM. Neonatal enterocolitis and short bowel syndrome. In: Fisher JE, Jones DB, Pomposelli FB, Upchurch GR (eds). *Mastery of Surgery*, 6th edn. Lippincott Williams and Wilkins, Philadelphia, 2012.

CHAPTER 29 NUTRITION OVERVIEW
1 American Society for Parenteral and Enteral Nutrition (ASPEN) Board of Directors and Task Force on Standards for Specialized Nutrition Support for Hospitalized Pediatric Patients, Wessel J, Balint J, Crill C, Klotz K. Standards for specialized nutrition support: hospitalized pediatric patients. *Nutr Clin Pract* 2005;**20**:103–116.

2 Baker SS, Baker RD, Davis AM (eds). *Pediatric Nutrition Support*. Jones and Barlett Publishers, Sudbury, 2007.
3 Bankhead R, Boullata J, Brantley S, *et al.*, and the American Society of Parenteral and Enteral Nutrition (ASPEN) Board of Directors. ASPEN Enteral Nutrition Practice Recommendations. *J Parenter Enteral Nutr* 2009;**33**:122–167.
4 Corkins MR (ed). *The ASPEN Pediatric Core Curriculum*. American Society for Parenteral and Enteral Nutrition, Silver Springs, 2010.
5 Lopez-Herce J, Mencia S, Sanchez C, Santiago MJ, Bustinza A, Vigil D. Postpyloric enteral nutrition in the critically ill child with shock: a prospective observational study. *Nutr J* 2008;**7**:6 doi10.1186/1475-2891-7-6.
6 Mehta NM, Compher C, and the American Society of Parenteral and Enteral Nutrition (ASPEN) Board of Directors. ASPEN Clinical Guidelines: nutrition support of the critically ill child. *J Parenter Enteral Nutr* 2009;**33**:260–276.
7 Zamberlan P, Delgado AF, Leone C, Feferbaum R, Okay TS. Nutrition therapy in a pediatric intensive care unit: indications, monitoring, and complications. *J Parenter Enteral Nutr* 2011;**35**:523–529.

Section 5 Pancreas

CHAPTER 30 CONGENITAL ANOMALIES OF THE PANCREAS

1 Agha FP, Williams KD. Pancreas Divisum: incidence, detection, and clinical significance. *Am J Gastroenterol* 1987;**82**:315–320.
2 Atlas A, Rosh J. Cystic fibrosis and congenital anomalies of the exocrine pancreas. In: Wyllie R, Hyams J (eds). *Pediatric Gastrointestinal and Liver Disease*, 4th edn. Saunders Elsevier, Philadelphia, 2011; Ch. 81, pp. 900–903.
3 Harrison E, Parks R. Congenital disorders of the pancreas: surgical considerations. In: Jarnagin WR (ed). *Blumgart's Surgery of the Liver, Pancreas and Biliary Tract*, 5th edn. Saunders Elsevier, Philadelphia, 2012; Ch. 51, pp. 817–828.
4 Klein SD, Affronti JP. Pancreas divisum, an evidence-based review: part I, pathophysiology. *Gastrointest Endosc* 2004;**60**:419–425.

5 Laughlin EH, Keown ME, Jackson JE. Heterotopic pancreas obstructing the ampulla of Vater. *Arch Surg* 1983;**118**:979–980.

6 Manfredi R, Costamagna G, Brizi MG, *et al*. Pancreas divisum and 'santorinicele': diagnosis with dynamic MR cholangiopancreatography with secretin stimulation. *Radiology* 2000;**217**:403–408.

7 Turkish A, Husain S. Pancreatic development. In: Wyllie R, Hyams J (eds). *Pediatric Gastrointestinal and Liver Disease*, 4th edn. Saunders Elsevier, Philadelphia, 2011; Ch. 80, pp. 878–881.

CHAPTER 31 EXOCRINE PANCREATIC INSUFFICIENCY

1 Borowitz D, Durie PR, Clarke LL, *et al*. Gastrointestinal outcomes and confounders in cystic fibrosis. *J Pediatr Gastroenterol Nutr* 2005;**41**:273–285.

2 Daneman A, Gaskin K, Martin DJ, Cutz E. Pancreatic changes in cystic fibrosis: CT and sonographic appearances. *Am J Roentgenol* 1983;**141**:653–655.

3 Durie PR. Pancreatic aspects of cystic fibrosis and other inherited causes of pancreatic dysfunction. *Med Clin North Am* 2000;**84**:609–620.

4 Rommens JM, Durie PR. Shwachman-Diamond syndrome. In: Pagon RA, Bird TD, Dolan CR, Stephens K, Adam MP (eds). *GeneReviews™*. University of Washington, Seattle, 2008;1993–2013.

5 Schibli S, Corey M, Gaskin KJ, *et al*. Towards the ideal quantitative pancreatic function test: analysis of test variables that influence validity. *Clin Gastroenterol Hepatol* 2006;**4**:90–97.

6 Tangpricha V, Kelly A, Stephenson A, *et al*. An update on the screening, diagnosis, management, and treatment of vitamin D deficiency in individuals with cystic fibrosis: evidence-based recommendations from the Cystic Fibrosis Foundation. *J Clin Endocrinol Metab* 2012;**97**:1082–1093.

7 Tumino M, Meli C, Farruggia P, *et al*. Clinical manifestations and management of four children with Pearson syndrome. *Am J Med Genet A* 2011;**155**A:3063–3066.

8 Wilschanski M, Durie PR. Patterns of GI disease in adulthood associated with mutations in the CFTR gene. *Gut* 2007;**56**:1153–1163.

9 Zenker M, Mayerle J, Lerch MM, *et al*. Deficiency of UBR1, a ubiquitin ligase of the N-end rule pathway, causes pancreatic dysfunction, malformations and mental retardation (Johanson–Blizzard syndrome). *Nat Genet* 2005;**37**:1345–1350.

CHAPTER 32 PANCREATITIS – ACUTE AND CHRONIC

1 Bai HX, Lowe ME, Husain SZ. What have we learned about acute pancreatitis in children? *J Pediatr Gastroenterol Nutr* 2011;**52**:262–270.

2 Morinville VD, *et al*. Definitions of pediatric pancreatitis and survey of current clinical practices: Report from Insppire (International Study Group Of Pediatric Pancreatitis: In Search For A Cure). *J Pediatr Gastroenterol Nutr* 2012;**55**(3):261–265.

3 Nievelstein RA, Robben SG, Blickman JG. Hepatobiliary and pancreatic imaging in children – techniques and an overview of non-neoplastic disease entities. *Pediatr Radiol* 2011;**41**(1):55–75.

4 Ooi CY, Dorfman R, Cipolli M, *et al*. Type of CFTR mutation determines risk of pancreatitis in patients with cystic fibrosis. *Gastroenterology* 2011;**140**:153–161.

5 Sultan M, Werlin S, Venkatasubramani N. Genetic prevalence and characteristics in children with recurrent pancreatitis. *J Pediatr Gastroenterol Nutr* 2012;**54**:645–650.

6 Sutherland DER, Radosevich DM, Bellin MD, *et al*. Total pancreatectomy and islet autotransplantation for chronic pancreatitis. *J Am Coll Surg* 2012;**214**:409–426.

CHAPTER 33 OTHER PANCREATIC DISORDERS

Pancreatic trauma

1 Buechter KJ, Arnold M, Steele B, *et al*. The use of serum amylase and lipase in evaluating and managing blunt abdominal trauma. *Am Surg* 1990;**56**(4):204–208.

2 De Blaauw I, Winkelhorst JT, Rieu PN, *et al*. Pancreatic injury in children: good outcome of nonoperative treatment. *J Pediatr Surg* 2008;**43**:1640–1643.

3 Holmes J, Sokolove P, Brant W, *et al*. Identification of children with intra-abdominal injuries after blunt trauma. *Ann Emerg Med* 2002;**39**:500–509.

4 Kumar S, Sagar S, Subramanian A, *et al*. Evaluation of amylase and lipase levels in

blunt trauma abdomen patients. *J Emerg Trauma Shock* 2012;**5**(2):135–142.

5 Makin E, Harrison P, Patel S, Davenport M. Pancreatic pseudocysts in children: treatment by endoscopic cystgastrostomy. *J Pediatr Gastroenterol Nutr* 2012;**55**(5):556–558.

6 Ramesh J, Bang JY, Trevino J, Varadarajulu S. Endoscopic ultrasound-guided drainage of pancreatic fluid collections in children. *J Pediatr Gastroenterol Nutr* 2013;**56**(1):30–35.

7 Wales PW, Shuckett B, Kim PC. Long-term outcome after nonoperative management of complete traumatic pancreatic transection in children. *J Pediatr Surg* 2001;**36**:823–827.

8 Wood JH, Partrick DA, Bruny JL, Sauaia A, Moulton SL. Operative versus nonoperative management of blunt pancreatic trauma in children. *J Pediatr Surg* 2010;**45**:401–406.

Pancreatic neoplasm

9 Dall'Igna P, Cecchetto G, Bisogno G, *et al*. Pancreatic tumors in children and adolescents: The Italian TREP project experience. *Pediatr Blood Cancer* 2009;**54**(5):675–680.

10 Nijs E, Callahan MJ, Taylor GA. Disorders of the pediatric pancreas: imaging features. *Pediatr Radiol* 2005;**35**:358–373.

11 Perez EA, Gutierrez JC, Koniaris LG, *et al*. Malignant pancreatic tumors: incidence and outcome in 58 pediatric patients. *J Pediatr Surg* 2009;**44**(1):197–203.

12 Yu DC, Kozakewich HP, Perez-Atayde AR, Shamberger RD, Weldon CB. Childhood pancreatic tumors: a single institution experience. *J Pediatr Surg* 2009;**44**:2267–2272.

Section 6 Hepatobiliary

CHAPTER 34 CHOLEDOCHAL MALFORMATION

1 Davenport M, Sinha CK. Congenital choledochal malformations – a European perspective. *Eur J Pediatr Surg* 2009;**19**(2):63–67.

2 De Angelis P, Foschia F, Romeo E, *et al*. Role of endoscopic retrograde cholangiopancreatography in diagnosis and management of congenital choledochal cysts: 28 pediatric cases. *J Pediatr Surg* 2012;**47**(5):885–888.

3 Goldman M, Pranikoff T. Biliary disease in children. *Curr Gastroenterol Rep* 2011;**13**(2):193–201.

4 Makin E, Davenport M. Understanding choledochal malformation (review). *Arch Dis Child* 2012;**97**:69–72.

5 Turowski C, Knisely AS, Davenport M. Role of pressure and pancreatic reflux in the aetiology of choledochal malformation. *Br J Surg* 2011;**98**:1319–1326.

CHAPTER 35 BILIARY ATRESIA

1 Davenport M. Biliary atresia: clinical aspects. *Semin Pediatr Surg* 2012;**21**:175–184.

2 Davenport M, Ong E, Sharif K, *et al*. Biliary atresia in England and Wales: results of centralization and new benchmark. *J Pediatr Surg* 2011;**46**:1689–1694.

3 Davenport M, Tizzard SA, Underhill J, Mieli-Vergani G, Portmann B, Hadzić N. The biliary atresia splenic malformation syndrome: a 28-year single-center retrospective study. *J Pediatr* 2006;**149**:393–400.

4 Feldman AG, Mack CL. Biliary atresia: cellular dynamics and immune dysregulation. *Semin Pediatr Surg* 2012;**21**:192–200.

5 Hartley JL, Davenport M, Kelly DA. Biliary atresia. *Lancet* 2009;**374**(9702):1704–1713.

CHAPTER 36 PEDIATRIC AUTOIMMUNE LIVER DISEASES

1 Davies YK, Cox KM, Abdulla BA, *et al*. Long-term treatment of primary sclerosing cholangitis in children with oral vancomycin: an immunomodulating antibiotic. *J Pediatr Gastroenterol Nutr* 2008;**47**:61–67.

2 Gregorio GV, Portmann B, Reid F, *et al*. Autoimmune hepatitis/sclerosing cholangitis overlap syndrome in childhood: a 16-year prospective study. *Hepatology* 2001;**33**:544–553.

3 Kerkar N, Hadzic N, Davies ET, *et al*. De-novo autoimmune hepatitis after liver transplantation. *Lancet* 1998;**351**:409–413.

4 Lindor KD, Kowdley KV, Luketic VA, *et al*. High-dose ursodeoxycholic acid for the treatment of primary sclerosing cholangitis. *Hepatology* 2009;**50**(3):808–814.

5 Mieli-Vergani G, Vergani D. Autoimmune liver disease in children. What is different from adulthood. *Best Pract Res Clin Gastroenterol* 2011;**25**:783–795.

6 Mieli-Vergani G, Heller S, Jara P, *et al*. Autoimmune hepatitis. *J Pediatr Gastroenterol Nutr* 2009;**49**:158–164.

7 Saadah OI, Smith AL, Hardikar W. Long-term outcome of autoimmune hepatitis in children. *J Gastroenterol Hepatol* 2001;**16**:1297–1302.

CHAPTER 37 VIRAL HEPATITIS

1 Friedman LS, Keefe EB. *Handbook of Liver Disease*, 2nd edn. Churchill Livingstone, Philadelphia, 2004.

2 Pickering LK, and the Committee on Infectious Diseases. *Red Book*, 30th edn. American Academy of Pediatrics, Elk Grove Village, IL, 2011.

3 Schwarz KB, Balistreri W. Viral hepatitis. *J Pediatr Gastroenterol Nutr* 2002;**35**:S29–S32.

4 Suchy FJ, Sokol RJ, Balistreri WF (eds). *Liver Disease in Children*, 3rd edn. Cambridge University Press, New York, NY, 2007.

CHAPTER 38 GALLBLADDER DISEASE

1 Chan S, Currie J, Malik AI, Mahomed AA. Paediatric cholecystectomy: Shifting goalposts in the laparoscopic era. *Surg Endosc* 2008;**22**(5):1392–1395.

2 Herzog D, Bouchard G. High rate of complicated idiopathic gallstone disease in pediatric patients of a North American tertiary care center. *World J Gastroenterol* 2008;**14**(10):1544–1548.

3 Goldman M, Pranikoff T. Biliary disease in children. *Curr Gastroenterol Rep* 2011;**13**(2):193–201.

4 Poffenberger CM, Gausche-Hill M, Ngai S, Myers A, Renslo R. Cholelithiasis and its complications in children and adolescents: update and case discussion. *Pediatr Emerg Care* 2012;**28**(1):68–76.

5 Svensson J, Makin E. Gallstone disease in childhood. *Semin Pediatr Surg* 2012;**21**:255–265.

CHAPTER 39 HEPATOTOXINS

1 Bond GR, Ho M, Woodward RW. Trends in hepatic injury associated with unintentional overdose of paracetamol (acetaminophen) in products with and without opioid: an analysis using the National Poison Data System of the American Association of Poison Control Centers, 2000–7. *Drug Saf* 2012;**35**:149–157.

2 Clarkson A, Choonara I. Surveillance for fatal suspected adverse drug reactions in the UK. *Arch Dis Child* 2002;**87**:462–466.

3 Dansette PM, Bonierbale E, Minoletti C, Beaune PH, Pessayre D, Mansuy D. Drug-induced immunotoxicity. *Eur J Drug Metab Pharmacokinet* 1998;**23**:443–451.

4 Dewit O, Starkel P, Roblin X. Thiopurine metabolism monitoring: implications in inflammatory bowel diseases. *Eur J Clin Invest* 2010;**40**:1037–1047.

5 Dourakis SP, Tolis G. Sex hormonal preparations and the liver. *Eur J Contracept Reprod Health Care* 1998;**3**:7–16.

6 Findor JA, Sorda JA, Igartua EB, Avagnina A. Ketoconazole-induced liver damage. *Medicina* (B Aires) 1998;**58**:277–281.

7 Fournier MR, Klein J, Minuk GY, Bernstein CN. Changes in liver biochemistry during methotrexate use for inflammatory bowel disease. *Am J Gastroenterol* 2010;**105**:1620–1626.

8 Giannattasio A, D'Ambrosi M, Volpicelli M, Iorio R. Steroid therapy for a case of severe drug-induced cholestasis. *Ann Pharmacother* 2006;**40**:1196–1199.

9 Hita EO, Ruiz-Extremera A, Garcia JA, *et al*. Amoxicillin-clavulanic acid hepatotoxicity in children. *J Pediatr Gastroenterol Nutr* 2012;**55**(6):663–667.

10 James LP, Mayeux PR, Hinson JA. Acetaminophen-induced hepatotoxicity. *Drug Metab Dispos* 2003;**31**:1499–1506.

11 Lheureux PE, Hantson P. Carnitine in the treatment of valproic acid-induced toxicity. *Clin Toxicol* (Phila) 2009;**47**:101–111.

12 Metushi IG, Cai P, Zhu X, Nakagawa T, Uetrecht JP. A fresh look at the mechanism of isoniazid-induced hepatotoxicity. *Clin Pharmacol Ther* 2011;**89**:911–914.

13 Roberts EA. Drug-induced hepatotoxicity. In: Kleinman RE, Goulet O-J, Mieli-Vergani G, Sanderson IR, Sherman PM, Schneider BL (eds). *Walker's Pediatric Gastrointestinal Disease*, 4th edn. Volume 2. BC Decker, Hamilton, Ontario, 2004; pp. 1219–1240.

14 Roberts EA. Drug-induced liver disease. In: Suchy FJ, Sokol RJ, Balistreri WF (eds). *Liver Disease in Children*, 3rd edn. Cambridge University Press, Cambridge, 2007; pp. 478–512.

15 Squires RH Jr, Shneider BL, Bucuvalas J, *et al*. Acute liver failure in children: the first 348 patients in the pediatric acute liver failure study group. *J Pediatr* 2006;**148**:652–658.

16 Tanaka E. *In vivo* age-related changes in hepatic drug-oxidizing capacity in humans. *J Clin Pharmacol Ther* 1998;**23**:247–255.

17 Stickel F, Patsenker E, Schuppan D. Herbal hepatotoxicity. *J Hepatol* 2005;**43**:901–910.

CHAPTER 40 METABOLIC DISORDERS I
Wilson disease

1 Ala A, Schilsky ML. Wilson disease: pathophysiology, diagnosis, treatment, and screening. *Clin Liver Dis* 2004;**8**:787–805.

2 Emerick, KM. Wilson's disease. In: Bishop, W (ed). *Pediatric Practice Gastroenterology*. McGraw-Hill, New York, 2011.

3 Franciosi JP, Loomes KM. Wilson disease. In: Liacouras CA, Piccoli DA (eds). *Pediatric Gastroenterology: The Requisites in Pediatrics*. Mosby Elsevier, Philadelphia, 2008.

4 Roberts EA, Schilsky ML. A practice guideline on Wilson disease. *Hepatology* 2003;**37**: 1475–1492.

5 Sanchez-Albisua I, Garde T, Hierro, L, *et al*. A high index of suspicion: the key to an early diagnosis of Wilson disease in childhood. *J Pediatr Gastroenterol Nutr* 1999;**28**(2):186–190.

6 Sokol RJ, Narkewicz MR. Copper and iron storage disorders. In: Suchy FJ, Sokol RJ, Balistreri WF (eds). *Liver Disease in Children*, 2nd edn. Lippincott Williams & Wilkins, Philadelphia, 2001.

Alpha1-antitrypsin deficiency

7 Bals R. Alpha-1-antitrypsin deficiency. *Best Pract Res Clin Gastroenterology* 2010;**24**(5): 629–633.

8 de Serres FJ. Worldwide racial and ethnic distribution of alpha-1-antitrypsin deficiency: summary of an analysis of published genetic epidemiologic surveys. *Chest* 2002;**122**:1818–1829.

9 Fairbanks KD, Tavill AS. Liver disease in alpha-1-antitrypsin deficiency: a review. *Am J Gastroenterol* 2008;**103**(8):2136–2141.

10 Perlmutter DH. Alpha-1-antitrypsin deficiency: Diagnosis and treatment. *Clin Liver Dis* 2004;**8**:839–859.

CHAPTER 41 METABOLIC DISORDERS II

1 Ali M, Rellos P, Cox TM. Hereditary fructose intolerance. *J Med Genet* 1998;**35**:353–365.

2 Bosch AM. Classical galactosaemia revisited. *J Inherit Metab Dis* 2006;**29**:516–525.

3 Bouteldja N, Timson DJ. The biochemical basis of hereditary fructose intolerance. *J Inherit Meta Dis* 2010;**33**:105–112. http://www.arup.utah.edu/database/GALT/GALT_welcome.php

4 Russo PA, Mitchell GA, Tanguay RM. Tyrosinemia: a review. *Pediatr Develop Pathol* 2001;**4**:212–221.

5 Sundaram SS, Alonso EM, Narkewicz MR, *et al*. Characterization and outcomes of young infants with acute liver failure. *Pediatrics* 2011;**159**(5):813–818.

6 Tang M, Odejinmi SI, Vankayalapati H, *et al*. Innovative therapy for classic galactosemia- tale of two HTS. *Mol Genet Metab* 2012;**105**(1):44–55.

CHAPTER 42 METABOLIC DISORDERS III

1 Kishnani PS, Austin SL, Arn P, *et.al*. Glycogen storage disease type III diagnosis and management guidelines. *Genet Med* 2010;**12**(7):446–463.

2 McGovern MM, Schuchman EH. Acid sphingomyelinase deficiency includes: Niemann–Pick disease Type A, Niemann–Pick disease Type B. In: Pagon RA, Bird TD, Dolan CR, *et al*. (eds). *GeneReviews* Internet: Initial posting: December 7, 2006; last update: June 25, 2009. 1993- Updated June 25, 2009.

3 Patterson MC, Hendriksz CJ, Walterfang M, Sedel F, Vanier MTA, Wijburg F. Recommendations for the diagnosis and management of Niemann–Pick disease type C: an update. On behalf of the NP-C Guidelines Working Group. *Mol Genet Metab* 2012;**106**(3):330–344.

4 Patterson MC, Vanier MT, Gibson KM, *et al*. Niemann–Pick disease Type C: a lipid trafficking disorder. In: Scriver CR, Beaudet AL, Sly WS, *et al*. (eds). *Metabolic and Molecular Bases of Inherited Disease*, 8th edn. www.ommbid.com, McGraw-Hill, New York, 2001.

5 Schuchman EH, Desnick, RJ. Niemann–
   Pick disease Types A and B: acid
   sphingomyelinase deficiencies. In: Scriver
   CR, Beaudet AL, Sly WS, *et al.* (eds).
   *Metabolic and Molecular Bases of Inherited
   Disease*, 8th edn. www.ommbid.com,
   McGraw-Hill, New York, 2001.
6 Vanier MT. Niemann–Pick disease type C.
   Orphanet J Rare Dis 2010;**5**:16.
7 Weinstein DA, Correia CE, Saunders AC,
   Wolfsdorf JI. Hepatic glycogen synthase
   deficiency: an infrequently recognized cause
   of ketotic hypoglycemia. *Mol Genet Metab*
   2006;**87**(4):284–288.
8 Weinstein DA, Roth KS, Wolfsdorf JI.
   Glycogen storage diseases. In: Sarafoglou
   K (ed). *Pediatric Endocrinology and Inborn
   Errors of Metabolism*, 1st edn. McGraw-Hill
   Medical, China, 2009; Ch. 6, pp. 71–81.
9 Wolfsdorf JI, Weinstein DA. Hypoglycemia
   in children. In: Lifshitz F (ed). *Pediatric
   Endocrinology Volume 1: Obesity, Diabetes
   Mellitus, Insulin Resistance, and Hypoglycemia*,
   5th edn. Informa Healthcare, New York,
   2007; Ch. 15, pp. 300–304.

CHAPTER 43 HEPATIC TUMORS

1 Boon LM, Burrows PE, Paltiel HJ, *et al.*
   Hepatic vascular anomalies in infancy: a
   twenty-seven-year experience. *J Pediatr*
   1996;**129**(3):346–354.
2 Brown J, Perilongo G, Shafford E, *et al.*
   Pretreatment prognostic factors for children
   with hepatoblastoma- results from the
   International Society of Paediatric Oncology
   (SIOP) study SIOPEL 1. *Euro J Cancer*
   2000;**36**(11):1418–1425.
3 Buetow PC, Buck JL, Ros PR,
   Goodman ZD. Malignant vascular tumors of
   the liver: radiologic-pathologic correlation.
   Radiographics 1994:**14**(1):153–166.
4 Burrows PE, Dubois J, Kassarjian A.
   Pediatric hepatic vascular anomalies. *Pediatr
   Radiol* 2001;**31**(8):533–545.
5 Carlson SK, Johnson CD, Bender CE, Welch
   TJ. CT of focal nodular hyperplasia of the
   liver. *Am J Roentgenol* 2000;**174**(3):705–712.
6 Christison-Lagay ER, Burrows PE, Alomari
   A, *et al.* Hepatic hemangiomas: subtype
   classification and development of a clinical
   practice algorithm and registry. *J Pediatr
   Surg* 2007;**42**(1):62–67.

7 Chung EM, Cube R, Lewis RB, Conran
   RM. From the archives of the AFIP:
   Pediatric liver masses: radiologic-pathologic
   correlation Part 1. Benign tumors.
   Radiographics 2010;**30**(3):801–826.
8 Chung EM, Lattin GE, Cube R, *et al.* From
   the archives of the AFIP: Pediatric liver
   masses: radiologic-pathologic correlation
   Part 2. Malignant tumors. *Radiographics*
   2011;**31**(2):483–507.
9 Crider MH, Hoggard E, Manivel JC.
   Undifferentiated (embryonal) sarcoma of the
   liver. *Radiographics* 2009;**29**(6):1665–1668.
10 Czauderna P. Adult type *vs.* childhood
   hepatocellular carcinoma – are they the same
   or different lesions? Biology, natural history,
   prognosis, and treatment. *Med Pediatr Oncol*
   2002;**39**(5):519–523.
11 Ferenci P, Fried M, Labrecque D, *et al.*
   World Gastroenterology Organisation
   Guideline. Hepatocellular carcinoma
   (HCC): a global perspective. *J Gastrointestin
   Liver Dis* 2010;**19**(3):311–317.
12 Giardiello FM, Petersen GM, Brensinger
   JD, *et al.* Hepatoblastoma and APC gene
   mutation in familial adenomatous polyposis.
   Gut 1996;**39**(6):867–869.
13 Grazioli L, Federle MP, Brancatelli G,
   Ichikawa T, Olivetti L, Blachar A. Hepatic
   adenomas: imaging and pathologic findings.
   Radiographics 2001;**21**(4):877–892.
14 Herzog CE, Andrassy RJ, Eftekhari F.
   Childhood cancers: hepatoblastoma.
   Oncologist 2000;**5**(6):445–453.
15 Kassarjian A, Zurakowski D, Dubois
   J, Paltiel HJ, Fishman SJ, Burrows PE.
   Infantile hepatic hemangiomas: clinical and
   imaging findings and their correlation with
   therapy. *Am J Roentgenol* 2004;**182**(3):785–
   795.
16 Keslar PJ, Buck JL, Selby M. From
   the archives of the AFIP: Infantile
   hemangioendothelioma of the liver revisited.
   Radiographics 1993;**13**(3):657–670.
17 Lyburn ID, Torreggiani
   WC, Harris AC, *et al.* Hepatic
   epithelioid hemangioendothelioma:
   sonographic, CT, and MR imaging
   appearances. *Am J Roentgenol*
   2003;**180**(5):1359–1364.
18 Makhlouf HR, Ishak KG, Goodman ZD.
   Epithelioid hemangioendothelioma of the
   liver: a clinicopathologic study of 137 cases.
   Cancer 1999;**85**(3):562–582.

19 McLarney JK, Rucker PT, Bender GN, Goodman ZD, Kashitani N, Ros PR. Fibrolamellar carcinoma of the liver: radiologic-pathologic correlation. *Radiographics* 1999;**19**(2):453–471.

20 Meyers RL. Tumors of the liver in children. *Surg Oncol* 2007;**16**(3):195–203.

21 Resnick MB, Kozakewich HP, Perez-Atayde AR. Hepatic adenoma in the pediatric age group. Clinicopathological observations and assessment of cell proliferative activity. *Am J Surg Pathol* 1995;**19**(10):1181–1190.

22 Spunt SL, Lobe TE, Pappo AS, *et al*. Aggressive surgery is unwarranted for biliary tract rhabdomyosarcoma. *J Pediatr Surg* 2000;**35**(2):309–316.

23 Steenman M, Westerveld A, Mannens M. Genetics of Beckwith–Wiedemann syndrome-associated tumors: common genetic pathways. *Genes, Chromosomes, Cancer* 2000;**28**(1):1–13.

24 Stocker JT. Hepatic tumors in children. *Clin Liver Dis* 2001;**5**(1):259–281.

25 Stringer MD, Alizai NK. Mesenchymal hamartoma of the liver: a systematic review. *J Pediatr Surg* 2005;**40**(11):1681–1690.

26 Van Tornout JM, Buckley JD, Quinn JJ, *et al*. Timing and magnitude of decline in alpha-fetoprotein levels in treated children with unresectable or metastatic hepatoblastoma are predictors of outcome: a report from the Children's Cancer Group. *J Clin Oncol* 1997;**15**(3):1190–1197.

27 Yu S-B, Kim H-Y, Eo H, *et al*. Clinical characteristics and prognosis of pediatric hepatocellular carcinoma. *World J Surg* 2006;**30**(1):43–50.

CHAPTER 44 LIVER TRANSPLANTATION

1 Alonso EM. Growth and developmental considerations in pediatric liver transplantation. *Liver Transplant* 2008;**14**:585–591.

2 Anonymous (no author listed). International Working Party. Terminology for hepatic allograft rejection. *Hepatology* 1995;**22**:648–654.

3 Avitzur Y, De Luca E, Cantos M, *et al*. Health status ten years after pediatric liver transplantation – looking beyond the graft. *Transplantation* 2004;**78**(4):566–573.

4 Guillen S, Black M, Thomas G, *et al*. *Liver Transplant*. EmedicineHealth, 2012.

5 Haddad E, McAlister V, Renouf E, *et al*. Cyclosporine versus tacrolimus for liver transplanted patients. *Cochrane Database of Systematic Reviews* 2006, Issue 4:CD005161.

6 Jain A, Nalesnik M, Reyes J, *et al*. Post transplant lymphoproliferative disorders in liver transplantation. A 20-year experience. *Ann Surg* **236**(4):429–437.

7 Kling K, Lau H, Colombani P. Biliary complications of living related pediatric liver transplant patients. *Pediatr Transplant* 2004;**8**(2):178–184.

8 Lu CH, Tsang LL, Huang TL, *et al*. Biliary complications and management in pediatric living donor liver transplantation for underlying biliary atresia. *Transplant Proc* 2012;**44**(2):476–477.

9 Moon JI, Jung GO, Choi GS, *et al*. Risk factors for portal vein complications after pediatric living donor liver transplantation with left-sided grafts. *Transplant Proc* 2010;**42**(3):871–875.

10 Verdonk RC, Buis CI, Porte RJ, Haagsma EB. Biliary complications after liver transplantation: a review. *Scand J Gastroenterol Suppl* 2006;**243**:89–101.

Section 7 Colonic Disease

CHAPTER 45 GASTROINTESTINAL TRACT POLYPS AND POLYPOSIS SYNDROMES

1 Allen BA, Terdiman JP. Hereditary polyposis syndromes and hereditary non-polyposis colorectal cancer. *Best Pract Res Clin Gastroenterol* 2003;**17**(2):237–258.

2 Bronner MP. Gastrointestinal polyposis syndromes. *Am J Med Genet* 2003;**122A**(4):335–341.

3 Corredor J, Wambach J, Barnard J. Gastro-intestinal polyps in children: advances in molecular genetics, diagnosis, and manage-ment. *J Pediatr* 2001;**138**(5):621–628.

4 Fargnoli MC, Orlow SJ, Semel-Concepcion J, Bolognia JL. Clinicopathologic findings in the Bannayan–Riley–Ruvalcaba syndrome. *Arch Dermatol* 1996;**132**(10):1214–1218.

5 Farooq A, Walker LJ, Bowling J, Audisio RA. Cowden syndrome. *Cancer Treat Rev* 2010;**36**(8):577–583.

6 Giardiello FM, Trimbath JD. Peutz–Jeghers syndrome and management recommendations. *Clin Gastroenterol Hepatol* 2006;**4**(4):408–415.

7 Huang SC, Erdman SH. Pediatric juvenile polyposis syndromes: an update. *Curr Gastroenterol Rep* 2009;**11**(3):211–219.

8 Hyer W. Pediatric polyposis syndromes. In: Wyllie R, Hyams J (eds). *Pediatric Gastrointestinal and Liver Disease*, 4th edn. Saunders Elsevier, Philadelphia, 2011.

9 Hyer W, Beveridge I, Domizio P, Phillips R. Clinical management and genetics of gastrointestinal polyps in children. *J Pediatr Gastroenterol Nutr* 2000;**31**(5):469–479.

10 Manfredi M. Hereditary hamartomatous polyposis syndromes: understanding the disease risks as children reach adulthood. *Gastroenterol Hepatol* 2010;**6**(3):185–196.

CHAPTER 46 ULCERATIVE COLITIS

1 Abramson O, Durant M, Mow W, *et al*. Incidence, prevalence, and time trends of pediatric inflammatory bowel disease in Northern California, 1996 to 2006. *J Pediatr* 2010;**157**(2):233–239.

2 Croft NM. Crohn's disease. In: Kleinman RE, Goulet O-J, Mieli-Vergani G, Sanderson IR, Sherman PM, Schneider BL (eds). *Walker's Pediatric Gastrointestinal Disease: Physiology, Diagnosis, Management*, 5th edn. McGraw-Hill, New York, 2008; pp. 545–558.

3 Eaden JA, Abrams KR, Mayberry JF. The risk of colorectal cancer in ulcerative colitis: a meta-analysis. *Gut* 2001;**48**(4):526–535.

4 Glickman JN, Bousvaros A, Farraye FA, *et al*. Pediatric patients with untreated ulcerative colitis may present initially with unusual morphologic findings. *Am J Surg Pathol* 2004;**28**(2):190–197.

5 Gower-Rousseau C, Dauchet L, Vernier-Massouille G, *et al*. The natural history of pediatric ulcerative colitis: a population-based cohort study. *Am J Gastroenterol* 2009;**104**(8):2080–2088.

6 Halfvarson J, Bodin L, Tysk C, Lindberg E, Järnerot G. Inflammatory bowel disease in a Swedish twin cohort: a long-term follow-up of concordance and clinical characteristics. *Gastroenterology* 2003;**124**(7):1767–1773.

7 Kugathasan S, Dubinsky M C, Keljo D, *et al*. Severe colitis in children. *J Pediatr Gastroenterol Nutr* 2005;**41**(4):376–385.

8 Lichtenstein GR, Abreu MT, Cohen R, Tremaine W; American Gastroenterological Association. American Gastroenterological Association Institute technical review on corticosteroids, immunomodulators, and infliximab in inflammatory bowel disease. *Gastroenterology* 2006;**130**(3):940–987.

9 Nemoto H, Kataoka K, Ishikawa H, *et al*. Reduced diversity and imbalance of fecal microbiota in patients with ulcerative colitis. *Dig Dis Sci* 2012;**57**(11):2955–2964.

10 Nguyen GC, Kaplan GG, Harris ML, Brant SR. A national survey of the prevalence and impact of *Clostridium difficile* infection among hospitalized inflammatory bowel disease patients. *Am J Gastroenterol* 2008;**103**:1443–1450.

11 Sartor RB. Mechanisms of disease: pathogenesis of Crohn's disease and ulcerative colitis. *Nat Clin Pract Gastroenterol Hepatol* 2006;**3**:390–407.

12 Sawczenko A, Sandhu BK, Logan RFA, *et al*. Prospective survey of childhood inflammatory bowel disease in the British Isles. *Lancet* 2001;**357**:1093–1094.

13 Schildkraut V, Alex G, Cameron D J, *et al*. Sixty-year study of incidence of childhood ulcerative colitis finds eleven-fold increase beginning in 1990s. *Inflamm Bowel Dis* 2013;**19**(1):1–6.

14 Van Limbergen J, Russell RK, Drummond HE, *et al*. Definition of phenotypic characteristics of childhood-onset inflammatory bowel disease. *Gastroenterology* 2008;**135**(4):1114–1122.

CHAPTER 47 INFECTIOUS COLITIS

1 Abreu MT, Harpaz N. Diagnosis of colitis: making the initial diagnosis. *Clin Gastroenterol Hepatol* 2007;**5**(3):295–301.

2 ARUP Laboratories: ARUPConsult Algorithms. *Diarrhea Acute Testing* (website): http://www.arupconsult.com/Algorithms/Diarrhea,%20Acute%20Testing.pdf. Accessed October 22, 2013.

3 Connor DH, Schwartz DA, Manz H. *Pathology of Infectious Diseases*, 1st edn. McGraw-Hill Professional, Blacklick, 1997.

4 Fry RD, Mahmoud NN, Maron DJ, Bleier J. Infectious colitis. In: Townsend CM (ed). *Sabiston Textbook of Surgery: the Biological Basis of Modern Surgical Practice*, 18th edn. Saunders Elsevier, Philadelphia, 2008; Ch. 50, pp. 1348–1432.

5 Giannella RA. Bacterial enteritis and proctocolitis and bacterial food poisoning. In: Feldman M, Friedman L, Brandt L (eds). *Sleisenger and Fordtran's Gastrointestinal and Liver Disease*, 9th edn. Elsevier, Philadelphia, 2010; Ch. 107, pp. 1843–1887.

6 Grossman AB, Baldassano RN. Inflammatory bowel disease. In: Kliegman R, Nelson WE (eds). *Nelson Textbook of Pediatrics*, 19th edn. Saunders Elsevier, Philadelphia, 2011; Ch. 328, pp. 1294–1303.

7 Lamps LW. Infectious diseases of the colon. In: Iacobuzio-Donahue CA, Montgomery EA (eds). *Gastrointestinal and Liver Pathology*. Saunders, Philadelphia, 2011; Ch. 9, pp. 297–351.

8 Lima A, Guerrant R. Inflammatory enterides. In: Mandell GL, Bennet JE, Dolin R (eds). *Mandell, Douglas, and Bennett's Principles and Practice of Infectious Diseases*, 7th edn. Churchill Livingstone Elsevier, Philadelphia, 2010; Ch. 97, pp. 1389–1398.

9 Osterman MT, Lichtenstein GR. Ulcerative colitis. In: Feldman M, Friedman L, Brandt L (eds). *Sleisenger and Fordtran's Gastrointestinal and Liver Disease*, 9th edn. Elsevier, Philadelphia, 2010; Ch. 112, pp. 1975–2013.

CHAPTER 48 DRUG, CHEMICAL, AND OTHER FORMS OF COLITIS

1 Aksoy DY, Tanriover MD, Uzun O, *et al*. Diarrhea in neutropenic patients: a prospective cohort study with emphasis on neutropenic enterocolitis. *Ann Oncol* 2007;**18**(1):183–189.

2 Elder K, Lashner BA, Al Solaiman F, Clinical approach to colonic ischemia. *Cleve Clin J Med* 2009;**76**(7):401–409.

3 Jain G, Scolapio J, Wasserman E, Floch MH. Chronic radiation enteritis: a ten-year follow-up. *J Clin Gastroenterol* 2010;**35**(3):214–217.

4 Kleinman RE, Goulet O-J, Mieli-Vergani G, Sanderson IR, Sherman PM, Shneider BL. *Walker's Pediatric Gastrointestinal Disease; Physiology, Diagnosis, Management*, 5th edn. McGraw-Hill, New York, 2008; Ch. 26 1.A.

5 Moran H, Yaniv I, Ashkenazi S, Schwartz M, Fisher S, Levy ISOJ. Risk factors for typhlitis in pediatric patients with cancer. *Pediatr Hematol Oncol* 2009;**31**(9):630–634.

6 Sheibani S, Gerson LB. Chemical colitis. *J Clin Gastroenterol* 2008;**42**(2):115–121.

CHAPTER 49 HIRSCHSPRUNG DISEASE AND DISORDERS OF INTESTINAL HYPOGANGLIONOSIS

1 Dingemann J, Prem P. Isolated hypoganglionosis: systematic review of a rare intestinal innervations defect. *Pediatr Surg Int* 2010;**26**(11):1111–1115.

2 De Lorijn, F, Reitsma, JB, Voskuiji, WP, *et al*. Diagnosis of Hirschsprung's disease: a prospective, comparative accuracy study of common tests. *J Pediatr* 2005;**146**:787–792.

3 Kim HJ, Kim AY, Lee CW, *et al*. Hirschsprung disease and hypoganglionosis in adults: radiologic findings and differentiation. *Radiology* 2008;**247**(2):428–434.

4 Kleinman RE, Goulet O-J, Mieli-Vergani G, Sanderson IR, Sherman PM, Schneider BL (eds). *Walker's Pediatric Gastrointestinal Disease: Physiology, Diagnosis, Management*, 5th edn. McGraw-Hill, New York, 2008.

5 Kobayashi H, Yamataka A, Lane G, Miyano T. Pathophysiology of hypoganglionosis. *J Pediatr Gastroenterol Nutr* 2001;**34**(2):231–235.

6 Martucciello G, Ceccherini I, Lerone M, Jasonni V. Pathogenesis of Hirschsprung's disease. *J Pediatr Surg* 2000;**35**:1017–1025.

7 Zhang HY, Feng J, Huang L, Wang G, Wei M, Weng Y. Diagnosis and surgical treatment of isolated hypoganglionosis. *World J Pediatr* 2008;**4**(4):295–300.

CHAPTER 50 CONSTIPATION

1 Constipation Guideline Committee of the North American Society for Pediatric Gastroenterology, Hepatology and Nutrition. Evaluation and treatment of constipation in infants and children: recommendations of the North American Society for Pediatric Gastroenterology, Hepatology and Nutrition. *J Pediatr Gastroenterol Nutr* 2006;**43**(3):e1–13.

2 Di Lorenzo C, Hillemeier C, Hyman P, *et al*. Manometry studies in children: minimum standards for procedures. *Neurogastroenterol Motil* 2002;**14**(4):411–420.

3 Mugie SM, Di Lorenzo C, Benninga MA. Constipation in childhood. *Nat Rev Gastroenterol Hepatol* 2011;**8**(9):502–511.

4 Scott SM, van den Berg MM, Benninga MA. Rectal sensorimotor dysfunction in constipation. *Best Pract Res Clin Gastroenterol* 2011;**25**(1):103–118.

CHAPTER 51 ANORECTAL MALFORMATIONS

1 Cuschieri A. Descriptive epidemiology of isolated anal anomalies: a survey of 4.6 million births in Europe. *Am J Med Genet* 2001;**103**:207–215.

2   Herman RS, Teitelbaum DH. Anorectal malformations. *Clin Perinatol* 2012;**39**(2):403–422.

3   Kluth D. Embryology of anorectal malformations. *Semin Pediatr Surg* 2010;**19**(3):201–208.

4   Pena A. Posterior sagittal anorectoplasty: results in management of 322 cases of anorectal malformations. *Pediatr Surg* 1988;**3**:94–104.

5   Spouge D. Imperforate anus in 700,000 consecutive liveborn infants. *Am J Med Genet* (Suppl) 1986;**2**:151–161.

Section 8 Gastrointestinal Bleeding and Therapeutics

CHAPTER 52 ESOPHAGEAL AND GASTRIC BLEEDING

1   Bak-Romaniszyn L, Małecka-Panas E, Czkwianianc E, Płaneta-Małecka I. Mallory-Weiss syndrome in children. *Dis Esophagus* 1999;**12**(1):65–67.

2   Brumbaugh DE, Colson SB, Sandoval JA, *et al*. Management of button battery-induced hemorrhage in children. *J Pediatr Gastroenterol Nutr* 2011;**52**(5):585–589.

3   Heyman MB, LaBerge JM. Role of transjugular intrahepatic portosystemic shunt in the treatment of portal hypertension in pediatric patients. *J Pediatr Gastroenterol Nutr* 1999;**29**(3):240–249.

4   Joint Recommendations of the North American Society for Pediatric Gastroenterology, Hepatology, and Nutrition (NASPGHAN) and the European Society for Pediatric Gastroenterology, Hepatology, and Nutrition (ESPGHAN). Pediatric Gastroesophageal Reflux Clinical Practice Guidelines. *J Pediatr Gastroenterol Nutr* 2009;**49**:498–547.

5   Molleston JP. Variceal bleeding in children. *J Pediatr Gastroenterol Nutr* 2003;**37**(5):538–545.

6   Reveiz L, Guerrero-Lozano R, Camacho A, Yara L, Mosquera PA. Stress ulcer, gastritis, and gastrointestinal bleeding prophylaxis in critically ill pediatric patients: A systematic review. *Pediatr Crit Care Med* 2010;**11**:124–132.

7   Savides TJ, Jensen DM. Gastrointestinal bleeding. In: Feldman M, Friedman LS, Brandt LJ (eds). *Sleisenger and Fordtran's Gastrointestinal and Liver Disease*, 9th edn.

Saunders Elsevier, Philadelphia, 2010; Ch.19.

8   Sharara AI, Rockey DC. Gastroesophageal variceal hemorrhage. *N Engl J Med* 2001;**30**;345(9):669–681.

9   Suskind D, Wahbeh G, Murray K, Christie D, Kapur RP. Collagenous gastritis, a new spectrum of disease in pediatric patients: two case reports. *Cases J* 2009;**10**(2):7511.

10 Zografos GN, Georgiadou D, Thomas D, Kaltsas G, Digalakis M. Drug-induced esophagitis. *Dis Esophagus* 2009;**22**(8):633–637.

CHAPTER 53 SMALL INTESTINAL BLEEDING

1   Barth BA. Enteroscopy in children. *Curr Opin Pediatr* 2011;**23**:530–534.

2   Bhargava SA, Putnam PE, Kocoshis SA. Gastrointestinal bleeding due to delayed perianastomotic ulceration in children. *Am J Gastroenterol* 1995;**90**(5):807–809.

3   Ell C, May A. Mid-gastrointestinal bleeding: capsule endoscopy and push-and-pull enteroscopy give rise to a new medical term. *Endoscopy* 2006;**38**(1):73–75.

4   Fox VL. Gastrointestinal bleeding in infancy and childhood. *Gastroenterol Clin North Am* 2000;**29**(1):37–66.

5   Lee KH, Yeung CK, Tam YH, Ng WT, Yip KF. Laparoscopy for definitive diagnosis and treatment of gastrointestinal bleeding of obscure origin in children. *J Pediatr Surg* 2000;**35**(9):1291–1293.

6   Lewis BS. Small intestinal bleeding. *Gastroenterol Clin North Am* 2000;**29**(1):67–95.

7   Pasha SF, Hara AK, Leighton JA. Diagnostic evaluation and management of obscure gastrointestinal bleeding: a changing paradigm. *Gastroenterol Hepatol* 2009;**5**(12):839–850.

8   Pennazio M. Enteroscopy in the diagnosis and management of obscure gastrointestinal bleeding. *Gastrointest Endosc Clin North Am* 2009;**19**(3):409–426.

CHAPTER 54 COLONIC BLEEDING

1   American Gastroenterological Association. American Gastroenterological Association medical position statement: diagnosis and care of patients with anal fissure. *Gastroenterology* 2003;**124**:233–234.

2   Drolet BA, Pope E, Juern AM, *et al*. Gastrointestinal bleeding in infantile hemangioma: a complication of segmental, rather than multifocal, infantile hemangiomas. *J Pediatr* 2012;**160**:1021–1026. e1023.

3   Eroglu Y, Emerick KM, Chou PM, Reynolds M. Gastrointestinal bleeding in Turner's syndrome: a case report and literature review. *J Pediatr Gastroenterol Nutr* 2002;.**35**:84–87.

4   Fishman SJ, Smithers CJ, Folkman J, *et al*. Blue rubber bleb nevus syndrome: surgical eradication of gastrointestinal bleeding. *Ann Surg* 2005;**241**:523–528.

5   Heaton ND, Davenport M, Howard ER. Incidence of haemorrhoids and anorectal varices in children with portal hypertension. *Br J Surg* 1993;**80**:616–618.

6   Hood B, Bigler S, Bishop P, *et al*. Juvenile polyps and juvenile polyp syndromes in children: a clinical and endoscopic survey. *Clin Pediatr* (Phila) 2011;**50**:910–915.

7   Kleinman RE, Goulet O-J, Mieli-Vergani G, Sanderson IR, Sherman PM, Schneider BL (eds). *Walker's Pediatric Gastrointestinal Disease; Physiology, Diagnosis, Management*, 5th edn. McGraw-Hill, New York, 2008.

8   Kokkonen J, Karttunen TJ. Lymphonodular hyperplasia on the mucosa of the lower gastrointestinal tract in children: an indication of enhanced immune response? *J Pediatr Gastroenterol Nutr* 2002;**34**:42–46.

9   Majowicz SE, Musto J, Scallan E, *et al*.; International Collaboration on Enteric Disease 'Burden of Illness' Studies. The global burden of nontyphoidal *Salmonella* gastroenteritis. *Clin Infect Dis* 2010;**50**:882–889.

10 Mansueto P, Iacono G, Seidita A, D'Alcamo A, Sprini D, Carroccio A. Review article: intestinal lymphoid nodular hyperplasia in children – the relationship to food hypersensitivity. *Aliment Pharmacol Ther* 2012 Mar 20 (Epub ahead of print).

11 Mantzaris G. Endoscopic diagnosis of infectious colitis. *Ann Gastroenterol* 2007;**20**(1):71–74.

12 Murray KF, Patterson K. *Escherichia coli* O157:H7-induced hemolytic uremic syndrome: histopathologic changes in the colon over time. *Pediatr Dev Pathol* 2000;**3**:232–239.

13 Nelson RL, Thomas K, Morgan J, Jones A. Non surgical therapy for anal fissure. The Cochrane Library, 2012 Feb 15;2:CD003431.

14 Perito ER, Mileti E, Dalal DH, *et al*. Solitary rectal ulcer syndrome in children and adolescents. *J Pediatr Gastroenterol Nutr* 2012;**54**:266–270.

15 Thakkar K, Alsarraj A, Fong E, Holub JL, Gilger MA, El Serag HB. Prevalence of colorectal polyps in pediatric colonoscopy. *Dig Dis Sci* 2012;**57**:1050–1055.

16 Vecchio Lo A, Zacur GM. *Clostridium difficile* infection: an update on epidemiology, risk factors, and therapeutic options. *Curr Opin Gastroenterol* 2012;**28**:1–9.

17 Yano T, Yamamoto H, Sunada K, *et al*. Endoscopic classification of vascular lesions of the small intestine (with videos). *Gastrointest Endosc* 2008;**67**:169–172.

18 Yoo S. GI-associated hemangiomas and vascular malformations. *Clin Colon Rectal Surg* 2011;**24**:193–200.

19 Yuksekkaya H, Ozbek O, Keser M, Toy H. Blue rubber bleb nevus syndrome: successful treatment with sirolimus. *Pediatrics* 2012;**129**: e1080–e1084.

Section 9 Miscellaneous Conditions

CHAPTER 55 ASCITES AND PERITONITIS

1   Aslam M, DeGrazia M, Gregory ML. Diagnostic evaluation of neonatal ascites. *Am J Perinatol* 2007;**24**(10):603–609.

2   Di Giorgio A, Agazzi R, Alberti D, Colledan M, D'Antiga L. Feasibility and efficacy of transjugular intrahepatic portosystemic shunt (TIPS) in children. *J Pediatr Gastroenterol Nutr* 2012;**54**(5):594–600.

3   Giefer MJ, Murray KF, Colletti RB. Pathophysiology, diagnosis, and management of pediatric ascites. *J Pediatr Gastroenterol Nutr* 2011;**52**(5):503–513.

4   Gines P, Cardenas A, Arroyo V, Rodés J. Management of cirrhosis and ascites. *N Engl J Med* 2004;**350**(16):1646–1654.

5   Gordon FD. Ascites. *Clin Liver Dis* 2012;**16**(2):285–299.

6   Haghighat M, Dehghani SM, Alborzi A, Imanieh MH, Pourabbas B, Kalani M. Organisms causing spontaneous bacterial peritonitis in children with liver disease and ascites in Southern Iran. *World J Gastroenterol* 2006;**12**(36):5890–5892.

7 Heyman MB, LaBerge JM, Somberg KA, *et al*. Transjugular intrahepatic portosystemic shunts (TIPS) in children. *J Pediatr* 1997;**131**(6):914–919.

8 Rimola A, Garcia-Tsao G, Navasa M, *et al*. Diagnosis, treatment and prophylaxis of spontaneous bacterial peritonitis: a consensus document. International Ascites Club. *J Hepatol* 2000;**32**(1):142–153.

9 Vieira SM, Matte U, Kieling CO, *et al*. Infected and noninfected ascites in pediatric patients. *J Pediatr Gastroenterol Nutr* 2005;**40**(3):289–294.

10 Wong CL, Holroyd-Leduc J, Thorpe KE, Straus SE. Does this patient have bacterial peritonitis or portal hypertension? How do I perform a paracentesis and analyze the results? *JAMA* 2008;**299**(10):1166–1178.

11 Kramer RE, Sokol RJ, Yerushalmi B, *et al*. Large-volume paracentesis in the management of ascites in children. *J Pediatr Gastroenterol Nutr* 2001;**33**(3):245–249.

CHAPTER 56 APPROACH TO PEDIATRIC DIARRHEA

1 Arvola T, Ruuska T, Keranen J, Hyoty H, Salminen S, Isolauri E. Rectal bleeding in infancy: clinical, allegological and microbiological examination. *Pediatrics* 2006;**117**:e760–e768.

2 Atia AN, Buchman AL. Oral rehydration solutions in non-cholera diarrhea: a review. *Am J Gastroenterol* 2009;**104**:2596–2604.

3 North American Society for Pediatric Gastroenterology, Hepatology and Nutrition, *et al*. Differentiating ulcerative colitis from Crohn disease in children and young adults: report of a working group of the North American Society for Pediatric Gastroenterology, Hepatology, and Nutrition and the Crohn's and Colitis Foundation of America. *J Pediatr Gastroenterol Nutr* 2007;**44**:653–674.

4 Gregorio GV, Dans LF, Silvestre MA. Early versus delayed refeeding for children with acute diarrhea. *Cochrane Database Syst Rev* 2011;**7**:CD007296.

5 Guandalini S. Probiotics for prevention and treatment of diarrhea. *J Clin Gastroenterol* 2011;**45**:S149–S153.

6 Hartling L, Bellemare S, Wiebe N, Russell K, Klassen TP, Craig W. Oral versus intravenous rehydration for treating dehydration due to gastroenteritis in children. *Cochrane Database Syst Rev* 2006;**3**:CD004390.

7 Hill DJ, Murch SH, Rafferty K, Wallis P, Green CJ. The efficacy of amino acid-based formulas in relieving the symptoms of cow's milk allergy: a systematic review. *Clin Exp Allergy* 2007;**37**(6):808–822.

8 Salvadori M, LeSaux N. Recommendations for the use of rotavirus vaccines in infants. *Paediatr Child Health* 2010;**15**(8):519–523.

9 Sherman PM, Mitchell DJ, Cutz E. Neonatal enteropathies: defining the causes of protracted diarrhea of infancy. *J Pediatr Gastroenterol Nutr* 2004;**38**(1):16–26.

10 Stormon MO, Durie PR. Pathophysiologic basis of exocrine pancreatic dysfunction in childhood. *J Pediatr Gastroenterol Nutr* 2002;**35**(1):8–21.

Index

T - #0795 - 101024 - C560 - 234/156/26 - PB - 9781840762020 - Gloss Lamination